T0181957

Register Now for Online Access to Your Book!

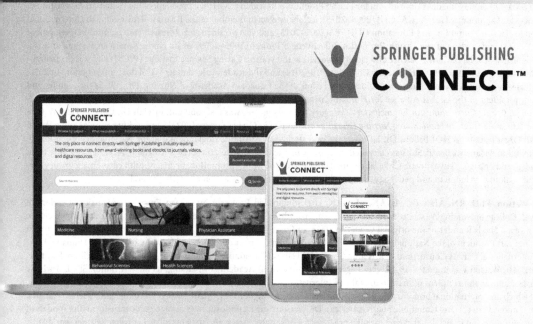

SPRINGER PUBLISHING
C**⏻**NNECT™

Your print purchase of *Creating a Caring Science Curriculum, Second Edition,* **includes online access to the contents of your book**—increasing accessibility, portability, and searchability!

Access today at:
http://connect.springerpub.com/content/book/978-0-8261-3603-9
or scan the QR code at the right with your smartphone and enter the access code below.

> **NNHVNRY0**

Scan here for quick access.

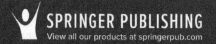

SPRINGER PUBLISHING
View all our products at springerpub.com

Marcia Hills, PhD, RN, FAAN, FCAN, is a professor at the School of Nursing, Faculty of Human and Social Development, University of Victoria, British Columbia (BC), Canada. She was the founding Director of the British Columbia Collaborative Nursing Program—the first Caring Science and collaborative nursing program in Canada (1989-94); founding director of the Centre for Community Health Promotion Research (2002-2009) at the University of Victoria; cochair (2002–04) and then president (2004–08) of the Canadian Consortium for Health Promotion Research (CCHPR); president of the Canadian Association of Teachers for Community Health (CATCH) (2004–2015); a globally elected member of the Board of Trustees for the International Union for Health Promotion and Education (IUHPE) (2001–2013) and vice president for Research and Technical Development (2010–2013) and cochair of the Health Promotion Effectiveness Project (2005–2009) of its North American Region; and is a Distinguished Scholar of Caring Science and faculty associate at the Watson Caring Science Institute (WCSI) and was the inaugural chair of its Faculty Executive and Faculty Council (2010–2014) and the academic lead of its WCSI doctoral program. In 2020, Dr. Hills was nominated and inducted as an inaugural Fellow of the Canadian Academy of Nursing. Dr. Hills is the founder and current president of the Global Alliance for Human Caring Education (2018–). She coauthored, with Dr. Jean Watson (2011), *Creating a Caring Curriculum: An Emancipatory Pedagogy for Nursing* and was a second author with Dr. Cara and Dr. Watson on *An Educator's Guide to Humanizing Nursing Education: Grounded in Caring Science* (2021). As a visiting Scholar and a World Health Organization (WHO) Fellow, Dr. Hills worked and studied in Australia, England, and at the National School of Public Health in Rio de Janeiro, Brazil. She has consulted extensively in: the United States, the United Kingdom, New Zealand, Australia, Trinidad, and Tobago, Kenya, Brazil, Chile, and Canada in the areas of: health promotion, primary health care, emancipatory caring curriculum development and pedagogy, women's health, and participatory action research and evaluation.

Jean Watson, PhD, RN, AHN-BC, FAAN, LL-AAN, is Distinguished Professor and Dean Emerita, University of Colorado Denver, College of Nursing Anschutz Medical Center campus, where she held the nation's first endowed chair in Caring Science for 16 years. She is founder of the original Center for Human Caring in Colorado and is a Fellow of the American Academy of Nursing; past President of the National League for Nursing; founding member of the International Association for Human Caring and International Caritas Consortium. She is founder and Director of the nonprofit foundation, Watson Caring Science Institute. In 2013 Dr. Watson was inducted as a Living Legend by the American Academy of Nursing, its highest honor. She is a widely published author and recipient of many national and international awards and honors, including 15 honorary doctoral degrees, 12 of which are International honorary doctorates (Sweden, United Kingdom (2), Spain, British Columbia and Quebec, Canada, Japan, Turkey, Peru (2), and Colombia, South America). Dr. Watson's caring philosophy is used to guide transformative models of caring education and professional caring–healing practices for hospitals, nurses, and patients alike, in diverse settings worldwide. As author/coauthor of over 30 books on caring, her latest books range from empirical measurements and international research on caring, to new postmodern philosophies of caring and healing, philosophy and science of caring, and Caring Science as sacred science, global advances in Caring Literacy. Her books have received the American Journal of Nursing's "Book of the Year" award and seek to bridge paradigms as well as point toward transformative models for this 21st century.

Chantal Cara, PhD, RN, FAAN, FCAN, is currently a professor at the Faculty of Nursing, Université de Montréal in Québec, Canada. She is a researcher at the Montreal's Centre for Interdisciplinary Research in Rehabilitation and at the Quebec Network on Nursing Intervention Research for humanistic practices. She received her Ph.D. in 1997 from the University of Colorado, under the directorship of Dr. Jean Watson. For more than 30 years, she has been actively involved in the advancement of Human Caring in both French and English communities. She is an internationally renowned scholar for creating and implementing the French Humanistic Model of Nursing Care and the Relational Caring Inquiry research methodology, both used in several countries. Dr. Cara's teaching, research activities, publications, and conferences reflect her disciplinary commitment to disseminate internationally her theory-guided research findings aimed at fostering humanistic nursing practices in the clinical, managerial, and educational domains. Dr. Cara has been actively involved for over 20 years as a member of the International Association for Human Caring, where she holds an editorial board position on the *International Journal for Human Caring* and is a current board member. In 2016, she was the first to be attributed the title Distinguished Caring Science Scholar by the Watson Caring Science Institute. In 2018, she was the first in Quebec to be inducted Fellow of the American Academy of Nursing. More recently, in 2020, she was invited to become a charter Fellow of the Canadian Academy of Nursing, representing the French nurses of Canada.

CREATING A CARING SCIENCE CURRICULUM

A Relational Emancipatory Pedagogy for Nursing

Second Edition

Marcia Hills, PhD, RN, FAAN, FCAN

Jean Watson, PhD, RN, AHN-BC, FAAN, LL-AAN

Chantal Cara, PhD, RN, FAAN, FCAN

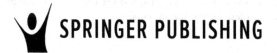 SPRINGER PUBLISHING

Springer Publishing Company, LLC
11 West 42nd Street, New York, NY 10036
www.springerpub.com
connect.springerpub.com/

Acquisitions Editor: Adrianne Brigido
Compositor: Exeter Premedia Services Private Ltd.

ISBN: 978-0-8261-3602-2
e-book ISBN: 978-0-8261-3603-9
DOI: 10.1891/9780826136039

20 21 22 23 24 / 5 4 3 2 1

The author and the publisher of this Work have made every effort to use sources believed to be reliable to provide information that is accurate and compatible with the standards generally accepted at the time of publication. The author and publisher shall not be liable for any special, consequential, or exemplary damages resulting, in whole or in part, from the readers' use of, or reliance on, the information contained in this book. The publisher has no responsibility for the persistence or accuracy of URLs for external or third-party Internet websites referred to in this publication and does not guarantee that any content on such websites is, or will remain, accurate or appropriate.

Library of Congress Control Number: 2020946258

Contact us to receive discount rates on bulk purchases.
We can also customize our books to meet your needs.
For more information please contact: sales@springerpub.com

Publisher's Note: **New and used products purchased from third-party sellers are not guaranteed for quality, authenticity, or access to any included digital components.**

Printed in the United States of America.

This book is dedicated to Dr. Em Olivia Bevis—mentor, colleague, master teacher, leader, visionary, loving person, and personal friend to us and thousands of others. A loving and provocative teacher, she dared you to reach the threshold of your own mind by challenging your taken-for-granted assumptions in a way that opened your heart and soul to new learning. Em often captured the imagination of hundreds of nurse educators crowded into a room to hear her speak. Her brilliance was in leading them back to themselves through critical questioning and dialogue with their colleagues, not necessarily with her.

She died too young and is deeply missed by her colleagues and friends and those in the nursing profession who did not have enough time to sit in her presence. Writing this book is a way to continue her legacy and a way to keep her vision for nursing and nursing education alive and vibrant.

Em loved nursing, and she loved nursing education more. Her words that follow echo her deep commitment to this wonderful profession. She writes:

There is a compelling splendor about both teaching and nursing that demands the highest forms of endeavor... a common core of caring about the human condition... a moral commitment to society's needs that requires... this trust will be steadfastly and excellently honored. (Bevis, 2000, p. 153)

Contents

Contributors

Lisa Bourque Bearskin, PhD, RN, MN, Indigenous Research Chair in Nursing, Canadian Institute of Health Research and Associate Professor, School of Nursing, Thompson Rivers University, Kamloops, British Columbia, Canada

Anne Boykin, PhD, RN, Professor and Dean Emerita, Christine E. Lynn College of Nursing, Florida Atlantic University, Boca Raton, Florida

Christina Chakanyuka, PhD Student, RN, MN, Assistant Professor, School of Nursing, University of Victoria, Victoria, British Columbia, Canada

Roberta Christopher, EdD, MSN, APRN, NE-BC, CAIF, CHTS-CP, Assistant Professor, Keigwin School of Nursing, Jacksonville University, Jacksonville, Florida

Lisa Lally, DNS, MS, RN, Associate Professor of Nursing and Director of the Baldwin Nursing Program, Siena College, Loudonville, New York

Piera Jung, BSN, RN, MALT, CCNE, Professor and Co-Chair, Bachelor of Science in Nursing, Faculty of Health and Human Services, Vancouver Island University, Nanaimo, British Columbia, Canada

Andrea Kennedy, PhD, RN, Associate Professor, School of Nursing and Midwifery, Mount Royal University, Calgary, Alberta, Canada

Leanne Poitras Kelly, MN, RN, Assistant Teaching Professor, School of Nursing, University of Victoria, Victoria, British Columbia, Canada

Lynn Rollison, PhD, RN, Professor, Bachelor of Science in Nursing, Faculty of Health and Human Services, Vancouver Island University, Nanaimo, British Columbia, Canada

Marlaine Smith, PhD, RN, AHN-BC, HWNC-BC, FAAN, Professor and Helen K. Persson Eminent Scholar, Christine E. Lynn College of Nursing, Florida Atlantic University, Boca Raton, Florida

Jennifer Thate, PhD, RN, CNE, Caritas Coach,   Assistant Professor of Nursing and Department Chair, Baldwin Nursing Program, Siena College, Loudonville, New York

Donnean Thrall, ND, RN, AHN-BC, Caritas Coach,   Assistant Professor of Nursing, Baldwin Nursing Program, Siena College, Loudonville, New York

Theris Touhy, DNP, GCNS-BC,   Emeritus Professor, Christine E. Lynn College of Nursing, Florida Atlantic University, Boca Raton, Florida

Foreword

In this important book, the authors and contributors provide a clear roadmap for nursing educators, leading to what I believe is essential if nurses of the future are to be equipped to make a real difference in healthcare in the future. I am writing this Foreword when all inhabitants of the globe are into the first few months of the global COVID-19 pandemic—an experience that is destined to have a lasting and dramatic effect on all aspects of human experience. This pandemic has laid bare the inadequacies and inequities of healthcare and the shameful neglect (in the United States) of public health. In these early days of the pandemic, the necessity of nurses as "essential" in caring for those who are hospitalized is clear. What is less obvious to those watching the unfolding of this experience through the eyes of public media, are the essential elements that come into play when nurses are there—when nurses stand at the bedside of those who are critically ill and dying, the only other human, in the absence of family and loved ones, who is there. Being there is of course in itself significant, but the manner of being there, the words of care and comfort, the touch of human hands even through protective equipment, and the skill to manage the technology surrounding the person—all of this comes together to constitute what means the most in times of need. Beyond the focus of the media on the tragic crisis experience is the fact that every nurse, including nurse educators, has become a vital source of support for our families and communities and as leaders and facilitators in the vital processes of prevention. We are all called on, perhaps daily, to translate, educate, and support those around us—as a member of our families, a friend and neighbor to those around us, the nurse at the chairside, roadside, or bedside.

Beyond this moment of crisis that has become so visible lies the foundation from which the best of nursing is born and the context in which the vital nature of nursing flourishes. The ideas and ideals that form a Caring Science curriculum set forth in this book point the way for nurse educators to envision our goals, our practices, and our expectations in ways that will sustain the essential elements of our discipline far into the future. The tragedy, in my view, is the fact that the power imbalances and traditions of nursing education have led educators down a path that, ironically, fails to live up to the caring ideals that are so essential to our discipline's foundation. For those who recognize that a new direction is not only possible, but necessary, this book points the way.

The great philosopher of education, Nel Noddings, advanced the idea many years ago that if we expect our students (in any discipline) to learn to care, they need to experience what it means to be cared for (Noddings, 1995). There is no discipline in which this admonition has more relevance (see nursology.net), nor is there a discipline in which this is more urgent.

Noddings outlined four essential characteristics/practices that educators need to enact to provide this experience for students. These are:

- Modeling: showing in our own behaviors what it means to care. The collection in this book provides a number of ways this can happen. In particular Chapter 16, "Indigenist Nursing: Caring Keeps Us Close to the Source" by Lisa Bourque Bearskin, Andrea Kennedy, Leanne Poitras Kelly, and Christina Chakanyuka, has content that points to the importance of authentic caring presence. They note that "Authenticity is an ongoing journey of self-discovery from a place of humility and respect" (Noddings, 1995, p. 20).
- Dialogue: making our caring manifest through illustrations, explanations, and discussions that deepen understanding of what it means to care. Noddings pointed out that a caring relationship requires that the cared-for person recognizes the caring, and it is through dialogue that you, as an educator, can nurture this recognition, and affirm your own understanding of what it means to care. As you read and use the wisdom contained in this volume, you are witness to this important dialogue.
- Practice: the deliberate focus on how the many batches of content in our curricula become mere vessels of knowledge that we use in the more vital, essential Caring Science practice that is detailed in this book. In essence, the ways of being, ways of relating, ways of skillfully working within each situation to meet the particular needs of the people in that situation—these are the essential practice elements of our teaching/learning. Everything else consists of those facts and theories that form the nurse's understanding that makes possible our core responsibility of "caring in the human health experience" (Newman et al., 1991).
- Confirmation: the acts of affirming and encouraging the best in our students. In this book, the authors provide the foundation for the creative process of "connoisseurship"— a model that moves beyond and transforms the processes traditionally known as "evaluation." The focus is on a process, not an outcome. The process, grounded in an authentic relationship between teacher and student, envisions, encourages, and supports students in their own path toward the best of nursing.

This book can lead to real transformation in nursing education at all levels. It is up to you, the reader, to answer the challenge and make the transformation real. We stand at a moment of unprecedented opportunity in the midst of the simultaneous triple challenges of a global COVID-19 pandemic, the world-wide exposure of racial and economic injustices and inequities, and ravages of global climate change. Let us join the authors and contributors to this volume to meet this challenge!

Peggy L. Chinn, PhD, DSc(Hon), RN, FAAN
Professor Emerita of Nursing
University of Connecticut

REFERENCES

Newman, M. A., Sime, A. M., & Corcoran-Perry, S. A. (1991). The focus of the discipline of nursing. *ANS. Advances in Nursing Science, 14*(1), 1–6. https://journals.lww.com/advancesinnursingscience/Citation/1991/09000/The_focus_of_the_discipline_of_nursing.2.aspx

Noddings, N. (1995). *Philosophy of Education.* Westview Press.

Preface

We wrote this book in response to a perception that the curriculum revolution, a hallmark event in nursing education in the late 1980s and early 1990s, had yet to fulfill its mandate to reform nursing education to embrace a Human Caring Science perspective. Some progress has been made, but there is still much to accomplish. This book is intended to provoke further debate and discussion about Caring Science as the foundation and philosophy of nursing, to explore emancipatory approaches to pedagogy, to provide a philosophical/theoretical framework, and a Caring Science curriculum development process as a way to move the nursing education agenda forward in its search for clarity of its foundation as a mature discipline.

We have attempted to present material in ways that inspire further and deeper thinking about Caring Science education topics. The purpose is to engage critical thinking and reflection and to assist both teachers and students to develop their own way of teaching and learning within the context of a Caring Science curriculum. The book is structured in five units consisting of several chapters each. Each unit overview introduces the chapters that are within it and the concepts covered in each chapter. Each chapter is structured to maximize student engagement by providing reflective exercises, called "Time Out for Reflection," and structured "Learning Activities" that encourage the integration of theory and practice into the learning process. Also, students are requested to create learning groups or partners so that they can engage in critical dialogue while learning from the book. Finally, students are encouraged to keep a learning/reflective journal that is intended to stimulate personal reflection within the learning process. Taken together, these processes kindle a deeper level of reflection and engagement that inspires and inspirits the intersection between the personal and the professional in teaching and learning.

Marcia Hills, PhD, RN, FAAN, FCAN
Jean Watson, PhD, RN, AHN-BC, FAAN, LL-AAN
Chantal Cara, PhD, RN, FAAN, FCAN

Acknowledgments

From Marcia

I want to acknowledge Em Olivia Bevis, my mentor, friend, and godmother to my son, Benji. She taught me to have courage in the face of adversity, and she inspired me to dedicate my career to nursing education and curriculum development and then she introduced me to my friend and colleague of 30 years, Jean Watson. Jean, thank you for the opportunity and the love we have shared in this endeavor, always keeping Em's and your vision from your original book, *Toward a Caring Curriculum*, close to our hearts so that we could contribute to the dream that nursing will claim its rightful place as a Caring Science. Thanks for the journey!

To my friend and colleague, Chantal Cara, who joined us for this edition of the book, thank you for your consistent and thoughtful work on this book, particularly your attention to detail and for your support of me through several versions of revisions. Thanks for joining us in this journey of commitment and love!

To my students and colleagues from whom I have learned so much, I thank you for your patience and for providing me space when I needed to work on this manuscript. I particularly want to acknowledge my director, Dr. Susan Duncan, whose leadership has encouraged me to continue to embrace Caring Science in my teaching, scholarship, and research. Thank you for *pondering* with me!

Also, I want to acknowledge all of the scholars who contributed to this book. Your willingness to make this commitment while we were in the midst of a pandemic is noteworthy. I asked and you answered eloquently. Thank you!

To John, my husband, thank you, not only for your support and encouragement, but also for your willingness to read and edit my work. To our children, Jenna and Benji, thanks for understanding when I had to miss time with you and our beautiful grandkids to work on this book.

Finally, I want to acknowledge Springer Publishing Company, especially Adrianne Brigido, executive director, for her support and encouragement.

From Jean

While this book and its energy are influenced, inspired, and dedicated to the early Em, this second edition, expands, elevates, and seeks to further humanize and liberate the human spirit, unleashing student and faculty creativity with emancipatory philosophies, pedagogies, and living exemplars that sustain integrity of what education and relational human caring are all about. Liberating and transformative educational and pedagogical practices during the '80s were a magical era of publications, workshops, seminars, conferences, and curriculum activities, especially throughout Canada, all sparked by the National League of Nursing and the '80s "curriculum revolution." Sadly, somewhere along the way during the '90s, nursing reverted backward and is now in a recovery mode. I bow to the passing of time and some educators who somehow sustained sparks of that original "curriculum revolution," against regressive institutional practices. Here at this time, in the midst of major pandemic worldview shifts, educators, practitioners, leaders, and systems alike are realizing how bereft both education and healthcare have become; how handicapped nursing has become by diluting its disciplinary foundation and core human-caring values. Now, we witness a call, a plea, a longing for a nursing education pedagogical/curriculum model that moves toward wisdom, transformation, and inclusion of human caring/healing/healthcare for all. This second edition seeks to address the call to help fill the empty disciplinary void, offering another way forward.

I am grateful for and to Marcia, and her devoted leadership in this book, bridging past with future, unleashing a Caring Science revolution; likewise I embrace Chantal for her dedicated and sustained history in living Caring Science throughout her career at Université de Montréal, Québec, contributing greatly to this edition. My continuing gratitude goes to Springer Publishing Company for its early support and guidance for the first edition, and enduring support toward transforming nursing curriculum and education, now and in the future, through Caring Science.

From Chantal

I would like to first thank Dr. Jean Watson, whom I am proud to call my teacher, my mentor, and my friend and who has continuously believed in me and supported my work since 1991. I am so grateful for her teachings and theories as they have guided my path to acting as one's own moral ideal and becoming a caring nurse educator, researcher, and scholar. I also want to thank Jean for introducing me to Dr. Marcia Hills, to whom I want to express my deepest gratitude for inviting me to participate in this book's second edition. Marcia's mentorship has truly inspired me to expand my knowledge on curriculum design, critical science theory, and relational emancipatory pedagogy. Needless to say that her passion for nursing education is uplifting.

I also want to express my appreciation to all my students, colleagues, and friends from whom I have learned so much and whose shared experience has allowed me to value the importance of a caring praxis in nursing education. I am also thankful to my late mentors from Université de Montréal, Dr. Georgette Desjean, Thérèse Doucet, and Suzanne Kérouac, who encouraged me to pursue my scholarship in Caring Science and without whom I would have never been introduced to Dr. Watson.

Finally, I wish to acknowledge my family, notably my loving and understanding husband, John, as well as my wonderful and amazing daughters, Stéphany and Émily. Without their unconditional love, unfailing support, tolerance, and ongoing presence, the possibility of pursuing this Caring Science journey would not have been a reality.

UNIT I

Foundations of a Caring Science Curriculum

[E]ducation that will teach persons to think as well as act; to know ... and to discourse about knowing; both to seek and doubt truth while developing a splendid sensitivity and devotion to it; to appreciate the enduring values that make nursing a moral activity... guided by a commitment to enlightened compassion and vigorous scholarship making the 21st century a renaissance for nursing.—Bevis, 2000, p. 81

In this first unit, we lay the foundations for a Caring Science curriculum. We argue that a Caring Science curriculum offers a new disciplinary discourse. This work offers the next evolution in professional nursing education; it places humanity, human evolution, human caring, health, and healing as its foundation. A Caring Science curriculum honors and celebrates diversity among the students–teachers and among approaches to teaching and learning. It is a revolution for whole-person teaching, learning, and knowing. It invites joy, a liberated human spirit, and passionate interest back into our lives and learning. It moves us toward a transformative consciousness of whole-person learning as the preferred pedagogical orientation and practices. Unit I has four chapters.

In Chapter 1, we describe the underlying philosophy and theory of Caring Science and its implications for developing a Caring Science curriculum. In addition, we introduce both the profession and discipline of nursing and articulate the differences between them.

In Chapter 2, we claim Caring Science as the disciplinary foundation of nursing. We further distinguish the *discipline* of nursing and the *profession* of nursing and describe why understanding these differences is critical in developing a Caring Science curriculum.

In Chapter 3, we articulate the underlying beliefs and assumptions that are intrinsic to a Caring Science curriculum.

Lastly, Chapter 4 introduces our philosophical/theoretical framework for Caring Science curriculum development. In addition, we discuss some key concepts that are explored in more depth in future chapters.

Bevis, E. O. (2000). Nursing curriculum as professional education: Some underlying theoretical models. In E.O. Bevis & J. Watson (Eds.), *Toward a caring curriculum: A new pedagogy for nursing* (pp. 67–106). National League for Nursing.

Caring Science: Curriculum Revolutions and Detours Along the Way

What about a model that inspires? That shows us what we would like to become, and infuses us with the ideas and strength needed to approximate it.
—Smith, 1982

INTRODUCTION

It has been more than 40 years since the National League of Nursing (NLN) began to call for reform in nursing education, a movement that has come to be known as the "Curriculum Revolution." This was a significant time in the history of nursing education in the United States as nursing leaders banded together to deinstitutionalize the long-standing behaviorist, Tylerian model of education that nursing education had been entrenched in for more than 40 years. This revolution called for a paradigm shift in nursing education from behaviorism and empiricism to human science and caring as foundations upon which to create nursing curricula (Bevis, 1988; Bevis & Watson, 1989/2000; Moccia, 1988; Munhall, 1988; Tanner, 1988; Watson, 1988). It demanded new pedagogies that created transformational learning and curriculum design that focused on critical thinking, creative solution-seeking attitudes, and learning, rather than on content to be transmitted. It challenged nursing educators to aspire to graduate nurses who were not only technically competent, but whose practice was steeped in the values and ethics of caring as the moral obligation of nursing to society.

Yet in 2003, the NLN confirmed that much of the innovation sought had focused instead on the addition or rearrangement of traditional content within the curriculum where we switch and swap the content around (Bevis, 1988). Tanner (2006) confirms this perspective when critiquing nursing educators using outdated models in clinical practice education. She makes several recommendations to rectify this situation.

In 2008, *Advances in Nursing Science* published a volume on the topic of the discipline of nursing. In this issue, it was noted by Newman et al. (2008) that the discipline is in a transformative phase. Moreover, it was reasserted here that within the *discipline of nursing*, "the concepts of health, caring, consciousness, mutual process, patterning, presence, and meaning" are essential to nursing (Newman et al., 2008, p. E18). Further, Smith and McCarthy's (2010) comprehensive review of seminal documents "guiding the development of baccalaureate and higher degree educational curriculum in nursing" (American Association of Colleges of Nursing [AACN], (2007, 2008, 2009) concluded: "nursing knowledge consisting of the philosophies, theories, research and practice models of the *discipline was mentioned tangentially, not centrally, and rarely explicitly*" ([our italics] p. 49). Others (Cowling et al., 2008; Willis et al., 2008) have defined similar meanings attesting to the disciplinary foundation of nursing, which include the human dimensions, consciousness, caring, relationships, and so on.

Furthermore, many reports, mainly in a reaction to the transformation in healthcare and health policy, continued to conclude that the need for curriculum transformation is still timely (Feller, 2018; Institute of Medicine, 2011; Mann, 2012) and some emphasize "the need to reconsider who we are teaching, what we are teaching, and how we are teaching" (Giddens et al., 2012, p. 67).

This curriculum revolution in the United States also had a significant impact on nursing education programs in Canada (Hills, 2016; Hills & Cara, 2019; Hills & Lindsey, 1994; Lewis et al., 2006, 2011), and other parts of the world (Lee et al., 2017; Rosa et al., 2019). *So, what happened to the curriculum revolution?*

DETOURS ALONG THE WAY

We examine three areas to explain the detours that drew us away from the caring curriculum revolution and inhibit nursing evolving within its disciplinary foundation:

- The false dichotomy of nursing as an art and a science
- The ambivalent and tormented relationship between nursing science and medical science
- Nursing's fascination with evidence-based practice (EBP)

Nursing as an Art and a Science: A False Dichotomy

> Nursing is an art, and if it is to be made an art, it requires as exclusive a devotion and as hard a preparation as any painter's or sculptor's work; for what is having to do with a dead canvas or cold marble, compared to having to do with the living body—the temple of God's spirit? It is one of the Fine Arts: I would say the finest of the Fine Arts. (Nightingale, 1871, p. 7)

As famous as Nightingale's quote of "nursing as an art . . . the finest of the Fine Arts" is, it has had a conflicting and paradoxical impact on nursing as a mature distinct discipline. Nursing's scientific evolution has tended to create an either/or approach to art and science—resulting in a false dichotomy between art and science: thus separating caring out as "art" and medical–empirical-procedural aspects as "science." This false dichotomy stands in contrast to a human Caring Science model within a disciplinary framework, which seeks to embrace and integrate both. As Smith (1993) states: "Science is considered as quantifiable, covering the nurse's science of curing and treating illness whereas arts are considered expressive, covering nurse's art of healing" (p. 42). This notion is explained further by Castledine (2010) when he states: "The scientific components of medicine have also become the scientific aspects of modern nursing, and have led us into a more dominant medical model of nursing care than ever before" (p. 937). Nurses also sustain this situation by wanting "to foster a professional, harder, rational, scientific and academic side" while maintaining the publicly held view of nursing as a *caring profession*. What is missing here from our perspective is the focus on nursing *qua* nursing, practiced as an expanded *human Caring Science*.

We argue that nursing's ethical, philosophical, and theoretical base can integrate caring and human phenomena within its disciplinary matrix, to become Caring Science, thus further differentiating nursing from medical science. Nursing scholars and theoretical discourses have demanded a shift to differentiate nursing from medicine, toward whole-person expanded views of science for several decades. For example, Newman (1986, 1992), Newman et al. (1991), Parse (1987, 1992), Rogers (1970, 1989), Sarter (1988), Watson (1979, 1988, 1995, 2012, 2018) all make a case for a different paradigm to differentiate nursing from medicine and Hills and Watson (2011) explore how to educate nurses within this perspective.

But even now it remains difficult to achieve this distinction due to competing dynamics and shifting priorities. Indeed, a position paper on *Nursing Knowledge—Impact on Nursing's Preferred Future* from an Expert Panel of the American Academy of Nursing (AAN; Jones & Wright, 2010) highlighted:

> The explosion of nursing theory in the . . . 1970s provided substance to the focus of the discipline, guided research and enhanced nursing's ability to articulate the substantive content of nursing and a professional vision. These works offered a worldview to guide knowledge development and expansion. . . . nursing, described as a science and a human practice discipline, uses scientific knowledge and values to promote a caring relationship with patients, families and communities. (p. 2)

As noted in this paper,

> [n]ursing theories, developed by academy leaders . . . and many others, have provided the discipline with innovative worldviews to guide practice, affect and sustain behavior change and enhance understanding of the human condition. *These approaches provide strategies to help providers move away from the prescriptive* . . . *'this is what you should do' strategies.* [emphasis added] (Jones & Wright, 2010, p. 2)

However, within education, emphasis on integrating nursing knowledge into the educational preparation of nurses remains inconsistent. Theory courses are often taught in isolation, frequently abandoned throughout the curriculum as a whole; some disciplinary courses are being eliminated or changed to emphasize new roles.

> More recently, the growth of the Doctorate in Nursing Practice (DNP) (in its current iteration), minimizes the inclusion and translation of nursing theory. Other trends include developing nursing research and scholarship framed in other disciplines, which further compromises disciplinary knowledge development and advancement of the discipline and profession of nursing. (Jones & Wright, 2010, p. 3)

In light of the historic advancements and developments in the discipline, the trends and detours, as noted in this AAN paper (Jones & Wright, 2010), are troubling, and call forth another phase in nursing's disciplinary evolution. However, this next phase requires a transformative way of thinking. It calls for nurses to think about the discipline of nursing as an integration of artistry within an expanded view of science. In other words, we recommend that creative artistry of our humanity be embodied within an expanded view of science. Once one places the *person* and *caring* into a model of science, there is no separation between art and science as they are one unitary field of human-planet existence. The model evolves, congruent with the timeless history, heritage, traditions, and practices of nursing. As Watson claims,

> As soon as one places Caring within its science model or as soon as one locates the science model within the Caring Ontology (which is relational) science automatically grounds

itself in it. Caring forces us as individuals and professions to Face our relation of the infinite responsibility of belonging to other human beings as well as to a unitary field of all-our-relations. Such an orientation becomes non-dualistic, relational and unified, wherein there is a connectedness of all. (Watson, 2005, p. 63)

NURSING'S AMBIVALENT, EVOLVING RELATIONSHIP WITH MEDICINE

Nursing has had, and continues to have, an ambivalent, evolving relationship with medicine. Nursing's current situation, in this regard, must include sorting out and clarifying its relationship with medicine. Certainly, the two professions overlap (Figure 1.1). There is no question that nurses need medical knowledge in order to care for people, just as physicians need bedside caring manners to treat diseases. However, nursing and medicine are not the same.

Medicine's main focus is on diagnosing, treating, and curing diseases (Figure 1.2), whereas nursing's main focus is on caring for people and their experience of health–illness, and healing (Figure 1.3). Nursing and medicine's knowledge and competencies overlap, yes, but the essence of what each profession does, and the knowledge base from within each, is quite different.

In addition to nurses having *medical* knowledge about disease processes, nurses also need *nursing* knowledge of caring and healing and the human health–illness experiences. As a result, a nurse's domain of practice is precise: caring for the individual (family or community) in relation to the person's/peoples' experience and meanings associated with health, recovery, and healing—not the disease process itself. Nurses use knowledge of anatomy and physiology, pharmacology, disease processes, and diagnoses to understand how a particular person is being affected by those processes. Nonetheless, that knowledge is background. In the foreground, there is focus on caring, relationships, and processes, and the health and healing

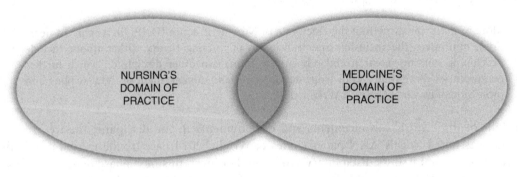

FIGURE 1.1 Complementary domains of practice.

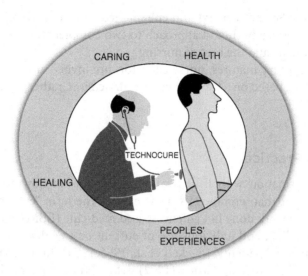

FIGURE 1.2 Medicine's domain of practice.

experiences of a person living with a disease. Nurses are not responsible for curing diseases; they are responsible for caring for people with diseases and health-illness-healing conditions and concerns. As a result, the disciplinary foundation for nursing incorporates the ethics, philosophy, and scientific knowledge of people and caring–healing health practices. Nursing is not a science of diseases. It is a science of people and their experiences.

For years nursing education has been dominated by medical–clinical orientations and conventional medical science, *not* nursing Caring Science as a complete discipline and profession. But now nursing is awakening to, and maturing within, its own human Caring Science foundation. As such, this awakening and this book reignite the caring curriculum, but now

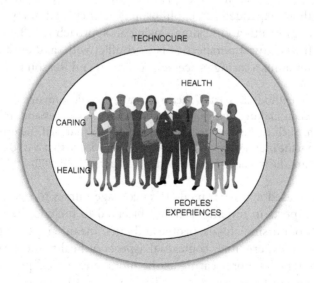

FIGURE 1.3 Nursing's domain of practice.

within a mature Caring Science context and enlightened views of caring pedagogies. It is not an either/or approach; it is a both/and approach to two complementary professions. Society needs the best of medicine and the best of nursing.

Now as the 21st century matures, nurse educators are invited anew to teach nursing as a more evolved discipline, based on a Caring Science curriculum, rather than a medically dominated one.

Evidence-Based Practice

Nursing's ongoing fascination with EBP is another example of how nursing continues to "follow" medicine rather than embrace its own science. The term "evidence-based nursing" evolved from the initial work done in evidence-based medicine (EBM), which was defined as "the conscientious, explicit, and judicious use of current best evidence in making decisions about the care of individual patients" (Sackett et al., 1996, p. 71). In their landmark paper, the Evidence-Based Medicine Working Group (1992) defined the primary source of evidence as randomized control trials (RCTs) and meta-analysis of RCTs. Despite a later effort to partially ameliorate this definition, the original definition eventually grew into the hierarchy of levels of evidence that underpin the concept of evidence-based medicine (Sackett et al., 1996). Here, the RCT remains the gold standard with a hierarchy of evidence entrenched in a positivist, reductionist ontology, epistemology, and methodology. Although this might work for medicine, many nursing scholars have recognized that the definitions of evidence espoused by the proponents of EBM are too narrow and exclusive to support the complexities of nursing practice (Estabrooks, 1998; Estabrook et al., 2005; Harvey & Kitson, 2015; Kitson et al., 1998; Madjar & Walton, 2001; Rycroft-Malone et al., 2004; Tarlier, 2005; Tracy & O'Grady, 2019). Furthermore, these hierarchy definitions of empiricism and objectivism as the dominant form of evidence, are incompatible with the complex and contextual knowledge of human health illness and human caring knowledge and processes (Estabrooks et al., 2005; Harvey & Kitson, 2015; Palmer, 2004; Thorne & Sawatzky, 2014).

For nursing, several limitations and contradictions arise when attempting to adapt to an EBM approach to practice. First, if nursing is to claim the core of its domain of practice as Caring Science—with an expanded ethic, philosophy, and epistemology, focused on people and their experiences of health and healing—using an approach to EBP that is situated in a limited, reductionistic, positivist perspective is in conflict with, and antithetical to, the very essence of nursing and human caring processes. As Heron and Reason (1997) state:

> Orthodox research methods, as part of their rationale, exclude human subjects from all the thinking and decision making that generates and designs, manages and draws conclusions from the research. Such exclusions treat the subject as less than self- determining persons, alienates them from the inquiry process and from the knowledge that is its outcome, and thus invalidates any claim the methods have to a science of persons. (p. 280)

Further, an evidence-based approach tends to encourage nurses to overly focus on technical and technocure aspects in nursing; it is not oriented to include the more complex and sophisticated aspects of nursing's focus: people and inner meaning, perceptions, feelings, and the complex, relational, experiential, contextual aspects of health and healing. In fact, EBP, as conventionally designed, ignores caring as the moral and ethical practice of nursing and denies nursing's science of human caring. As Baumann (2010) suggests, "outcome-oriented

EBP often fails to fully respect the primacy of the individual or to consider the importance of the meaning of the experience for the person" (p. 229).

Finally, nurses who base their practice exclusively on results from conventional evidence-based research through RCTs perhaps unknowingly reinforce the dichotomy of nursing—separating art from science, further compromising nursing's standing as a legitimate discipline and perpetuating nursing's ambivalent, tormented relationship with medicine.

For nursing to continue to evolve as a unique discipline, we need to critically examine our caring knowledge and practices and develop ways of revealing evidence that are consistent with the philosophical and theoretical foundation of a mature discipline and profession distinct from, but complementary to, medicine and all health professions. As Chinn (2019) claims "it is time to recognize that our own disciplinary perspective can all to easily get lost unless we ourselves recognize, value and strengthen our ontology" (p. 26). Smith (2019) also affirms that:

> First, the discipline of nursing must be an integral part of all levels of nursing education. There is an urgent need to develop curricula in baccalaureate, masters, and doctoral programs that educate students about the focus of the discipline and nursing knowledge including theory-guided practice. Without a grounding in the discipline, nursing appears to be an applied science in which nurses use the knowledge of other disciplines in the care of patients. Nursing has its own science, and this body of knowledge needs to be the foundation of the next generations' socialization into the discipline. (p. 13)

CARING SCIENCE: THE NEXT ENTRANCE AHEAD

"Caring Science can be defined as an evolving ethical-epistemic field of study that is grounded in the discipline of nursing and informed by related fields" (Watson & Smith, 2002, p. 456). Throughout this book, we make Caring Science explicit as the disciplinary foundation of the nursing profession. In this chapter, we also explore the question, *What is Caring Science and why is it important in nursing education, practice and research?*

The discipline of nursing and the profession of nursing are not synonymous, and it is important for teachers and students alike to know and understand the difference between them. Understanding this difference is fundamental to designing and implementing a Caring Science curriculum.

The disciplinary foundation provides the moral and intellectual blueprint for education, practice, research, and leadership. It is the starting point for a professional orientation. More specifically, within the discipline of nursing are its knowledge and research traditions. The discipline offers the metanarrative, worldview, historical heritage, theories, principles, assumptions, traditions, values, and the lens to view human and caring-healing-health phenomena. The discipline bridges the moral, philosophical, ethical, and theoretical foundations with practice demands and conventional expectations.

The disciplinary foundation guides the profession and the professional from the inside out, in contrast to outside in. Nonetheless, professional practice expectations and demands often result in the profession and the professional being whiplashed by the changing circumstances and external forces of our high-paced practice healthcare (sick care) system. Without disciplinary clarity, nursing can lose its way in the outer world of compromise and conformity, modeling itself on other developments (often originating from medical technology, industry, business, and economics), rather than maturing as a distinct discipline in its own right. Witness the historical detours we have already noted in succumbing to outer forces: the dichotomy of art and science; the lingering, ambivalent relationship with medical science; and the limited approaches of EBP. Thus, we make explicit that there is a difference between nursing maturing within its own Caring Science paradigm and nursing maturing within medicine's paradigm. The two paths exist but they are divergent.

Indeed, we can now acknowledge that as soon as nursing identifies its science as encompassing the *human* and the phenomena of *human caring* and *human health-illness experiences*—and their *meaning, relations,* and *context*—then we must make a case for a different model for nursing science, that is, Caring Science. Incorporating caring and human experiences in a model of science demands a relational and ethical starting point and a relational worldview, which differs from medical science.

Caring Science provides this deep underpinning for a scientific-philosophical-moral context from which to explore, describe, and research human caring–healing phenomena as integral to our humanity. As the disciplinary foundation for nursing, Caring Science clarifies for the profession, and the professional, the question of ontology, that is, *what is our worldview of reality? What is the nature of Being and Becoming human in relation to the larger infinite universal field of life itself?*

Here, the starting point and underlying ontology is one of *relation* in contrast to *separation.* Caring Science does not separate mind from body, heart from head, person from environment–community, the human from the ecosystem. Caring Science also addresses a core question: what does it mean to be human? It acknowledges the unity of mindbodyspirit-environment-universe, as one entity; it makes explicit that we all *belong* to the wider universal field of planet Earth, the universe, the cosmos, the mystery, the void (Watson, 2005, 2008, 2018).

Caring Science helps us reflect upon what it means to be whole, to be healed, and to be caring. It reminds us—as we place, or replace, human caring and the human experiences within a model of science—that we have a distinctive model of science that informs and inspires the discipline and profession of nursing; a model of science underpinned by a cosmology and ethic of unity, of belonging, of relations, of connectedness with the great circle, and of the web of life itself.

In terms of more concrete practicalities, Caring Science, ethically and philosophically, seeks to avoid reducing any human, whether student or patient or any other, to the moral status of object. For example, in the conventional world of daily nursing practice, a scenario, such as the following, can be quite common:

- Person is reduced to patient.
- Patient is reduced to body physical.
- Body physical is reduced to machine; thus, the human is reduced to the moral status of an object.

Once a human being has been reduced to the moral status of object, we professionals can separate ourselves from one another, can justify doing things to the *other-as-object* that we would never do to the other as a fully functioning human like ourselves (Watson, 2005, influenced by Gadow, previous personal communication). Furthermore, we know from humanity (including our own unique experiences) and the wisdom traditions across time that one person's level of humanity is reflected on another. If the person/patient/student is reduced to object status, then so is the nurse, the practitioner, and the teacher, even if they are not precisely aware of it. Therefore, it is the disciplinary lens, the values and the moral imperatives located within

Caring Science philosophies and theories of nursing, which guide and sustain nursing in its covenant with humanity across time and space, worlds and change.

DISCIPLINARY FOUNDATION AS GUIDE TO ACTION

As teachers and students engage the consciousness of Caring Science, the moral-ethical-epistemic-spiritual dimensions of caring (and healing and humanity) become more explicit as a formal guide to action. Caring Science as a disciplinary foundation acknowledges

- a philosophy of human freedom, choice, responsibility, and human consciousness evolution;
- a biology and psychology of holism; a unity of *Being/Becoming*;
- an epistemology that allows not only for empirics, but also for the advancement of aesthetics, ethical values, intuition, personal-emotional knowing, spiritual insights, a process of discovery, creative imagination, joy, passion, and evolving forms of inquiry;
- an ontology of time and space;
- a context of inter-subjective human experiences, events, processes, and relationships that connect with/are at-one-with the environment and the wider universe;
- caring knowledge is, as a serious epistemic endeavor, not to be assumed or taken for granted;
- a scientific worldview that is open, guided by ethics as first principle and starting point for humans and Being-in-the-world (Levinas, 1969; Watson, 1985/2007, p. 16; Watson, 2008).

A Caring Science orientation differs from conventional science and invites qualitatively different aspects of our shared humanity in the universe that are to be honored as legitimate and necessary. This is especially true when working with humanity, human experiences, human caring–healing, life phenomena, and all the vicissitudes of human living:

> *Facing ourself and our humanity . . .*
> *Is a moral act*
> *And comes before clinical knowledge;*
> *. . . the value-laden human condition . . .*
> *Vulnerability, pain, suffering and discomfort,*
> *Are value-laden phenomena;*
> *They are moral realities*
> (Nortvedt, 2000, p. 2, as cited in Watson, 2005, p. 44)

It is imperative to be explicit about one's starting point and core values, since one's moral–ethical starting point determines where one ends up. For example, if one starts with a professional, clinical-medical lens regarding humanity and one's phenomena of focus, then that medical professional lens guides one's approach to teaching, learning, and practicing nursing.

If we start with a disciplinary lens in Caring Science that values, honors, and acknowledges the wholeness of humanity, our oneness with each other and all aspects of humanity, and our place in the wider universe, then we can be open to unknowns and the fullness of our humanity, dwelling in paradox, ambiguity, mystery, and even miracles. The overall Caring Science disciplinary lens allows for our own and others' evolution and for transformation of consciousness. Thus, personal growth, change, insight, humility, spirit-guided inner resources, and wisdom are present in the moment in human-to-human caring relationships. This allows for *caring moments* to occur between student and teacher or between nurse and patient. The disciplinary foundation helps the nursing profession to sustain and enact its deep values, its *raison d'etre* in the world, and its commitment to humanity itself. As one of our colleagues in England put it:

> *Any profession which loses its values becomes Heartless;*
> *Any professional who becomes heartless, becomes Soulless;*
> *Any profession that becomes heartless and soulless becomes Worthless!*
> (Eagger, 2001, personal communication)

Again, Caring Science differs from conventional science in several significant ways as identified in Table 1.1.

We can see from Table 1.1 that a Caring Science disciplinary starting point informs and guides our approach to given phenomena. It is important for us to clarify our disciplinary

TABLE 1.1 Differences Between Conventional and Caring Science

CONVENTIONAL SCIENCE	CARING SCIENCE
ONTOLOGY: Worldview Neutrality of Values Paternalistic–External Control A separatist worldview as starting point A stance toward clinical distance, separation, control—attempt to be neutral or value-free with objective assumptions	ONTOLOGY AS ETHIC Ethic/ontology of Belonging as first principle Connectedness, Interdependence; Inner control A relational unitary worldview as starting point Values: preserving humanity, human caring, dignity, human spirit, wholeness, integrity, unity
EPISTEMOLOGICAL RESTRICTIONS Limited Epistemology Knowledge: Objective–factual procedural, outer knowledge—empirics as starting point; reductionistic epistemology	EPISTEMOLOGICAL PLURALISM Expanded Epistemology Honoring all ways of Knowing/Being/Becoming; diversity of knowledge development, cocreated from inside out and outside in; move from information to knowledge to understanding to meaning to wisdom to inner knowing. Multiple forms of "evidence" from empirics to aesthetic, noetic, poetic, personal, intuitive, ethical, mystical and even spiritual knowing . . . allowing for "elegance, beauty, simplicity and parsimony as alternative theoretical-scientific explanatory models" (Watson, 2005, p. 28).
METHODOLOGY Experimental scientifically controlled research methods; largely quantitative objective data are what count as "evidence," as knowledge	CARING INQUIRY Caring Science methodology allows for multiple forms of "evidence" and diverse methods, forms of inquiry, open to creative-artistic-visionary, narrative, performance, expanded epistemological approaches to research and knowledge development, while incorporating empirical data

(continued)

TABLE 1.1 Differences Between Conventional and Caring Science (*continued*)	
CONVENTIONAL SCIENCE	**CARING SCIENCE**
PRACTICE Professional scientific, clinicalized/medicalized views of humanity and human conditions; efforts to "fix the parts," control human processes and environment, treat disease and body physical (often at all costs) from external treatments mechanisms; outer curing focus	PRAXIS Practice shifts to *praxis*—that is, reflective practice informed by disciplinary foundational values, theories, philosophical, ethical stance; informed by meaning, context, relations, and knowledgeable caring/healing practices; honoring deeply spirit-filled dimensions of humankind

starting point to make explicit the focus and direction of nursing education, of a caring curriculum, of approaches to knowledge development, of learning–teaching, of teaching strategies, and of pedagogy. Other disciplines such as social work or child and youth care may claim to be human sciences in contrast to natural sciences and they are entitled to this claim. However, Caring Science, as a human science, is what sets nursing apart from these other human sciences. In turn, our entire intellectual consciousness of Caring Science informs our nursing professional practices and development of the profession and the discipline itself. This consciousness affects our approaches to self-knowledge and to humanity in general.

A Caring Science curriculum provides the disciplinary map for teaching–learning nursing. It may be in contrast to, or even in conflict with, conventional nursing models and blueprints of education and practice that are guided by a historical, medicalized, technical, or more established professional focus. It is time for nursing to claim its societal mandate for addressing inequities, advocacy, social justice, as well as health and healing for all.

WHAT IS A CARING SCIENCE CURRICULUM?

> It is time for the nursing educational system to question the impact our current curricular and pedagogical approaches might be having on nurses' ability to work effectively beyond the demand for technical competence at the bedside; nurses need to be politically active, work autonomously, and create the sort of caring-healing practices that first attracted most nurses into the profession. (Clark, 2010, p. 42)

This quote, although written initially in 2001, remains as relevant and significant today in 2020.

A Caring Science curriculum lays a solid foundation for reconnecting the heart, soul, mind, emotions, and the human spirit of students and teachers alike; it invites passion, intellect, moral ideals, and love into our classrooms and curriculum, restoring humanity and human caring–healing knowledge and practices for now and the future. Danish philosopher Logstrup helps make explicit that educators, quite literally and metaphorically, hold other people's lives in their hands.

> By our value/attitude to the other person, we help to determine the scope and hue of his/her world; we make it larger or smaller, bright or drab, rich or dull, threatening or secure. We help to shape his/her world, not by theories and views but by our very being and attitude toward other. Herein lies the unarticulated and, one might say, anonymous demand that we take care of life which trust has placed in our hands. (Logstrup, 1997, p. 18)

Core Ingredients of a Caring Science Curriculum

A Caring Science curriculum seeks to create authentic, egalitarian, human-to-human relationships. This assumption is based on the notion that there is reciprocity between power, knowledge, and control, and that, in order for there to be more equitable relationships, those with power need to give up and share control, so that others may benefit and share their knowledge, thus their power. Authentic power is shared power; it is power with, not power over. It does not negate faculty or nurses' responsibilities, skills, or knowledge. It also means standing in one's own power, one's own truth and integrity, and authenticity without succumbing to another's position of power, authoritarian control, and so on.

We can still acknowledge the reality that there is a difference between having authority and being authoritarian; the teacher has authority by the nature of their position; however, that does not justify an authoritarian, power-control stance toward knowledge, toward students, and toward control of knowledge. In a Caring Science curriculum, students also have authority in their own knowing and experiences that can be shared and jointly critiqued for deeper knowledge, understanding, integrative insights, and wisdom, ultimately resulting in transformation of consciousness.

To create such a visionary Caring Science curriculum for human caring–healing, Hills and Cara (2019) identified at least five curriculum processes and pedagogical practices that are essential to advance a Caring Science Curriculum. They are the following:

- Claiming Caring Science as the moral, theoretical, and philosophical foundations of the discipline of nursing and, therefore, nursing education
- Using Caring Science language to articulate nursing education and practice
- Teaching and learning in caring collaborative relationships
- Creating Caring Science curriculum design and structure
- Evaluating student's practice experiences on the basis of Caring Science rather than on reductionistic methods such as behavioural objectives, competencies or standards (p. 200)

These five processes and practices are philosophical and ethical, as well as practical orientations to hold in our framework for implementing and living out a Caring Science curriculum. These ingredients flow from underlying beliefs and values that can be made explicit in a Caring Science context. Once we are clear about the disciplinary direction for nursing, then curricular issues and directions become more consistent; we are less compromised by conventional mind-sets and the status quo. We are less tied to or caught up within previously established, limiting approaches to education, to teaching–learning, and to traditional pedagogical issues. A new horizon of moral ideals, inspiration, creativity, human spirit, liberation, intellectual passion, joy, and even spiritual freedom is available to all.

Time Out for Reflection

How would you define a Caring Science curriculum?
What does Caring Science offer for nursing education and practice?
What is the difference between the discipline of nursing and the profession of nursing? Why is this difference important to understand?

What are the factors that distinguish a Caring Science curriculum from another type of nursing curriculum?

Evolution of Curriculum Directions: Current Dilemmas

Nurse educators continue to face challenges in addressing curriculum reform from nursing's disciplinary foundation. For example, recent AACN national reports (i.e., white paper on the education and role of the Clinical Nurse Leader; the essentials of doctoral education for advanced nursing practice; the essentials of baccalaureate education for professional nursing practice, AACN, 2007, 2008, 2009) have been critiqued as having *"insufficient emphasis . . . on the disciplinary knowledge of nursing* [emphasis added]" (Smith & McCarthy, 2010, p. 44). This gap between educational recommendations and the need for disciplinary knowledge as foundation makes it all the more important that we, as scholars of nursing education, review and critique such documents and reports for their strengths and shortcomings. As part of nursing maturing as a health and caring profession, distinct from, but complementary to, medicine, it is important that major educational blueprints are critiqued within the most contemporary scholarly discourse. Thus, the work of creating a Caring Science curriculum requires nursing educators and progressive educational programs and curricula to acknowledge, benefit from, and critique current reports and documents, to incorporate the most current scholarly discourse of nursing.

A Caring Science curriculum seeks to move beyond conventional blueprints and relocate all generalist and advanced specialist nursing education within the philosophies, ethics, theories, research, and practice models that originate from the disciplinary foundation of nursing.

Indeed, our challenge and request is that you, as nurse educators, critique these, and any other documents, explore educational scholarship that ensures that our future nurses will be prepared, educated, informed, inspired, and passionate about nursing maturing as a Caring Science. By doing so, you help to assure that the disciplinary ground is established to distinguish and guide education, practices, and research in nursing (*qua* nursing) for future generations.

Traditionally, curriculum has been thought of as a planned program of studies or a blueprint for learning, focusing largely on content and dissemination of objective clinical data, information, procedural knowledge for technological competencies, and skills. Important as these dimensions are, a Caring Science orientation to curriculum takes a marked shift from those past, conventional, views. As Bevis and Watson (1989, 2000) explained, conventional nursing educators have typically shuffled content around within the curriculum structure declaring this *swapping and switching as curriculum change*, when no real change has actually taken place.

Despite the shortcoming and critiques of the aforementioned documents and reports, and while we are inviting still another evolutionary turn, it is important to acknowledge that curricular changes have occurred in nursing education over the past decade or so toward more humane and humanitarian approaches to teaching, learning, and practice.

At least in part, these changes have occurred due to the NLN's *caring curriculum revolution* series of programs, publications, and conferences held during the 1980s, and were further influenced by Bevis and Watson's (2000) redefinition of curriculum as "the interactions and transactions that occur between and among teachers and students with the intent that learning occur" (p. 5), with curriculum linked more than ever to a view of the person as whole. As Bevis and Watson indicated, the teacher's pedagogical skills encompassed student/faculty learning relationships and sought inspired teaching/learning within the context of these relationships.

This reorientation to the relationship between and among teachers and students, and teachers' pedagogical skills, has had a tremendous impact on the teaching of nursing over the last 30 plus years.

Of course, pedagogy is discussed at length in later chapters. We agree that it is the heart of curriculum development and the space that invites learning. In the meantime, we can point to inspired pedagogical changes that have spilled over from the curriculum revolution and which represent the heart of curriculum change.

Progressive nurse educators responded to pedagogical challenges identified by the curriculum revolutionaries, and, as a result, we see hopeful current changes in relational learning; a renewed interest in active learning; student-centered learning (Diekelmann, 2004; Duffy, 2018; Hunt, 2018; Jillings & O'Flynn-Magee, 2007; Young & Paterson, 2007); interactive learning (Hills & Cara, 2019; Middleton, 2013); context-based learning (Williams & Day, 2007); story-based learning (Young, 2007); narrative pedagogy (Brown & Rodney, 2007; Diekelmann, 2005; Hunt, 2018); esthetics pedagogy (Rockwood Lane & Samuels, 2011); and transformative virtual pedagogy (Enzman Hines, 2011; Sitzman & Watson, 2017; Smith, 2019; Watson, 2002).

Benner et al. (2010) make 26 recommendations as they call for a radical transformation for nursing education. It is noteworthy that many of these recommendations address the critical need to increase the entry level of nursing education to be a baccalaureate degree rather than an associate degree, which is an important issue in the United States. Because Canada requires a baccalaureate degree to enter nursing practice, many of these recommendations do not apply in Canada. While we support these recommendations, we propose that developing a Caring Science curriculum and pedagogical practices meet these recommendations.

Although these developments represent important progress in articulating innovative *pedagogical* approaches for nursing education, only a few authors (Boykin & Schoenhofer, 2001; Boykin, Touhy, & Smith, 2011; Giddens & Brady, 2007; Hills & Cara, 2019; Hills & Lindsey, 1994; Horton-Deutch et al., 2019; Iwasiw et al., 2020; Smith, 2019) have attempted to outline different approaches to the *structure and organizational aspects of curriculum development*. Perhaps the most significant development in the last decade is the emergence of concept-based curriculum (CBC) (Erickson, 2002; Hendricks & Wangerin, 2017; Lewis et al., 2011). All of these historic and contemporary trends and turns in nursing education are evolutionary in the sense that they each contribute to a new dimension in curriculum thinking and pedagogical processes. However, there is still another turn to be made that underpins these curricular processes and structures.

For example, other, earlier reports from national professional organizations and educational foundations reflect the authentic, evolutionary spiral still needed. The 1994 Pew-Fetzer Task Group Report on Relationship-Centered Care for all health professions, the new essentials of nursing education: BS, MS, DNS document of the AACN (2009), and the early Boyer report (1990) addressed the need for serious reform. This need was highlighted again in the Carnegie Report on Nursing Education by Benner et al. (2010). This Carnegie report specifically recommended dramatic changes in how nurses are educated: "immersing nursing students in the *discipline* [emphasis added] of nursing during the first two years of study" (2010, p. 218). Each of these reports in some way critiques the status quo for nursing and health science professional education and makes a case for caring relationships and foundational basics as the essential core of educational reform. One nursing education reform that has occurred in Canada (with the exception of Quebec) and that has not yet happened in the United States, is the requirement that nurses have a baccalaureate degree to enter nursing practice. Having a BSN as "entry to practice" addresses many of the issues and recommendations outlined in the Carnegie Report (Benner et al., 2010).

Although many nursing educators today seek to embrace expanded views of professional education and curriculum, nursing education on the whole has yet to actualize this broader vision proposed by earlier and more recent reports and recommendations. Indeed, in the publications by Caring Science scholars (Smith, 2019; Smith & McCarthy, 2010), faculty are encouraged to "go beyond these earlier and recent blueprints to educate generalist, advanced generalist, and advanced specialty nurses who are grounded in the philosophies, theories, research, and practice models within the *discipline* [emphasis added]) of nursing" (Smith & McCarthy, p. 44). Still, despite reports, recommendations, and specific changes to make the necessary shift from teaching knowledge, techniques, procedures, and content toward authentic disciplinary learning (between and among faculty and students), there remains a gap between the status quo and creating a caring curriculum and one that is explicitly based within its most mature, evolved disciplinary foundation—in this instance: Caring Science.

There are notable exceptions, especially the curriculum work of Lewis et al. (2011), who describe their efforts at York University, Ontario, Canada, within a human science/caring paradigm. Their work is guided by an explicit focus on human/Caring Science, which is evolutionary in itself, moving, as it has, beyond the Bevis and Watson text that emphasized the educative paradigm of critical thinking and Critical Social Theory. Dr. Anne Boykin, with her visionary, sustained Caring Science leadership and successes with her colleagues and the college-wide programs at Florida Atlantic University, is another noteworthy exception. They have also contributed a chapter to this book (see Chapter 13). The Collaborative Nursing Program of British Columbia (CNPBC) in Canada is a third example in which a collaborative curriculum was based on a philosophy of caring and health promotion. You will find this program discussed in Chapter 11 to highlight different frameworks and processes for curriculum development. More recently the Siena Program in New York (see Chapter 14) have developed nursing programs based in Caring Science.

These current successful programs and projects serve as hopeful models and exemplars of movement toward a mature Caring Science educational model for nursing.

NEXT TURN IN CURRICULUM EVOLUTION: EMBRACING A RENAISSANCE

The need remains to move more explicitly toward a curriculum that is grounded in, and builds upon, Caring Science as a more evolved disciplinary guide for structural organization, content, context, pedagogical strategies, and meaningful relationships. For now and the near future, the requirement is to prepare nurses as mature caring-healing-health practitioners of nursing, informed by their distinct discipline.

At the heart of the curriculum revolution, Watson wrote an evocative article that remains relevant to this day (Watson, 1991). She used the lyrics of Tracy Chapman's famous song "Talking 'bout a Revolution" to call for a shift from a *revolution* to a *renaissance* for nursing, and nursing education to move forward with its Caring Science curriculum agenda. As Watson (1991) states,

> the time is now for a renaissance—a commitment to an expanded human caring consciousness, as well as toward the possible and what ought to be. It is time to create what might be: a new social and scientific order in a techno-cure system that has lost its way. (p. 99)

Hills and Cara (2019) support this shift and suggest "renaissance ... means conceiving a rebirth of nursing's historical claim to *caring* [emphasis added] for people and their health and healing experiences as its foremost contribution to healthcare in our current society" (p. 202).

In this book, we offer a guide to creating a nursing curriculum that is grounded in this renaissance movement with the disciplinary matrix of Caring Science, going beyond the conventional blueprints, offering a model that serves as an emancipatory, even passionate, ethical–philosophical, educational, and pedagogical learning guide for both teachers and students, and the caring relationship for both teaching and learning. The next chapter moves us further into this territory.

REFERENCES

American Association of Colleges of Nursing. (2007). *White paper on the education and role of the clinical nurse leader*. Author. https://nursing.uiowa.edu/sites/default/files/documents/academic-programs/graduate/msn-cnl/CNL_White_Paper.pdf

American Association of Colleges of Nursing. (2008). *The essentials of baccalaureate education for professional nursing practice*. https://www.aacnnursing.org/portals/42/publications/baccessentials08.pdf

American Association of Colleges of Nursing. (2009). *The essentials of doctoral education for advanced nursing practice*. https://www.aacnnursing.org/Portals/42/Publications/DNPEssentials.pdf

Baumann, S. (2010). The limitations of evidence-based practice. *Nursing Science Quarterly, 23*(93), 226–230. https://doi.org/10.1177/0894318410371833

Benner, P., Sutphen, M., Leonard, V., & Day, L. (2010). *Educating nurses: A call for radical transformation. The Carnegie report for the advancement of teaching*. Jossey-Bass.

Bevis, E. O. (1988). *Curriculum building in nursing. A process* (3rd ed.). National League of Nursing.

Bevis, E. O., & Watson, J. (1989). *Toward a caring curriculum. A new pedagogy for nursing*. National League of Nursing.

Bevis, E. O., & Watson, J. (2000). *Towards a caring curriculum: A new pedagogy for nursing*. Jones & Bartlett.

Boyer, E. (1990). *Scholarship reconsidered: Priorities for the professoriate*. Carnegie Foundation for the Advancement of Teaching.

Boykin, A., & Schoenhofer, S. (2001). *Nursing as caring: A model for transforming practice*. Jones & Bartlett Publishers.

Boykin, A., Touhy, T., & Smith, M. (2011). Evolution of a caring-based College of nursing. In M. Hills & J. Watson, *Creating a Caring Science curriculum: An emancipatory pedagogy for nursing* (1st ed., pp. 157–184). Springer Publishing Company.

Brown, H., & Rodney, P. (2007). Beyond case studies in practice education: Creating capacities for ethical knowledge through story and narrative. In L. Young & B. Paterson (Eds.), *Teaching nursing: Developing a student-centered learning environment* (pp. 141–163). Lippincott Williams & Wilkins.

Castledine, G. (2010). Creative nursing: Art or science? *British Journal of Nursing, 19*, 937–938. https://doi.org/10.12968/bjon.2010.19.14.49056

Chinn, P. L. (2019, March). *Keynote Address: The Discipline of Nursing: Moving Forward Boldly*. Presented at "Nursing Theory: A 50 Year Perspective, Past and Future," Case Western Reserve University Frances Payne Bolton School of Nursing. https://nursology.net/2019-03-21-case-keynote

Clark, C. S. (2010). The nursing shortage is a community transformational opportunity. *Advances in Nursing Science, 33*(1), 35–52. https://doi.org/10.1097/ANS.0b013e3181c9e1c4

Cowling, W. R., Smith, M. C., & Watson, J. (2008). The power of wholeness, consciousness and caring: A dialogue on nursing science, art, and healing. *Advances in Nursing Science, 31*, e41–e51. https://doi.org/10.1097/01.ANS.0000311535.11683.d1

Diekelmann, N. (2004). Class evaluations: Creating new student partnerships in support of innovation. *Journal of Nursing Education, 43*(10), 436–439. https://doi.org/10.3928/01484834-20041001-06

Diekelmann, N. (2005). Engaging the students and the teacher: Co-creating substantive reform with narrative pedagogy. *Journal of Nursing Education, 44*(6), 249–252. https://doi.org/10.3928/01484834-20050601-02

Duffy, J. (2018). *Quality caring in nursing and health systems: Implications for clinicians, educators, and leaders* (3rd ed.). Springer Publishing Company.

Enzman Hines, M. (2011). Caring in advance practice education: A new view of the future. In M. Hills & J. Watson (Eds.), *Creating a Caring Science curriculum: An emancipatory pedagogy for nursing* (1st ed., pp. 203–216). Springer Publishing Company.

Erickson, H. (2002) *Concept-based curriculum and instruction: Teaching beyond the facts.* Sage.

Estabrooks, C. (1998). Will evidence-based nursing practice make practice perfect? *Canadian Journal of Nursing Research, 30*, 15–36. https://cjnr.archive.mcgill.ca/article/view/1422

Estabrooks, C. A., Rutakumwa, W., O'Leary, K., Profetto-McGrath, J., Milner, M., Levers, M. J., & Scott-Findlay, S. (2005). Sources of practice knowledge among nurses. *Qualitative Health Research, 15*(4), 460–476. https://doi.org/10.1177/1049732304273702

Feller, F. (2018). Transforming nursing education: A call for a conceptual approach. *Nursing Education Perspectives, 39(2), 105–106. https://doi.org/10.1097/01.NEP.0000000000000187*

Giddens, J., & Brady, D. (2007). Rescuing nursing education from content saturation: The case for a concept-based curriculum. *Journal of Nursing Education, 46*(2), 65–70. https://doi.org/10.3928/01484834-20070201-05

Giddens, J. F., Wright, M., & Gray, I. (2012). Selecting concepts for a concept-based curriculum: Application of a benchmark approach. *Journal of Nursing Education, 51*(9), 511–515. https://doi.org/10.3928/01484834-20120730-02

Harvey, G., & Kitson, A. (2015). *Implementing evidence-based practice in healthcare: A facilitation guide.* Routledge.

Hendricks, S., & Wangerin, V. (2017). Concept-based curriculum changing attitudes and overcoming barriers. *Nurse Educator, 42*(3), 138–142. https://doi.org/10.1097/NNE.0000000000000335

Heron, J., & Reason, P. (1997). A participatory inquiry paradigm. *Qualitative Inquiry, 3*(3), 274–294. doi /10.1177/107780049700300302

Hills, M. (2016). Emancipatory and collaborative: leading from beside. In W. Rosa (Ed.), *Nurses as leaders: Evolutionary visions of leadership* (pp. 293–309). Springer Publishing Company.

Hills, M., & Cara, C. (2019). Curriculum development processes and pedagogical practices for advancing Caring Science literacy. In W. Rosa, S. Horton-Deutsch, & J. Watson (Eds.), *A handbook for caring science: Expanding the paradigm* (pp. 197–210). Springer Publishing Company.

Hills, M., & Lindsey, E. (1994). Health promotion: A viable framework for nursing education. *Nursing Outlook, 42*(4), 465–462. https://doi.org/10.1016/0029-6554(94)90003-5

Hills, M., & Watson, J. (2011). *Creating a Caring Science curriculum: An emancipatory pedagogy for nursing* (1st ed.). Springer Publishing Company.

Horton-Deutsch, S., Oman, K., & Sousa, K. (2019). Nurturing doctorally prepared caring scientists. In W. Rosa, S. Horton-Deutsch, & J. Watson, (Eds.), *A handbook for caring science: Expanding the paradigm* (pp. 277–284). Springer Publishing Company.

Hunt, D. D. (2018). *The new nurse educator: Mastering academe* (2nd ed.). Springer Publishing Company.

Institute of Medicine. (2011). *The future of nursing: Leading change, advancing health.* National Academies Press.

Iwasiw, C. L., Andrusyszyn, M.-A., & Goldenberg, D. (2020). *Curriculum development in nursing education* (4th ed.). Jones & Bartlett Publishers.

Jillings, C., & O'Flynn-Magee, K. (2007). Barriers to student-centered teaching: Overcoming institution and attitudinal obstacles. In L. Young & B. Paterson (Eds.), *Teaching nursing: Developing a student-centered learning environment* (pp. 467–483). Lippincott Williams & Wilkins.

Jones, D., & Wright, B. (2010). Nursing knowledge—Impact on nursing's preferred future. Position paper: Expert panel on nursing theory-guided practice. *American Academy of Nursing* (Unpublished paper).

Kitson, A., Harvey, G., & McCormack, B. (1998). Enabling the implementation of evidence-based practice: A conceptual framework. *Quality in Health Care, 7*, 149–158. https://doi.org/10.1136/qshc.7.3.149

Lee, S., Palmieri, P., & Watson, J. (Eds). (2017). *Global advances in human caring literacy.* Springer Publishing Company.

Levinas, E. (1969). *Totality and infinity.* Duquesne University.

Lewis, S., Rogers, M., & Naef, M. R. (2006). Caring-human science philosophy in nursing education: Beyond the curriculum revolution. *International Journal of Human Caring, 10*(4), 31–37. https://doi.org/10.20467/1091-5710.10.4.31

Lewis, S., Rogers, M. & Naef, M. R. (2011). Caring-human science philosophy in nursing education: Beyond the curriculum revolution. In M. Hills & J. Watson (Eds.), *Creating a Caring Science curriculum: An emancipatory pedagogy for nursing* (1st ed., pp. 185–202). Springer Publishing Company.

Logstrup, K. (1997). *The ethical demand.* University of Notre Dame.

Madjar, I., & Walton, J. (2001). What is problematic about evidence? In J. Morse, J. Swanson, & A. Kuzel (Eds.), *The nature of qualitative evidence* (pp. 28–45). Sage.

Mann, J. (2012). Critical thinking and clinical judgment skill development in baccalaureate nursing students. *The Kansas Nurse, 87*(1), 26–31.

Middleton, R. (2013). Active learning and leadership in undergraduate curriculum: How effective is it for student learning and transition to practice? *Nurse Education Practice, 13*(2), 83–88. https://doi.org/10.1016/j.nepr.2012.07.012

Moccia, P. (1988). Curriculum revolution: An agenda for change. In the National League for Nursing (Eds.), *Curriculum revolution: Mandate for change* (pp. 53–64). National League of Nursing.

Munhall, P. (1988). Curriculum revolution: A social mandate for change. In the National League for Nursing (Eds.), *Curriculum revolution: Mandate for change* (pp. 217–230). National League of Nursing.

Newman, M. A. (1986). *Health as expanding consciousness.* Mosby.

Newman, M. A. (1992). Prevailing paradigms in nursing. *Nursing Outlook, 40*(1), 10–13. https://doi.org/10.1097/00152193-199207000-00005

Newman, M. A., Sime, A. M., & Cororan-Perry, S. A. (1991). The focus of the discipline of nursing. *Advances in Nursing Science, 14*(1), 1–6. https://doi.org/10.1097/00012272-199109000-00002

Newman, M. A., Smith, M. C., Pharris, M. C., & Jones, D. (2008). The focus of the discipline revisited. *Advances in Nursing Science, 8*(31), e16–e27. https://doi.org/10.1097/01.ANS.0000311533.65941.f1

Nightingale, F. (1971). *Una and the Lion.* Riverside Press. https://en.wikisource.org/wiki/Una_and_the_Lion

Nortvedt, P. (2000). Clinical sensitivity: Inseparability of ethical perceptiveness and clinical knowledge. *Scholarly Inquiry for Nursing Practice, 14*(3), 1–19.

Palmer, P. (2004). *The violence of our knowledge. Toward a spirituality of higher education. 21st learning initiative.* Fetzer Institute.

Parse, R. R. (1987). *Nursing science: Major paradigm, theories and critiques.* Saunders.

Parse, R. R. (1992). Human becoming: Parse's theory of nursing. *Nursing Science Quarterly, 5*, 35–42. https://doi.org/10.1177/089431849200500109

Rockwood-Lane, M., & Samuels, M. (2011). Introduction to caring as a pedagogical approach to nursing education. In M. Hills, & J. Watson (Eds.), *Creating a Caring Science curriculum: An emancipatory pedagogy for nursing* (1st ed., pp. 217–244). Springer Publishing Company.

Rogers, M. E. (1970). *An introduction to the theoretical basis of nursing.* FA Davis.

Rogers, M. E. (1989). Nursing: A science of unitary human beings. In J. Riehl Sisca (Ed.), *Conceptual models for nursing practice* (pp. 181–188). Appleton and Lange.

Rosa, W., Horton-Deutsch, S., & Watson, J. (Eds). (2019). *A handbook for caring science: Expanding the paradigm.* Springer Publishing Company.

Rycroft-Malone, J., Seers, K., Titchen, A., Harvey, G., Kitson, A., & McCormack, B. (2004). What counts as evidence in evidence-based practice? *Journal of Advanced Nursing, 47*, 81–90. https://doi.org/10.1111/j.1365-2648.2004.03068.x

Sackett, D., Rosenberg, W., Gray, J., & Haynes, R. (1996). Evidence-based medicine: What it is and what it isn't. *British Medical Journal, 312*, 71–72. https://doi.org/10.1136/bmj.312.7023.71

Sarter, B. (1988). Philosophical sources of nursing theory. *Nursing Science Quarterly, 1*, 52–59. https://doi.org/10.1177/089431848800100205

Sitzman, K., & Watson, J. (2017). *Watson's caring in the digital world.* Springer Publishing Company.

Smith, H. (1982). *Beyond the postmodern mind.* Crossroads Publications.

Smith, L. (1993). The art and science of nursing. *Nursing Times, 89*(25), 42–43. https://doi.org/10.1097/00000446-199312000-00024

Smith, M. C. (2019). Regenerating nursing's disciplinary perspective. *Advances in Nursing Sciences, 42*(1), 3–16. https://doi.org/10.1097/ANS.0000000000000241

Smith, M., & McCarthy, P. (2010). Disciplinary knowledge in nursing education: Going beyond the blueprints. *Nursing Outlook, 58*, 44–51. https://doi.org/10.1016/j.outlook.2009.09.002

Tanner, C. (1988). Curriculum revolution: The practice mandate. *Nursing & Health Care, 9*(8), 426–430.

Tanner, C. (2006). The next transformation: Clinical education. *Journal of Nursing Education, 45*(4), 99–101. https://doi.org/10.3928/01484834-20060401-01

Tarlier, D. (2005). Mediating the meaning of evidence through epistemological diversity. *Nursing Inquiry, 12*(2), 126–134. https://doi.org/10.1111/j.1440-1800.2005.00262.x

Thorne, S., & Sawatzky R. (2014). Particularizing the general: Sustaining theoretical integrity in the context of an evidence-based practice agenda. *Advanced in Nursing Sciences, 37*(1), 5–18. https://doi.org/10.1097/ANS.0000000000000011

Tracy, M. F., & O'Grady, E. T. (2019). *Hamric and Hanson's advanced practice nursing: An integrative approach* (6th ed.). Elsevier Saunders.

Watson, J. (1979). *Nursing the philosophy and science of caring.* Little Brown.

Watson, J. (1988). New dimensions of human caring theory. *Nursing Science Quarterly, 1,* 175–181. https://doi .org/10.1177/089431848800100411

Watson, J. (1991). From revolution to renaissance. *Revolution: Journal of Nurse Empowerment, 1*(1), 94–100.

Watson, J. (1995). Postmodern knowledge development in nursing. *Nursing Science Quarterly, 8*(2), 60–64. https:// doi.org/10.1177/089431849500800207

Watson, J. (2002). Metaphysics of virtual caring communities. *International Journal of Human Caring, 6*(1), 41–45. https://doi.org/10.20467/1091-5710.6.1.41

Watson, J. (2005). *Caring science as sacred science.* F. A. Davis.

Watson, J. (2007). *Nursing: Human science and human care.* Jones & Bartlett. (Original work published 1985)

Watson, J. (2008). *Nursing: The philosophy and science of caring* (rev. ed.). University Press of Colorado.

Watson, J. (2012). *Human caring science: A theory of nursing.* Jones & Bartlett Learning.

Watson, J. (2018). *Unitary caring science: The philosophy and praxis of nursing.* University Press of Colorado.

Watson, J., & Smith, M. (2002). Caring science and the science of unitary human beings: Trans-theoretical discourse. *Journal of Advanced Nursing, 37*(5), 452–461. https://doi.org/10.1046/j.1365-2648.2002.02112.x

Williams, B., & Day, R. (2007). Context-based learning. In L. Young & B. Paterson (Eds.), *Teaching nursing: Developing a student-centered learning environment.* Lippincott Williams & Wilkins.

Willis, D. G., Grace, P. J., & Roy, C. (2008). A central unifying focus for the discipline: Facilitating humanization, meaning, choice, quality of life and healing our living and dying. *Advances in Nursing Science, 31,* e28–e40. https://doi.org/10.1097/01.ANS.0000311534.04059.d9

Young, L. (2007). Story-based learning: Blending content and process to learn nursing. In L. Young & B. Paterson (Eds.), *Teaching nursing: Developing a student-centered learning environment.* Lippincott Williams & Wilkins.

Young, L., & Paterson, B. (Eds.). (2007). *Teaching nursing: Developing a student-centered learning environment.* Lippincott Williams & Wilkins.

Caring Science Disciplinary Evolution

CARING SCIENCE DISCIPLINARY DISCOURSE

We are witnessing in our time the undermining and erosion of the discipline of nursing; its values and unique lens on knowledge, what counts as knowledge and nursing's global gift to humanity and the world. There are clarion calls for nursing to assume more responsibility for sustaining and advancing nursing's disciplinary values, theories, phenomena, and importance (e.g., Barrett, 2002, 2016; Chinn, 2019; Fawcett, 2020; Fitzpatrick et al., 2019; Smith, 2019; Turkel et al., 2018; Watson, 2018; Willis et al., 2008), and, discourse and debates within the American Academy of Nursing (AAN) Expert Panel on Nursing Theory and Knowledge Development (AAN Annual Meeting, Washington, DC, personal experiences, 2017, 2018, 2019).

DEFINITION OF DISCIPLINE

In light of the importance of this issue, it is helpful to clarify the meaning of "discipline." The most common reference of "discipline" in nursing literature is the classic Donaldson and Crowley (1978) article: The Discipline of Nursing. They were clear that the discipline informs the profession, rather than the other way around. Being inspired by Donaldson and Crowley's (1978) definition of "discipline," Smith (2019) defines it as "a field of study, grounded in higher education, that delineates its unique phenomena of concern, the context in which they are viewed, its relevant questions and methods of inquiry" (p. 5). Fawcett (2020) acknowledged that "nursing as a discipline and practice profession—or the disciplinary focus—continues to evolve" (p. 97).

Another view of "discipline" is "a field of study, or activity concerned with theory, rather than method, or requiring the knowledge and systematic application of principles, rather than relying on traditional rules, acquired skill, or intuition" (Fawcett, 2020, p. 97). This perspective is also supported by Fitzpatrick et al. (2019). Chinn (2019) and others (Fawcett, 2019; Smith, 2019) now are introducing "nursology" as a new term to define nursing as a discipline. This latest focus is an attempt to further identify nursing as a distinct discipline, meriting its scholarly standing as a defined field of study.

The disciplinary foundation of nursing transcends individual theories; however, the need to advance and clarify discipline—specific knowledge and practices—is essential to nursing education, research, management, sociopolitical, and practice. Indeed, the discipline provides the epistemological lens, moral–ethical values, ontological and philosophical lens to knowledge and to theory and to professional practice.

DISCIPLINE VERSUS PROFESSION

By way of review, at this crossroads, it is important to clarify the difference between the "discipline of nursing" and the "profession of nursing." When people have difficulty articulating, "why nursing?" or "what is nursing?" or "what is nursing science?" (Barrett, 2002, 2016), we realize there continues to be a void, even within the Academy itself and the nature and direction of its programs and priorities. To be more specific, based on Watson's latest works (2018), we have outlined some essentials regarding the nature of discipline:

- The discipline of nursing is what holds the timeless values, nursing's heritage and traditions and knowledge development toward sustaining humanity as well as health and healing for all.
- The discipline is what holds and honors an ontology of whole person—the unity of oneness of Being/Becoming and a relational unitary worldview.
- The discipline is what adheres to nursing's philosophical orientation toward humanity and nursing's ethical global covenant with humanity to sustain human caring-healing-health for all.
- The discipline is what holds the theories, the orientation toward knowledge development and what counts as knowledge—expanding conventional medical science/Western science epistemologies.
- The discipline is what holds nursing's research traditions and diverse and evolving approaches to knowledge development; the discipline-specific orientation to knowledge critiques "what counts as knowledge."
- The discipline addresses expanded, diverse, creative and innovative curriculum development processes, pedagogical practices, as well as methodologies and methods consistent with human caring-healing health–illness experiences and phenomena (Hills & Cara, 2019; Watson, 2018).
- The discipline holds grand, middle range, and situation-specific theories to provide a shared evolved, unitary worldview, whereby health is related to social-moral justice, whole person/whole system processes and outcomes; acknowledging human caring and eco-caring are one (e.g., people and planet are connected).
- Theories and philosophies of science frame disciplinary knowledge; they transcend specific circumstances and events and seek to provide universal explanations that reflect the ethical/philosophical foundation and values for the entire field of study (Reed et al., 2003, p.12, as cited in Watson, 2018, p. 38).
- Likewise, theories contain underlying ontological/philosophical/ethical assumptions about knowledge and values for humanity, human caring health experiences, environment, and science (Watson, 2018).
- This underlying orientation to core dimensions of nursing reflects a distinct disciplinary position. All nursing theories hold an underlying ontology—take a position on disciplinary knowledge—and this collective building leads to professional identity and visibility of nursing knowledge. Without identity, disciplinary clarity and commitment, to support, promote and develop substantive nursing knowledge and diverse theories, nursing will not continue to exist.
- Without adhering to nursing's core disciplinary foundation, without advancing nursing theory as a guide toward knowledge, nursing education, research, and practice will fail to meet its global covenant with humankind.

DISCIPLINARY EVOLUTION

It is also true that the discourse on core aspects of the discipline evolves and changes as knowledge advances and dynamic scholarly critiques uncover new horizons. For example, the most common view of the original disciplinary metaparadigm was posed by Fawcett (1984); but it has been challenged over the past several decades. The challenge includes three major critiques (Watson, 2018):

- Tautology of 'nursing' as a concept within its own paradigm
- Caring as a missing core concept
- Lack of clarity of philosophical ontological assumptions related to the worldview concepts, and confusion as to which paradigm concepts are located (e.g., particulate-deterministic; interactive-integrative; or unitary transformative; Watson, 2018, p. 32)

Scholars have also posited that while nursing phenomena are a unified whole, our paradigm worldview is often parts-focused, inconsistent with the phenomenon of human caring, health, healing, and wholeness, and intellectually inconsistent with an evolved unitary worldview and a relational ontology (Newman et al., 2008; Watson, 2018). This also has implications for nursing education both in terms of curriculum development and pedagogical practices. It is timely to revisit caring as a core concept within the discipline of nursing.

CARING AS CORE DISCIPLINARY CONCEPT

Through critiques of nursing's disciplinary maturity, the current and most contemporary scholarly discourse includes caring as one of the core disciplinary phenomena, along with concepts such as "human wholeness," "health, healing, well-being," and "human-environment–health relationship" (Smith, 2019, p. 10).

In addition to Watson's (1979, 1985, 1999, 2008, 2018) early focus on caring as philosophy and science of nursing, prominent caring scholars and nursing theorists include stellar theorists, researchers, and pioneer-caring scholars, educators, and authors, such as Leininger (1977), Boykin (1994), Boykin and Schoenhofer (1993/2001), Ray (1989, 2016), Roach (2002), Wolf (2013), and Swanson (1991). Others include Bevis and Watson (1989/2000), Stevenson and Tripp-Reimer (1989), Halldorsdottir (1990), Newman et al. (1991), Smith (1992, 2019), Cowling et al. (2008), Newman et al. (2008), Hills and Watson (2011), Cara et al. (2016), Turkel et al. (2018), Hills and Cara (2019), Cara et al. (2021), Willis et al. (2008), Litchfield and Jonsdottir (2008), and Meleis (1992, 2018).

Nevertheless, there continues to be concern about nursing preserving, sustaining, and advancing its disciplinary foundation, its unique knowledge and human-universe phenomena, social relevance and value orientation in education and research. To sustain and advance nursing, there is a continuing contemporary call "to be diligent about disseminating it through education and socialization of students, and to preserve and advance it in our research and practice traditions" (Smith, 2019, p. 3).

Further, nursing-discipline scholars and think tanks (e.g., 50th Anniversary Theory Conference "A 50-year Perspective, Past, and Future" at Case Western Reserve University, Frances Payne Bolton School of Nursing, March, 2019) are challenging the American Association College of Nursing (AACN) "Essentials" document, advocating for critiquing and going beyond established norms; acknowledging as Smith proclaimed, "it is time to revise [AACN] Essentials documents, and go beyond them to reflect the importance of the legacy of knowledge development in the discipline" (Smith, 2019, p.14).

In order to preserve and advance nursing and Caring Science, the disciplinary foundation must be an integral part of all levels of nursing education, research, scholarly professional practice, especially doctoral studies.

A commitment to a Caring Science curriculum requires study, philosophical–ethical knowledge, theories, diverse forms of inquiry, and a distinct focus within the curricular course structure of the program. A Caring Science curriculum will be evident in the worldview of faculty; the philosophy and theories of teaching/learning; and the nature of creative, authentic, pedagogical relations between faculty and students, including outcomes of students in their advancement of caring (Cara et al., 2020; Hills & Cara, 2019; Hills & Watson, 2011). All will make a distinct contribution to maturing the discipline of nursing into the future.

THE PROFESSION–CARING CURRICULUM

The nursing profession, along with other professions, can get caught up with rise of external crises of global economics, management science, technology, medicalized, hospital-based practices, artificial intelligence, humanoid nurse robotics, and institutional depersonalized policies, and negative political discourse, thus detoured from its disciplinary foundation. Without a clear disciplinary orientation and foundation to guide the development of the profession, it is easy to lose the way.

- The nursing profession, without the disciplinary foundation for knowledge and practice, can easily be guided by pressure of a separatist, externalized, professional worldview, versus a unitary internal disciplinary worldview (e.g., a committed worldview based on timeless values and knowledge that sustains global humanity). You cannot have a discipline without knowledge, substance, and content informed by assumptions, values, philosophy, principles, and purpose.
- Without disciplinary ontological, ethical, epistemological, methodological guidance, educational and clinical systems tend to adhere to pressures of distancing and objectifying knowledge, informed by techniques, tasks, and technology to control and manipulate care, humans, and health.

In closing, the good news is: Outdated policies and administrative practices, based on the dominant conventional separatist worldview, are crumbling and broken, and now there are shifts toward a relational global unitary caring–healing and health worldview—essential for human and planet survival. This also needs to be part of nursing educators' commitment.

Visionary Caring Science scholars, academic and clinical leaders, grounded in the discipline of nursing, are leading the way forward, even in midst of outdated mindsets. As educators, adhering to core values and informed moral–theory-guided practice, a new world of nursing science/Caring Science is unfolding in global service to humankind.

In creating a Caring Science curriculum, Caring Science is considered a core disciplinary concept, based upon an "Ethic of Belonging" (Watson, 2005), a relational ontology, expanded epistemology invoking curiosity and exploration of human-universe caring as a formidable philosophical-ethical-epistemic endeavor for our world. This disciplinary focus for sustaining nursing and caring requires commitment, courage, language, study, and guidance from history, as well as imagination of what might be, rather than adhering to what is and no longer is working for our world, our people (including students and educators), and our planet.

REFERENCES

Barrett, E. M. (2002). What is nursing science? *Nursing Science Quarterly, 15*(1), 51–60. https://doi.org/10.1177/08943180222108778

Barrett, E. M. (2016). Again; What is nursing science? *Nursing Science Quarterly, 30*(2), 129–133. https://doi.org/10.1177/0894318417693313

Bevis, E. O., & Watson, J. (1989). *Toward a caring curriculum: A new pedagogy for nursing.* National League for Nursing.

Bevis, E. O., & Watson, J. (2000). *Toward a caring curriculum. A new pedagogy for nursing* (2nd ed.). Jones & Bartlett.

Boykin, A. (Ed.). (1994). *Living a caring based program.* National League for Nursing.

Boykin, A., & Schoenhofer, S. O. (2001). *Nursing as caring: A model for transforming practice.* Jones & Bartlett Publishers & National League for Nursing. (Original work published 1993)

Cara, C., Gauvin-Lepage, J., Lefebvre, H., Létourneau, D., Alderson, M., Larue, C., Beauchamp, J., Gagnon, L., Casimir, M., Girard, F., Roy, M., Robinette, L., & Mathieu, C. (2016). Le Modèle humaniste des soins infirmiers—UdeM: perspective novatrice et pragmatique. *Recherche en soins infirmiers, 125*, 20–31. https://doi.org/10.3917/rsi.125.0020

Cara, C., Hills, M., & Watson, J. (2021). *An educator's guide to humanizing nursing education: Grounded in caring science.* Springer Publishing Company.

Chinn, P. L. (2019, March). *Keynote address: "The Discipline of Nursing. Moving forward boldly." Presented at Nursing Theory: A 50 Year Perspective. Past and Future.* Case Western Reserve University, Frances Bolton School of Nursing. https://nursologycom.files.wordpress.com/2019/03/2019-03-21-case-keynote-7.pdf

Cowling, W. R., Smith, M. C., & Watson, J. (2008). The power of wholeness, consciousness, and caring: A dialogue on caring science, art and healing. *Advances in Nursing Science, 31*, E41–E51. https://doi.org/10.1097/01.ANS.0000311535.11683.d1

Donaldson, S. K., & Crowley, D. M. (1978). The discipline of nursing. *Nursing Outlook, 26*(2), 113–120. PMID: 245616.

Fawcett, J. (1984). The metaparadigm of nursing: Present status and future refinements for theory development. *Journal Nursing Scholarship, 16*(3), 84–87. https://doi.org/10.1111/j.1547-5069.1984.tb01393.x

Fawcett, J. (2019). Nursology revisited and revived [Editorial]. *Journal of Advanced Nursing, 75*, 919–920. https://doi.org/10.1111/jan.13925

Fawcett, J. (2020). Thoughts about nursing science and nursing sciencing revisited. *Nursing Science Quarterly, 33*(1), 97–99. https://doi.org/10.1177/0894318419882029

Fitzpatrick, J. J., Reed, P. G., Smith, M. C., Smith, M. J., & Roy, C. (2019). Guest editorial: The nursing disciplinary perspective—50 years ago and the view forward. *Advances in Nursing Science, 42*(1), 2. https://doi.org/10.1097/ANS.0000000000000251

Halldorsdottir, S. (1990). The essential structure of a caring and uncaring encounter with a teacher: The perspective of the nursing student. In M. Leininger & J. Watson (Eds.), *The Caring imperative in nursing education* (pp. 95–108). National League for Nursing Press.

Hills, M., & Cara, C. (2019). Curriculum development processes and pedagogical practices for advancing caring science literacy. In W. Rosa, S. Horton-Deutsch, & J. Watson (Eds.), *A handbook for caring science: Expanding the paradigm* (pp. 197–210). Springer Publishing Company.

Hills, M., & Watson, J. (2011). *Creating a Caring Science curriculum: An emancipatory pedagogy for nursing* (1st ed.). Springer Publishing Company.

Leininger, M. (1977). Caring: The essence and central focus of nursing. *American Nurses Foundation. Nursing Research Rep, 12*(10), 2. PMID: 584383

Litchfield, M., & Jonsdottir, H. A. (2008). A practice discipline, here and now. *Advances in Nursing Science, 31*(1), 79–91. https://doi.org/10.1097/01.ANS.0000311531.58317.46

Meleis, A. (1992). Directions for nursing theory development in 21st Century. *Nursing Science Quarterly, 5*(3), 112–117. https://doi.org/10.1177/089431849200500307

Meleis, A. (2018). *Theoretical nursing: Development and progress* (6th ed.). Wolters Kluwer.

Newman, M. A., Sime, A. M., & Corcoran-Perry, S. A. (1991). The focus of discipline of nursing. *Advances in Nursing Science, 14*(1), 1–6. https://doi.org/10.1097/00012272-199109000-00002

Newman, M. A., Smith, M. C., Pharris, M. D., & Jones, D. (2008). The focus of the discipline of nursing revisited. *Advances in Nursing Science, 31*, E16–E27. https://doi.org/10.1097/01.ANS.0000311533.65941.f1

Ray, M. A. (1989). The theory of bureaucratic caring for nursing practice in the organizational culture. *Nursing Administrative Quarterly, 13*(2), 31–42. https://doi.org/10.1097/00006216-198901320-00007

Ray, M. A. (2016). *Transcultural caring: Dynamics in nursing and health care* (2nd ed.). FA Davis.

Reed, P. G., Sheaver, N. B., & Nicholl, L. (2003). *Perspectives on nursing theory* (4th ed.). Lippincott Williams and Wilkins.

Roach, M. S. (2002). *Caring, the human mode of being: A blueprint for the health professions* (2nd ed.). Canadian Hospital Association Press.

Smith, M. C. (1992). The distinctiveness of nursing knowledge. *Nursing Science Quarterly, 5*(4), 148–149. https://doi.org/10.1177/089431849200500402

Smith, M. C. (2019). Regenerating nursing's disciplinary perspective. *Advances in Nursing Science, 42*(1), 3–16. https://doi.org/10.1097/ANS.0000000000000241

Stevenson, J. S., & Tripp-Reimer, T. (Eds.). (1989). *Knowledge about care and caring: State of the art and future developments. Proceedings of a Wingspread Conference.* American Academy of Nursing.

Swanson, K. M. (1991). Empirical development of a middle range theory of caring. *Nursing Research, 40*, 161–166. https://doi.org/10.1097/00006199-199105000-00008

Turkel, M., Fawcett, J., Amankwaa, L., Clark, P. N., Dee, V., Eustache, R., Hansell, P. S., Jones, D. A., Smith, M. C., & Zahourek, R. (2018). Thoughts about nursing curricular: Dark clouds and bright lights. *Nursing Science Quarterly, 31*(2), 185–189. https://doi.org/10.1177/0894318418755734

Watson, J. (1979). *Nursing the philosophy and science of caring.* Little Brown.

Watson, J. (1985). *Nursing: Human science and human care.* Appleton-Century-Crofts.

Watson, J. (1999). *Postmodern nursing and beyond.* Churchill-Livingstone.

Watson, J. (2005). *Caring science as sacred science.* F. A. Davis.

Watson, J. (2008). *Nursing the philosophy and science of caring. New Revised Edition.* University Press of Colorado.

Watson, J. (2018). *Unitary caring science: The philosophy and praxis of nursing.* University Press of Colorado.

Willis, D. G., Grace, P. J., & Roy, C. A. (2008). A central unifying focus for the discipline: Facilitating humanization, meaning, choice and quality of life, and healing on living and dying. *Advances in Nursing Science, 31*(1), E28–E40. https://doi.org/10.1097/01.ANS.0000311534.04059.d9

Wolf, Z. (2013). *Exploring rituals in nursing: Joining art and science.* Springer Publishing Company.

Beliefs and Assumptions: The Hidden Drivers of Curriculum Development

[A] philosophical belief in human freedom—a "Wide Awakeness" that is paradigm shattering and emancipatory . . . calls for encouragement, self-reflection . . . educators come in touch with their own humanity . . . encourage the release of the human spirit.—From Maxine Greene (1978) cited in Jean Watson (1989a, p. 37)

INTRODUCTION

The purpose of this chapter is to highlight the important role that beliefs, values, and assumptions play in guiding our thinking, behaviors, and actions in general, as we engage in the curriculum development process, and, specifically, the influence they have on our pedagogical practices, ultimately student–teacher relationships and knowing. We address the underlying beliefs and assumptions of a Caring Science curriculum in order to help faculty and students gain clarity about just what Caring Science is and why, we argue, it must form the foundation of the *discipline* of nursing. This foundation of beliefs and assumptions opens up the heart and mind to the beauty and manifestation of Caring Science as a serious and emancipatory epistemic, ethical, ontological, pedagogical, methodological, and praxis endeavor.

IMPACT OF BELIEFS ON WORLDVIEW AND BEHAVIORS

Beliefs and assumptions are embedded in and deeply influence our worldview, our perceptions, and our actions in everyday experiences. It is important to be aware of our beliefs and assumptions because they influence our thinking, our learning, and our ways of interacting as we encounter experiences. In fact, they determine the meaning that we give a specific situation at any moment in time; they reflect our level of consciousness and our own evolution, which in turn affects our very view of reality.

Our beliefs are convictions that we hold as "truths." They may not actually be true but, within ourselves, they are the "facts" that we hold as "Truth." For example, we may believe that "we cannot teach anyone anything." This may not be "true" but, because it is a belief we hold, we will act as if it were true. We all have many beliefs, and, although they may change from time to time, many of us operate in the world unaware of the beliefs we hold. Many of these beliefs may have been with us since childhood and may, in fact, no longer be relevant to one's current circumstances and context. For example, we may unconsciously hold the belief "people can't be trusted"; thus, this embedded belief from childhood will affect our interactions and ability to relate to others. We also have many conflicting beliefs and, at times, may have difficulty making decisions because of these conflicting beliefs.

Although our beliefs have an epistemic status (i.e., they make assumptions about what is "true"), often they are more deeply embedded in and determined by our "values," or those things to which we attach worth. This makes some of our beliefs difficult to change and even highly resistant to change. Combs (1982) as well as Egan and Reese (2019) suggest that if you want to understand what your values are, you should monitor how you spend your time. For example, if you say that you value reading but when asked: When was the last time that you read a book? you respond that you do not have time to read, we would say that reading is not a value for you. Similarly, if you say that you value patient-centered care but you say that you do not have time to talk to your patients because there is too much to do, your behavior does not support your stated values. So, think about how you spend your time. This process can be thought of as learning to read your behavior backwards.

The most important idea to take away from this discussion about beliefs and assumptions is to appreciate how these fundamental aspects of human nature affect your behavior, your consciousness, and in turn your very worldview, particularly in relation to curriculum development and pedagogical practices. To demonstrate this point, we share this classic story that Combs (1979) shared when talking to a group of educators. Consider your experiences with teaching/learning situations as you read the story.

> In a school in the outskirts of Atlanta there was a young woman teaching the first grade who was a very beautiful young woman with a beautiful head of blonde hair that she was accustomed to wearing in a ponytail that hung down to the middle of her back. The first few days of school she wore her hair this way. Then on Thursday, she decided she wanted to do it differently, so she did it all up in a bun on the top of her head. One of the little boys in her class looked into her room but he didn't recognize his teacher, you know that happens sometimes when a woman changes her hairdo, because she doesn't look like the same person. So here he was, lost and the bell rang and school started and he didn't know where to go. Along came the supervisor and found this little boy in the hall crying and she said to him, "What is the trouble?" and he said, "I can't find my teacher." So she said, "What is your teacher's name?" And he didn't know, so she said, "What room are you in?" and he didn't know that either. He had looked in there and it was the wrong place. So she said, "Well come on. Let's see if we can find her." And they started down the hall opening one door after another without much luck. Finally, they came to the room where this young woman was teaching and she opened the door and she saw the supervisor and the little boy and she said, "Why Joey, it is so good to see you. We have been wondering where you were. Come on in. We have missed you so." And the little boy pulled out of the supervisor's hand and threw himself into the teacher's arms. She gave him a hug and patted him on the fanny and he ran down to his seat. Now the supervisor was telling me this story and said to me, "You know, I said a prayer for that teacher. She thought little boys were important."
>
> As the supervisor was telling me this story we were riding along in a car. We began to play a game, you know. We said, "Well suppose she hadn't thought that little boys were important." Suppose for instance, she thought supervisors were important. Well in that case she might have said, "Why, good morning Miss Cheeves. We have been hoping that you would come by and see us, haven't we boys and girls?" or she might have thought that discipline was important.

And in that case she might have said, "Joey you know very well when you are late you must go to the office and get a permit, now run right down there." or she might have thought the lesson was important. In that case she might have said, "Joey, for heaven's sake where have you been, get your books and get to work." But she didn't, she thought that little boys were important and she behaved in terms of what she thought WAS important. So it is with all of us. We are discovering that this is what makes the difference between a good counsellor and a poor one, or a good teacher and a poor one, or a good nurse and a poor one, or a good priest and a poor one.

What Do You Believe Is Important?

This story provides an excellent illustration of how our beliefs, values, and assumptions are apparent in our behavior, affecting our consciousness, our worldview, and our response to any given situation.

LEARNING ACTIVITY: ACTIONS SPEAK LOUDER THAN WORDS

ENDS IN VIEW

The purpose of this learning activity is to become aware of how our beliefs, values, and assumptions are present in our behaviors.

In your journal, divide the page by drawing a line down the middle of it. In the left-hand column, write five beliefs that you have that are consistent with a Caring Science curriculum. In the right-hand column, write a corresponding action that you take that demonstrates that belief or value. Over the next week, monitor your behaviors, your awareness of your thoughts and state of your consciousness, and views toward any given situation. Reflect in your journal about what beliefs and values seem evident to you based on your behaviors and evolving consciousness related to beliefs and values.

TIME OUT FOR REFLECTION

Reflect on your beliefs, values, and corresponding actions. Share your reflections with your learning partner or group. Consider the following questions:

Did you have similar beliefs or values but different actions?
Was the relationship between your beliefs or values and your actions apparent?
What is your understanding of the relationship between your beliefs or values and your actions?

Becoming aware of your beliefs and assumptions, particularly in relation to how they "show up" in your behavior, can prove to be a very insightful exercise. Many of us behave without really being aware of what is driving our behavior, not being aware of how we "see the world" through our own value lens.

Learning to monitor your beliefs, values, and assumptions will assist you in discarding those that are no longer relevant or that do not fit with your desire to develop a Caring Science worldview. Such a shift in beliefs and assumptions reflects a change in, or evolution of consciousness, affecting your very view of the world.

Learning to do so will assist you in becoming a much more critically reflective practitioner and teacher. For example, one definition of "theory" goes back to the Latin word "theoria," which literally means "to see"; as we engage in this simple exercise, we find new lenses "to see" our reality in new ways. When one can critique one's own beliefs and "see" things differently, then one can act differently (Watson, 2008a).

The following is a synopsis of a fascinating study conducted a number of years ago but which remains relevant to this day. Combs (1971, 1993) examined the factors that influence a teacher's effectiveness. He was interested in knowing what the differences were between effective and ineffective teachers. At first, he thought it might be the knowledge that teachers had about a certain subject, but he discovered that knowledge was not a critical factor in teacher effectiveness. As you may have experienced, many teachers are knowledgeable about their subject matter but are not effective teachers! In this initial work, he also discovered that the methods teachers used did not influence their effectiveness, nor did their theoretical perspectives.

As Combs pursued his research, *he discovered that it was not the knowledge, methods, or theoretical perspective that made a teacher effective, but rather the nature of the interaction and the beliefs that teachers held that were of paramount importance in determining teaching effectiveness* (our emphasis). Combs (1971) tested 12 hypotheses in five different areas regarding the beliefs held by teachers that made them effective or not effective. These are summarized in Table 3.1. In her meta-analysis of caring within nursing science, Swanson (2013) also highlights that the impacts of beliefs that nurses hold as well as caring relationships nurses develop with others are significant and consequential.

TABLE 3.1 Differences Between Effective and Ineffective Teachers

EFFECTIVE TEACHERS	INEFFECTIVE TEACHERS
Beliefs About Frame of Reference	
Other-oriented	Self-oriented
Focus on people	Focus on things—rules, regulations, test results
Beliefs About People	
People are able: they have the capacity to handle their own problems	People are not able: it would be unethical to let someone do something if you didn't believe they were able to do it
People are friendly	
People are worthy of dignity and integrity	People are basically unfriendly
People are dependable	People are unworthy of dignity and integrity
	People are not dependable
Beliefs About Self	
Identify with others	Feel apart (different) from others
Feel they are "enough" the way they are	Feel they are not "enough"—feel inadequate
Positive self-image	Negative self-image
Reveal "self" to others	Conceal "self" from others

(continued)

TABLE 3.1 Differences Between Effective and Ineffective Teachers (*continued*)

EFFECTIVE TEACHERS	INEFFECTIVE TEACHERS
Purposes	
Approach to issues is freeing—working with others to understand issues and change them—solution-focused vs. problem-focused, strength exploration vs. weakness Focus on larger goals; search for authentic meaning; inner truth/purpose/vision	Approach to problem is "problem" emphasis; controlling "fix it" orientation Focus on smaller goals

BELIEFS THAT MAKE A DIFFERENCE

LEARNING ACTIVITY: WALKING THE WALK: BELIEFS THAT MAKE A DIFFERENCE

ENDS IN VIEW

This learning activity will provide you with opportunities to consider how your beliefs impact on your pedagogical practices. Using the format set out by Combs (1982) in his study on teaching effectiveness, try to identify where your beliefs fit within these categories. Create a blank table using his headings, and fill it in using your knowledge about yourself in teaching/learning situations. Consider your readings, thoughts, and discussions about beliefs and values. Using the framework you developed based on Combs's work, identify areas where you need to reconsider your beliefs. Using this same framework, write goals for yourself for the remainder of the course. Your journal is a great place to consistently reflect on your progress.

TIME OUT FOR REFLECTION

Think about the following questions:

What is your reaction to Combs's study? Does it resonate with you?
What did you discover about your beliefs in relation to Combs's findings?
What is the orientation you bring to your own teaching/learning issues? To others' issues?

BELIEFS AND ASSUMPTIONS ABOUT CARING SCIENCE CURRICULUM

The purpose of this section is to highlight the important role that beliefs, values, and assumptions play in guiding our thinking, behaviors, and actions in general as we engage in the curriculum development process in general and, specifically, the influence they have on our pedagogical practices.

Beliefs and Assumptions About Humanity

Certain assumptions about humanity underlie a Caring Science curriculum. These assumptions acknowledge the following:

- People are unitary holistic beings and *cannot* be broken down into component parts. People experience the world as whole human beings and make meaning of the world as they experience it.
- People are able and evolving and everyone has their own learning journey. This assumption is based on the belief that people have the ability to identify their own needs, have inner wisdom to solve their own problems, and generally know what is best for them in a given situation. This assumption also recognizes that people are their own best resource and often need only support and/or understanding to better understand and respond to their health issues.
- People are always situated. This assumption is closely related to the existential-phenomenological perspective that people are always situated in time and space and can best be understood within their own context. This refers to people's social, cultural, spiritual, political, and historical background and experiences; it recognizes the impact of this context in relation to health choices.
- Individual and social responsibility for health, well-being, and social justice regarding inequities are increasingly highlighted in local and global health discourses, as well as acknowledging that expanded notions of health and well-being are distinct from the historical medical-technocure orientation to health as the absence of disease.

Beliefs and Assumptions Related to Health and Healing

A Caring Science curriculum is based on the following assumptions about health and healing:

- Health is individually and subjectively defined and best understood by the person experiencing it. The person experiencing a health issue is in the best position to name it. Nurses cannot assume that all people experience health issues in the same way. Health and illness coexist and are not points on a continuum. People who are experiencing health issues or an illness often consider themselves healthy. This is particularly relevant for those people who experience chronic health challenges such as living with diabetes.
- There is a difference between curing and healing; curing seeks to eliminate disease, treat, remove, and diagnose. Curing is largely focusing on the body physical. Healing represents wholeness, oneness, unity of mind-body-spirit; healing is *"being-in-right-relation"* (Quinn, 1989, 2019); it honors and incorporates the human spirit, transcending the body/physical/material/medicine mind-set.
- Intersectionality (Hill & Bilge, 2016) is understood, valued, and celebrated. Respect for differences is inherent in one's assumptions and beliefs, honoring differences of race, culture, sexual orientation, political orientation, or ways of thinking about or being-in-the-world.

- One of the greatest human needs is to be authentically heard and to authentically listen to another's story; thus, persons are more able to hear and listen to their own inner wisdom, to detect their own best solutions for health and healing.

From these broader philosophical, scientific, and spiritual perspectives, one realizes that someone may be cured of a disease but not be healed. Healing, in contrast to curing, is based upon the internal meaning, the inner subjective experiences, and held by the individual person and all the processes and thoughts held in relation to the disease, the treatment, and outcomes. Healing is an inner process, whereas curing is an outer treatment process. With this level of awareness, someone may, in the process of dying, experience the ultimate healing. That is, if they are helped to die peacefully, having taken care of "unfinished business" and *"being-in-right-relation"* with self and other, their dying is a peaceful and sacred transition. Perhaps, it is the ultimate healing.

Teachers' Beliefs Reflected in a Caring Science Curriculum

A Caring Science curriculum reflects a teacher's belief in:

- the power and primacy of people in-relation, power of human consciousness, human imagination, and human spirit;
- the inner resources, the individual interests, and passionate scholarly questions and wonderings as key components in teaching/learning and in health/illness processes and outcomes;
- all student questions are considered sacred; no question is treated as trivial; as any and all questions reflect the inner learning processes of the student;
- wholeness, harmony, and beauty; connectedness/oneness of all; beauty inner truth;
- the unitary wholeness of humanity and environment and the larger universe;
- ways of knowing and teaching/learning that incorporate not only rational, cognitive, and technical empirics but also call upon aesthetic values, moral ideals, intuition, personal knowing, joy of process discovery, passion, and spiritual-metaphysical dimensions;
- the context of intersubjectivity, interhuman events, processes, relationships; and human-environment energetic patterns within a universal field;
- an ontology of evolving consciousness, human freedom, release of human spirit—while adhering to caring as a moral ideal and absolute value for sustaining human dignity; and authentic relationships in education and practice; and
- a worldview for human-evolutionary destiny that is open (Adapted from Watson, 1989b, p. 52, and Watson, 2000b, p. 52)

In summary, these basic, identified beliefs and assumptions underlie a Caring Science curriculum. Making explicit such basic assumptions provides the disciplinary foundation for education and professional practice, as well as for scholarly inquiry. This explicit disciplinary Caring Science orientation to education and teaching/learning seeks to release and tap into inner resources, the human spirit; in order to inspire, invite, empower, and emancipate students and educators, as well as patients. Accordingly, for Cara et al. (2021), being grounded in Caring Science can assist nurse educators to perceive their role as creating a caring/trusting teaching/learning environment that will support and nurture students' growth and emancipation. Finally, Caring Science seeks to preserve human dignity and honor the whole person for learning and healing; it is open to inner exploration for meaning and personal knowing, and, thus, the transformation and evolution of human consciousness.

As noted by Clark (2010):

> As we heal our individual selves, [our classrooms], small workplaces, communities, and our larger systems, we can partake of the great Awakening universal change process in the nursing profession . . . realize our interconnectedness and take our profession into a place of sacred autonomous practices. (p. 50)

EMANCIPATORY KNOWING: STUDENT–TEACHER DYNAMICS

The next section uncovers how deeply held beliefs and assumptions play out in student–teacher–student dynamics, in turn affecting classroom relations, emancipatory learning, and knowing.

> It is vital to de-professionalize the public debate on matters that vitally affect the lives of ordinary people. (Arundhati Roy, Indian writer-activist, 2001)

Chinn and Kramer (2018), in their classic work on theory and knowledge development, point out that through *emancipatory knowing* (our emphasis), nurses gain the ability to critique and analyze barriers of unfair and unjust conditions, and the complexity of social and political contexts, thus becoming agents of change to improve human life.

A Caring Science curriculum holds underlying beliefs and assumptions about power–control dynamics. The core assumption is based on the notion that there is reciprocity between power, knowledge, and control, and that, in order for there to be more equitable relationships, there is shared power. Thus, everyone benefits as they share their knowledge and in turn hold authentic power with others. Authentic power is shared power; it is power with, not power over. It does not negate faculty or nurses' responsibilities, skills, or knowledge. It also means standing in one's own power, one's own truth and integrity, without succumbing to other's power position, authoritarian control, and so on. We still acknowledge the reality that there is a difference between having authority and being authoritarian; the teacher has authority by the nature of their position; however, that position does not justify an authoritarian, power/control stance toward knowledge, toward students, and toward control of knowledge. In a Caring Science curriculum, students also have authority in their own knowing and experiences that can be shared and jointly critiqued for deeper knowledge. As Canales and others emphasize, "emancipatory learning helps to situate ourselves in the center of another's experience, while recognizing and respecting our differences" (in Canales, 2010, p. 31; Aptheker, 1989, p. 60)—not as separate, but as a reflection of the diversity of our shared human condition.

Issues of differences and power can be thought through and further critiqued within a Caring Science curriculum. As Mohanty (2003) points out, there is a need to think relationally (e.g., Caring Science is about honoring each individual as a unique person, embracing a relational ethical–ontological worldview and starting point) about questions of power, equality, justice, and the need to be inclusive. We know from our shared life experiences, as well as from the wisdom traditions across time, that we are all connected through our shared humanity and our sharing the planet Earth and its precious resources. Once again it is helpful to remind ourselves that everyone is situated in a given personal, relational, historical, cultural, deep phenomenal life-experience context. This backdrop needs to be considered, as each context of self and other is deeply rooted in a personal inner life contextual phenomenal field of history and meaning. In a Caring Science framework, the basic tenet is that one person's level of humanity reflects on the other and at the deeply human level; we are all one and connected through our shared humanity (Watson, 2006, 2008a, 2012, 2018). As the poet Maya Angelou reminds us in a major address, "I am a Human Being and nothing Human is alien to me" (in Watson, 2008b, p. 55)—thus if one person is put down, so am I; "likewise if the other person's human spirit is lifted up, so is mine" (Watson, 2008b, p. 56).

Within a Caring Science curriculum, it is important to uncover more pervasive issues of power/control/knowledge/social justice. What is of deeper concern regarding power relations in education and clinical care practices are the more fundamental issues of knowledge/ epistemology as power and, thus, epistemology as ethic (Palmer, 2004).

EPISTEMOLOGY AS ETHIC: ANOTHER TURN IN POWER RELATIONS IN EDUCATION AND PEDAGOGY*

Within a critique of knowledge and education, curriculum and learning, we have a new awareness, an awakening to the fact that every epistemology (ways of knowing and what counts as knowledge) becomes an ethic (Palmer, 2004). A fundamental conflict has prevailed within our institutions of higher learning that has already caught up with us in the Western world of science and professionalism. Everything has consequences. The types and ways of teaching and learning that have prevailed at the cognitive, intellectual, rational level alone are formative to our human development; they are shaping the lives of human beings and forming, informing, or deforming our mind-sets and actions as people and as professionals. As Palmer (2004, p. 2) profoundly asked, "What ethical formation and deformation has this approach to education created in our lives?" suggesting overtly a relationship between our knowledge and violence: the violence of knowledge (and language of power, control, domination, superiority). This form of knowledge development as often practiced in institutions of higher learning has "lent itself to subtle and pervasive forms of violence," to our personal, social, and professional ontological being, our epistemology informing our ethics, our human mode of living (2004, p. 2).

By "violence," Palmer means more subtle forms than dropping a bomb or hitting someone physically. Rather, he refers to violence associated with "violating the integrity" of the other, whether the other is the Earth, another human being, or another culture. This mode of learning and knowledge is tied up with the Western academy emphasis on three dominant ways of thinking, teaching, and learning, which according to Palmer (2004) are intended to guide our professional and personal lives: "objective, analytic, and experimental."

Each of these three dominant ways of learning, of valuing, of teaching, of knowing is critiqued by Palmer in his classic paper presented at the 2004 U.S. Fetzer Institute–sponsored conference, "21st Century Learning Initiatives." He points out the misguided myth that one cannot know anything truly well unless it is held at arm's length, at a distance, at great remove from self—thus perpetuating a chasm between the knower and the known. This myth reinforces the belief that knowledge is tainted, distorted, and untrustworthy if close to the individual; thus, one cannot possibly generate valid knowledge from a personal connection with the data or information.

---

*excerpt reprinted from Watson, 2008a, chapter 20.

OBJECTIVISM AS MYTHIC EPISTEMOLOGY—EPISTEMOLOGY-AS-ETHIC

Within this mythic epistemological system of knowledge, of learning, of valuing, of teaching as objective, Palmer (2004) reminds us that we create a profound fear of subjectivity, a fear of relatedness, of entering into a relationship with that which we know. Using the metaphors of war, he points out different explanations of the approaches related to objectivity and subjectivity. For example, we can try to detach ourselves from what is happening in an objective medical diagnosis, making disease a war of conquest to fight against the body, the disease. Further, it is safer to detach and separate one's self from the other person who is experiencing the disease. However, the subjective experience cannot be held at emotional–spiritual arm's length from the medical impersonal analysis; our world may be turned upside down, but the medical–clinical gaze is on the disease, the fight to win the war through correct diagnosis and treatment with cure the ultimate end, often at all costs. We all eventually come face to face with subjective evidence of our vulnerability and connectedness with our inner life world, our very humanity.

With the thin line of separation and connectedness between objective and subjective clinical professional relationships, one can begin to see how our limited view of how we think about objective knowledge crosses over into ethics. We cannot therefore justify "turning our face away" from self or others who are different from us or distant from us. Objectivity for its own sake and the mythology of rightness from a clinical (distanced) point of view can create cruelty if we are not able to accurately acknowledge and portray how events, knowledge, and experiences really exist/coexist in our world.

For its part, the objectivist mythology, whether in medical science per se or in terms of clinical war metaphors used for personal life events, is a distortion both of reality and knowledge—certainly a distortion of values and a distortion of science and how science is done. Palmer (2004) helps us remember: great knowing and great learning are not simply done objectively. Paradoxically, great knowing and learning constitute a dance between the objective and subjective, between intimacy and distance, between the personal, inner-life world and the outer, professional/political domain. This is true in all disciplines, not just nursing or "nursology" (Fawcett & Chinn, 2019). The mythology of objectivism is "more about [power] and control over the world, or over each other [or a given phenomenon], more a mythology of power than a real epistemology that reflects how real knowing proceeds" (Palmer, 2004, p. 4). As such, perpetuating this mythology of objectivism does not help us to see that "every epistemology becomes an ethic" (Palmer, 2004, p. 2) and affects how we value and see the different phenomena in our world.

Nightingale as Exemplar of Understanding "Epistemology as Ethic"

The story of Nightingale and her hands-on approach to knowing is a historic as well as a modern example of the "dance" of great knowing, the paradoxical integration of the subjective and objective. She skillfully wove together objective data and subjective visions, a personal sense of calling for her mission and outer-world life's work that transcended any objectivist logic of her era. Yet her internal ethics guided her approach to knowing, to valuing, to teaching, and to learning. She is arguably an exemplar of living the paradox of oneness with her being, knowing, doing in the world. This is not to say that we must agree with everything she said and did, but it is worth remembering that her underlying beliefs, assumptions, and weltanschauung (worldview) was largely what motivated her actions as one of the founders of modern nursing.

The Analytic and Experimental as Mythic Epistemology

Just as objectivism is a mythology yet can destructively become our ethic, ethos, and mind-set for teaching, learning, scholarship, and so on, Parker Palmer (2004) pointed out the same misstep with the notion that "analytic" and "experimental" mean "being scientific." Analytic, as he makes explicit, means that once you have objectified a phenomenon as something to be studied, you are then free to cut it into little pieces to see how it works; to break it down into parts, hold it at a distance, analyze it, and thus understand it. Palmer used this cutting-things-up phenomenon in order to look at, to understand, something "objectively," as a metaphor for what education often does to the human mind and human heart and human soul—the human experience in its totality. This cutting-up approach is the same as trying to describe and appreciate a rose, by cutting it up into little pieces. The same is true about humans and any human phenomena. The pieces never can depict and capture understanding, beauty, appreciation, majesty, or even knowledge of the whole "rose."

Palmer argues that this great facility for taking things apart, dissecting them to the point that one cannot know the original, is a form of violence in that it cultivates a lack of sensitivity and little capacity for putting things back together, including the human heart.

The same is true for the myth of "experimental," in that the mythology of objectivity, analytic, sets up mythological imprints that suggest that once things are objectified, dissected into parts, we are free to experiment. This focus in turn leads us to justify reducing a human to the moral status of object so we can objectively know, study, experiment, and conduct science.

This form of experimentation with humans and nature leads us to seek designs with what we think the world should be like, to control and dominate the outcome, so to speak, with our logic, our distant data, and our moving things around from their original form. We do this without paying attention to potentially destructive outcomes for self, society, humanity, the environment, and nature alike.

In summary, this section has introduced beliefs and assumptions as the starting point that underpins curriculum, approaches to humanity, to relations, to knowledge, power, and emancipatory education. We made more explicit what is meant by Caring Science, its assumptions, beliefs, and nature of the politics, policies, and dynamics that affect and can alter educational practices. Conventional myths identified by Parker Palmer (2004), world-renowned educator, helped us reveal how set beliefs both subtly, and overtly, permeate our approaches toward self and other, toward teaching/learning, toward education, and curriculum. This Caring Science critique shifts the discourse from conventional minds and mind-sets of education, of nursing, of caring, of teaching to learning, to emancipatory approaches, to knowledge, and all ways of knowing. This shift offers a new turn in nursing education; and ultimately invites the human spirit, the head/heart, soul, and love of nursing, a love of humanity, back into nursing, back into our educational programs, and back into our world.

REFERENCES

Aptheker, B. (1989). *Tapestries of life: Women's work, women's consciousness and the meaning of daily life*. The University of Massachusetts Press.

Canales, M. (2010). Othering: Difference understood?? A 10-year analysis and critique of the nursing literature. *Advances in Nursing Science, 33*(1), 15–34. https://doi.org/10.1097/ANS.0b013e3181c9e119

Cara, C., Hills, M., & Watson, J. (2021). *An educator's guide to humanizing nursing education: Grounded in caring science*. Springer Publishing Company.

Chinn, P. L., & Kramer, M. K. (2018). *Integrated theory and knowledge development in nursing* (10th ed.). Mosby Elsevier.

Clark, C. S. (2010). The nursing shortage as a community transformational opportunity. *Advances in Nursing Science, 33*(1), 35–52. https://doi.org/10.1097/ANS.0b013e3181c9e1c4

Combs, A. (1971). *Helping relationships: Basic concepts for the helping professions.* Allyn & Bacon.

Combs, A. (1979). *Myths in education.* Allyn & Bacon.

Combs, A. (1982). *Personal approach to teaching: Beliefs that make a difference.* Allyn & Bacon.

Combs, A. (1993). *Helping relationships: Basic concepts for the helping professions* (4th ed.). Allyn & Bacon.

Egan, G., & Reese, R. J. (2019). *The skilled helper* (11th ed.). Cengage Learning.

Fawcett, J., & Chinn, P. (2019). *About.* https://nursology.net/about

Hill, P., & Bilge, S. (2016). *Intersectionality.* Polity Press.

Mohanty, C. T. (2003). *Feminism without borders: Decolonizing theory, practicing solidarity.* Duke University Press.

Palmer, P. (2004). *The violence of our knowledge: Toward a spirituality of higher education.* 21st learning initiative. Fetzer Institute.

Quinn, J. F. (1989). On healing, wholeness and the Haelan effect. *Nursing and Health Care, 10*(10), 553–556. PMID: 2616056.

Quinn, J. F. (2019). The integrated nurse: Way of the healer. In M. J. Kreitzer & M. Koithan (Eds.), *Integrative nursing* (2nd ed., pp. 40–54). Oxford University Press.

Roy, A. (2001). *Power politics.* South End Press.

Swanson, K. M. (2013). What is known about caring in nursing science: A literary meta-analysis. In M. C. Smith, M. C. Turkel & Z. R. Wolf (Eds.), *Caring in nursing classics. An essential resource* (pp. 59–102). Springer Publishing Company.

Watson, J. (1989a). A new paradigm of curriculum development. In E. O. Bevis & J. Watson (Eds.), *Toward a caring curriculum* (pp. 37–49). National League for Nursing.

Watson, J. (1989b). Transformative thinking and a caring curriculum. In E. Bevis & J. Watson (Eds.), *Toward a Caring Curriculum: A New Pedagogy for Nursing* (p. 51–60). National League for Nursing.

Watson, J. (2000a). A new paradigm of curriculum development. In E. O. Bevis & J. Watson (Eds.), *Toward a caring curriculum: A new pedagogy for nursing* (2nd ed., pp. 37–49). Jones & Bartlett.

Watson, J. (2000b). Transformative thinking and a caring curriculum. In E. Bevis & J. Watson (Eds.), *Toward a Caring Curriculum: A New Pedagogy for Nursing* (p. 51–60). National League for Nursing.

Watson, J. (2006). *Caring science as sacred science.* F. A. Davis.

Watson, J. (2008a). *Nursing: The philosophy and science of caring* (New rev. ed.). University Press of Colorado.

Watson, J. (2008b). Social justice and human caring: A model of caring science as a hopeful paradigm for moral justice for humanity. *Creative Nursing, 14*(2), 54–61. https://doi.org/10.1891/1078-4535.14.2.54

Watson, J. (2012). *Human caring science: A theory of nursing* (2nd ed.). Jones & Bartlett.

Watson, J. (2018). *Unitary caring science: The philosophy and science of praxis.* University Press of Colorado.

A Theoretical/Philosophical Framework for a Caring Science Curriculum

If graduating nurses are presented with a cohesive and comprehensive curriculum [framework] that meets the need for competent and critically reflexive nurses, the discipline of nursing can continue to expand in function and voice. . .As nursing educators we are left with the challenge to prepare our students not only with nursing skills and knowledge but also with the internal skills of self-evaluation, reflexivity, awareness of thinking and decision-making processes, and instilling of the values of the discipline which include social justice and health care equity.—Josephsen, 2014, p. 5

INTRODUCTION

With the shift away from reductionist curriculum development models such as Tylerian behaviorism (Tyler, 1949), there has been a void in curriculum development frameworks that support more holistic, liberating, empowering, educative platforms. In this void, concept-based education has emerged as a possible alternative (Hendricks & Wangener, 2017). Another trend that has occurred is a curriculum drift to competency-based programs that use provincial/state standards that are set by colleges or provincial nursing associations. The difficulty with most of these approaches is that they are not grounded in nursing per se or nursing theories in particular. Most of these approaches emerged to deal with the over-saturation of content within nursing education (Giddens & Brady, 2007; Herinckx et al., 2014). However, there seems to be no overall theoretical perspective that guides the selection of which concepts to use when building a curriculum. As Josephsen (2014) suggests, "it may be warranted to develop a nursing curricular theory that employs several theories in a cohesive manner, rather than focusing nursing curriculum on a particular nursing theory or a solely competency based curriculum" (p.3).

We offer a framework that anchors several concepts that are essential in a Caring Science curriculum and pedagogy in a theoretical/philosophical base. This theoretical/philosophical framework is grounded in the perspectives outlined in the first three chapters of this book. It is a conceptual framework that unifies our beliefs, values, and assumptions with underlying concepts that arise from significant theories for nursing *and* education. Its most significant contribution is to provide "paradigmatic consistency" or "cohesiveness" that aligns beliefs, values, ontology, epistemology, methodology, and evaluation in curriculum design. This framework transcends reductionist frameworks that historically have often been used in nursing curriculum development and pedagogical practices. In summary, it provides a curriculum development structure and design that is congruent with nursing as a human Caring Science that transcends reductionistic frameworks such as the behavioural education theory.

ESSENTIAL COMPONENTS OF CARING SCIENCE CURRICULUM

We present a framework based on three different but congruent and complementary theories/philosophies and identify the concepts that arise from these theories/philosophies as a guide for Caring Science curriculum development and pedagogical practices. The three theories/philosophies that we have identified as being central in a Caring Science curriculum are *Caring Science* (Bevis & Watson, 1989/2000; Boykin, 1994; Boykin & Schoenhofer, 1993/2001, 2013b; Cara et al., 2021; Hills & Cara, 2019; Hills & Watson, 2011; Ray, 2010; Roach, 2002, 2013; Watson, 1979, 2005, 2008, 2012, 2018b; Watson & Smith, 2002), *Phenomenology* (Heidegger, 1927/2011; Husserl, 1970; Merleau-Ponty, 1962; van Manen, 2014), and *Critical Social Theory* and particularly Critical Pedagogy (Darder et al., 2009; Freire, 1972, 1993, 2009; Kincheloe, 2008; see Table 4.1).

This framework provides a platform for the development of nursing education programs that want to ground their programs in nursing rather than medicine (which often happens); with people and their experiences of health and healing including the meaning people make of their experiences (instead of diseases); and to develop nursing students' critical consciousness, reflective praxis, and understanding of their sociopolitical context.

TABLE 4.1 Integration of Three Theories/Philosophies for the Caring Science Curriculum

THEORIES/PHILOSOPHIES	AUTHORS
Caring Science	Bevis and Watson (1989/2000) Boykin (1994) Boykin and Schoenhofer (1993/2001, 2013b) Cara et al. (2021) Hills and Cara (2019) Hills and Watson (2011) Ray (2010) Roach (2002, 2013) Watson (1979, 2005, 2008, 2012, 2018b) Watson and Smith (2002)
Phenomenology	Husserl (1970) Heidegger (1927/2011) Merleau-Ponty (1962) van Manen (2014)
Critical Social Theory	Freire (1972, 1993, 2009) Kincheloe (2008) Darder et al. (2009)

While it is beyond the scope of this chapter and book to describe these philosophical/ theoretical positions in detail, we will highlight the essential contributions—the concepts that each theory makes to nursing education, particularly in the areas of curriculum development and pedagogical practices.

Caring Science

In addition to the beliefs outlined in Chapter 3 that underpin the transformative worldview of Caring Science curriculum, this curriculum framework embraces the moral ideals of Caring Science such as a relational ontology, "relational, subjective inner experiences, while honoring intuition, personal, spiritual, cognitive, and physical senses alike" (Watson, 2000, p. 53) within teacher/student relationships.

Historically, nursing was considered a human science as opposed to a natural science like physics or chemistry. Although nursing is still a human science, Watson (1979, 1988) advanced this human science ideal by promoting nursing as a Caring Science (Watson, 2008, 2012, 2018b) with human caring being the ethical, philosophical, theoretical, epistemic, and practical foundation of Caring Science. Along the way, others (Benner, 1984; Benner & Wrubel, 1989; Boykin & Schoenhofer, 1993/2001, 2013a, 2013b; Cara et al., 2016; Cara et al., 2021; Chinn & Falk-Raphael, 2018; Duffy, 2018; Eriksson, 2013; Halldorsdottir, 1991, 2013; Leininger, 1981, 2013; Newman et al., 1991; Newman et al., 2008; Ray, 2010; Ray & Turkel, 2019; M. C. Smith, 2013, 2019; Roach, 2002, 2013; Swanson, 2013; Wolf et al., 2013) have joined Watson's journey to advance human caring and Caring Science as nursing's core foundation.

Many schools of nursing, even with the best intentions, continue to use an outdated reductionistic, behavioural, biomedical, technocure perspective and theory to educate nurses (Forbes & Hickey, 2009). Recently, concept-based teaching has become a popular approach in many nursing education programs (Giddens & Brady, 2007; Herinckx et al., 2014; Hendricks & Wangener, 2017). Although this approach advances the Caring Science agenda to embrace nursing rather than biomedical, technocure perspective, it usually fails to appropriately ground concepts within theories from which they arise. That is, concepts are chosen and taught as a strategy to overcome content-laden curricula. While we support the need to teach more conceptually and less from a biomedical perspective, we recommend a theory-based approach to curriculum development. This theory-based approach requires that particular theories are identified and the concepts within those theories that contribute to a Caring Science curriculum are illuminated, highlighting the contribution they make to curriculum development. As mentioned by Chinn and Falk-Rafael (2018), "practices of teaching and learning grounded in nursing perspectives will prepare nurses to practice with a firm nursing theoretical foundation and advance the discipline of nursing as one that supports dignity, humanization, and human flourishing" (p. 693).

This framework recognizes the teaching/learning experience as a fully human-to-human experience based on caring and love while embracing a unitary worldview based on holism, intersubjectivity, intentionality, and authenticity (Watson, 2000). Furthermore, Caring Science curricula claim caring as the moral imperative to act ethically and justly. Linked to an extended epistemology, the following concepts, the building blocks of Caring Science theories, are also essential to Caring Science curriculum development. They are: caring, relational ontology, caring relationships, wholeness and holism, love, and caring consciousness. Each of these concepts inform a Caring Science curriculum and must be evidenced throughout the program. Again, it is not intended to discuss these concepts in nursing but rather we intend to discuss the contribution they make to a Caring Science curriculum.

CARING

Caring is the primary theory that grounds a Caring Science curriculum in nursing *qua* nursing (Watson, 2008). It forms the disciplinary knowledge for educating nurses, especially prelicensed undergraduate nurses. For too many years, as outlined in Chapter 1, nurses have been educated within a biomedical, technocure, and a behavioral educational reductionistic theoretical framework. In this 21st century, nurses must be educated within their own disciplinary knowledge in order to take their rightful leadership role within the evolving complex healthcare and education systems. "Developing knowledge of caring cannot be assumed; it is a philosophical–ethical–epistemic endeavour that requires ongoing explication and development of theory, philosophy, and ethics, along with diverse methods of caring inquiry that inform caring–healing practices" (Watson & Smith, 2002, p. 456). There are feelings associated with caring, for example compassion and empathy, *but* caring is not just a feeling, it is a moral imperative to act ethically and justly. When nurses understand this deeper notion of caring they have no choice: caring becomes their moral compass for action.

As Ray (2010) states: "[c]aring forms the foundation for an ethical commitment to uphold the good of the other. . . . [it] promotes a social and ethical obligation, responsibility, and accountability" (p. 49). A moral imperative is "to sustain human caring, wholeness, dignity, and integrity of the human-universe–health-healing process" (Watson, 2018b, p. 10). In other terms, caring awakens and stimulates nurses' hearts to engage with imputability in social action towards our social mandate, the very survival of our communities across the globe, against injustices and inequities.

Throughout the last decades, the importance of the concept "caring" has been acknowledged by many authors in the clinical realm (Boykin & Schoenhofer, 1993/2001, 2013a, 2013b; Cara et al., 2016; Duffy, 2018; Eriksson, 2013; Leininger, 2013; Ray, 2010; Ray & Turkel, 2019; Roach, 2013; Swanson, 2013; Watson, 2012, 2018b; Watson & Smith, 2002), hence, supporting its added value to curriculum development.

More specifically to nursing education, Whelan (2017) believes that, as a moral imperative, nursing educators must facilitate students' development of caring literacies since caring is the essence of nursing. Indeed, embracing such an important concept will invite nursing teachers to value their relationships with students, nurturing their growth and emancipation, by accompanying them in their journey to develop their own moral imperative, essential to become caring nurses.

RELATIONAL ONTOLOGY

Ontology is the philosophical study of the nature of existence or being in the world. A relational ontology means to move beyond an objective view of the world, as posited by empiricism and orthodox science, to an understanding of interconnected, intersubjective relationships, as well as wholeness. As Hills and Carroll (2017) explain,

> [T]he world is constituted as relational; it assumes a subjective-objective duality, an always ready world for consciousness that spreads out before us and enlists us, throws us into its being. Before we analyze and separate, before we fall into a world of subjective–objective dualism (and mind-body-human-cosmos separation), we are part of one thriving, living cosmos, a unitary being that confronts us as our source and embeds us within its spiritual–ethical demand for caring. It is in the face of the other that we find an absolute obligation to be empathic, to recognize our connection, our oneness. (pp. 121–122)

Accordingly, a relational ontology also implies that the nurse will *be in relation* with the patient or, in the nursing education domain, with the student, sharing meaning and understanding of the person's lived experience. Inviting patients or students to share their meaning implies "honoring their voice . . . to remain 'true' to their perceptions, beliefs, meanings, and stories pertaining to their lived experience" (Cara et al., 2017, p. 104). Moreover, from a relational ontology, nurses' practice would be guided by a moral imperative grounded in an interconnectedness with the world, rather than a reductionist view of the person, exposing a patient or a student to dehumanizing practices.

Moreover, a relational ontology is deeply linked to Caring Science. As Watson and Smith (2002) explain,

> Caring science is grounded in a relational ontology of unity within the universe (in contrast to a separatist ontology that guides conventional science models); this relational ontology of caring establishes the ethical–moral relational foundation for [Caring Science] (and for nursing) and informs the epistemology, methodology, pedagogy and praxis of caring in nursing and related fields. (p. 456)

In a Caring Science curriculum, a relational ontology guides the development of all aspects of curricula development, the pedagogical framework (see Chapters 5, 6, 7, and 8) and the structure and design of the curriculum (see Chapter 10), including the courses that are developed and how they are taught. Indeed, Watson et al. (2019) acknowledge that such ontology can assist nurses to understand various nursing phenomena, such as diverse human health/healing lived experiences, from an interconnected and wholeness perspective. Hence, this relational ontology appears essential to include in curriculum development.

This relational ontology also informs the development of caring relationships between nurse educators and students in their quest for learning and teaching the discipline of nursing. These committed, authentic, caring relationships (see the following section), which nurse educators and students develop, are based on trust, mutual respect, and integrity. Students who experience this type of relationship also learn how to develop these types of relationships with patients, clients, and communities. We live immersed in relationships, with ourselves, others, communities, environment, society, and the world.

CARING RELATIONSHIPS

This concept, "caring relationships," corresponds to a human-to-human connection between nurses and their patients and families, or in the nursing education domain, between teachers and their students. A caring relationship is a special kind of relationship. Such humanistic relationships are grounded on humanistic values, such as respect for all human life, preserving human dignity, acknowledging a person's freedom of choice and action, and so on.

It also emphasizes the importance of considering all individuals as unique and holistic (recognizing the person's unitary being and multidimensional dimensions). Hence, it aims to avoid any judgmental attitude towards the person and necessitates a conscious commitment to develop such trusting relationships in order to promote health, healing, safety, meaning, emancipation, as well as transformation, while preserving equity and human dignity of the person cared-for. As claimed by Watson (2018b), "[c]aring is being aware of holding intentions for well-being, healing, peace; for enfolding loving-kindness and compassion in our hearts" (p. 39). In other words, this special kind of relationships involves a conscious engagement and responsibility towards assisting the patient or the students in their journey. In fact, according to Halldorsdottir (1991, 2013), a "life-giving mode of being" is created by having a caring relationship, grounded on "loving benevolence, responsiveness, generosity, mercy and compassion" (2013, p. 206).

Ultimately, several authors (Boykin & Schoenhofer, 1993/2001, 2013b; Cara et al., 2016; Duffy, 2018; Eriksson, 2013; Ray & Turkel, 2019; Roach, 2013; Swanson, 2013; Watson, 2012, 2018b; Watson & Smith, 2002) in the domain of Caring Science also consider "caring relationships" to be of utmost importance in the clinical domain, supporting its added value to curriculum development. These are exactly the same concepts that must be present in the nurse-educator/student and student-to-student relationships. If students experience these caring relationships with their educators, they are more likely to create these relationships with their patients and colleagues.

As explained by Cara et al. (2021),

> [T]he relational nature of the nurse educators' work with students is crucial to humanize nursing education, as nurse educators' engagement and commitment in getting to know, understand, and accompany their students are required to develop these teaching/learning caring relationships. (p. 104)

The "lived experience" of these caring relationships builds confidence and courage for students to be guided by their moral imperative to act ethically and justly in their daily practice.

THE PERSON: WHOLENESS AND HOLISTIC

In a unitary worldview, based on Martha Rogers's fundamental work, the term "unitary" refers to the view that "humans and the environment are irreducible and integral" (Watson et al., 2019, p. 25). Such worldview is central to the relational ontology discussed previously as an interconnectedness exists between the persons and their environment.

With that in mind, the concepts "wholeness" and "holistic" are inextricably linked to this perspective. The notion of "wholeness" implies that the person is complete, whole, and in harmony, whereas, the notion of "holistic" acknowledges the interconnectedness of the various dimensions of a person (physical, psychological, social, cultural, developmental, spiritual, etc.) understood as whole. Reviewing with students those concepts helps them understand that, as nurses, we cannot separate the individual from their environment, nor can we consider only the physical dimension of the cared-for person. As a master of nursing student explains in her weekly online discussion forum;

> I felt compelled to discuss ensuring that we, as people, and our patients are not broken down into parts—that we strive to keep wholeness. Beginning this course, I was so challenged by this concept because I prided myself on my understanding of the "parts" and mastering each system, each category of health and even compartmentalizing social needs of my patients. I was totally broken of this pride when I learned about caring science, and how we need to be inclusive of all areas of health of our patients and to also include the personal and loving relationships that nurses embody each day. I had to give myself permission to not be so reliant on science, or the biomedical model of viewing health. Since then I have become a better nurse, relating better to the mothers and fathers of the infant's care and have been more conscious of the stages of the development of the infants and facilitating bonding. The personal is professional because we are all human—we all need love and care and we strive for acceptance. It is very easy to fall into the trap of maintaining a boundary with our patients and families, to

spare ourselves of the reality of what they are experiencing and how difficult hospitalization is or separation between a mother and her infant. I think it is important to sensitize, rather than desensitize from our patients and families during this time to really care, to listen, and to strive to see them in their whole state. This course has taught me to see the nursing world differently, in a much more complete, positive, and whole view. I do not know if I will ever truly be able to articulate all that I have learned or what caring science means to me, but I am forever changed. (personal communication, 2015, cited in Hills, 2016)

In fact, when students are learning about health and healing, it is impossible to exclude these concepts, acknowledging the importance of including them in curriculum development.

As explained by Boykin and Schoenhofer (2013b),

Our understanding of person as caring centers on valuing and celebrating human wholeness, the human person as living and growing in caring, and active personal engagement with others. This perspective of what it means to be human is the foundation for understanding nursing as a human endeavor, a person-to-person service . . . a human science. (p. 227)

As a nursing teacher, these concepts are also important in the way to consider our students, celebrating them as unitary, whole, unique, and holistic human beings, accompanying them in their learning journey of becoming caring nurses.

Love

In 1999, Watson expanded her concept of carative factors to the concept of Caritas processes. In doing so, Watson (2018b) captured the essence of love to be included with the concept of caring. As she states,

Love is the highest level of consciousness and the greatest source of healing in the world. . . . When we include and bring together caring and Love in our work and our lives, we discover and affirm that nursing, like teaching, is more than a job. . . . It is maturing in an awakening and an awareness that nursing has much more to offer humankind than simply an extension of an outdated model of medicine and medical-techno-cure science. (pp. 45–46)

Similarly, Goldin's (2016, 2017, 2019) results from her hermeneutical/phenomenological study realised that clinical nurses highlight the meaning of love in their day-to-day critical care practice. Love "is a dynamic human energy, which touches soul and spirit of both the patient and the nurse. Omitting love from human caring threatens the very foundation of the nursing profession" (Goldin, 2019, p. 445).

Despite the fact that this concept is rarely covered in curriculum, a few authors (Eriksson, 2013; Goldin, 2016, 2017, 2019; Roach, 2001, 2013; Stickley & Freshwater, 2002; Thorkildsen et al., 2013, 2015; Watson, 2012, 2018a, 2018b) in the domain of Caring Science also suggest "love" to be of uttermost importance in the clinical domain or nursing education, hence endorsing its added worth to curriculum development.

From our point of view, this concept of "love" is linked to the nurses' highest moral imperative, a profound passion to act ethically and justly to assist patients, families, and communities towards health, healing, and emancipation, while unfailingly fostering human dignity.

As nursing teachers, it is the passion to act ethically and justly to accompany and inspire students, contributing to their learning and academic success. It is sharing their learning journey of being and becoming caring nurses to serve the population. Moreover, ultimately, love is what gives meaning to one's work. This sense of achievement provides the energy to boost one's passion. Pertaining to the nursing education domain, we also wrote that "teaching from the heart is an act of love." This definition of "love" invites nursing teachers to consider "their teaching role as *a virtuous driving force giving purpose, meaning, and well-being in accomplishing oneself as a nurse educator to contribute to students' learning and success*" (Cara et al., 2021, p.74).

Caring Consciousness

We believe that "caring consciousness" is another important concept to include in curriculum development. In fact, Watson (2012, p. 41) points out that, caring consciousness . . . becomes an intentional commitment . . . "seeing" and being with loving/caring consciousness, manifesting in concrete doing and being. Watson (2018b) explains that: "In this awakening of the unitary field, the personal is the professional. We practice who we are, we teach who we are, we live who we are as a person—thus, this work requires a personal transformation for our own journey to a higher level of consciousness" (p. 46).

In order to raise one's own consciousness, Watson (2008, 2017) has specifically suggested caring literacy to facilitate nurses' personal caring consciousness. This caring literacy may find itself to be useful in the realm of nursing education (see Table 4.2). For instance, this concept of "caring consciousness" means that the nurse educators must truly be conscious of having the intention to assist the students in their learning journey while preserving their human dignity in the class. Being conscious, from a Caring Science perspective, also means to actively listen to students without judgment, being totally open, present, and compassionate to them, and their lived experience, as well as to their meanings they attribute to their learning journey.

We therefore suggest that this concept of caring consciousness is relevant to Caring Science curriculum development.

TABLE 4.2 Watson's Caritas Literacy Pertaining to Caring Consciousness Adapted to Nursing Education

CULTIVATE PERSONAL CARING CONSCIOUSNESS AND INTENTIONALITY WITH THE PATIENT	CULTIVATE PERSONAL CARING CONSCIOUSNESS AND INTENTIONALITY WITH STUDENTS
Nurse suspending role and status–honor each person's unique diversity–their gifts, talents, and contributions–as essential to the whole	Teacher and students suspending role and status –engaging human-to-human as colearners and coteachers
Nurse speaking and listening without judgment– know the difference between discerning, and judging	Teacher and students speaking and listening without judgment–"owning" perspectives and encouraging others to do the same
Nurse working from heart-centered consciousness with others–seek shared meaning and common values	Teacher and students working from heart-centered consciousness and common humanistic caring values cocreating shared meaning
Nurse listening with compassion and an open heart–do not interrupt	Teacher and students listening with compassion and an open heart–do not interrupt. . .stay within the others' frame of reference

(continued)

TABLE 4.2 Watson's Caritas Literacy Pertaining to Caring Consciousness Adapted to Nursing Education (*continued*)

CULTIVATE PERSONAL CARING CONSCIOUSNESS AND INTENTIONALITY WITH THE PATIENT	CULTIVATE PERSONAL CARING CONSCIOUSNESS AND INTENTIONALITY WITH STUDENTS
Nurse learning to be still, to center self while holding a "still point" inside the midst of turmoil	Teacher and students learning to be still, to center *self* while holding a "still point" inside the midst of turmoil of their daily teaching/learning practice. Assisting others to "pause" when they are anxious–to take a breath and slow down to be opened to new ways of knowing
Nurse welcoming and cultivating silence for reflection, contemplation, and clarity	Teacher and students welcoming and cultivating silence for reflection, contemplation, and clarity in their daily teaching/learning experience
Nurse realizing that Caritas transcends ego and connects with others human-to-human, spirit-to-spirit–life and work are divided no more; personal becomes professional	Teacher and students realizing that Caritas transcends ego and connects with each other human-to-human, spirit-to-spirit–life, learning, and work are divided no more; personal becomes professional

Source: Adapted from Watson, J. (2017). Global advances in human caring literacy. In S. M. Lee, P. A. Palmieri, & J. Watson, (Eds). *Global advances in human caring literacy* (pp. 3–11). Springer Publishing Company.

Claiming Health and Health Promotion as Synergistic Perspectives With Nursing's Caring Science

Health promotion was originally created to bolster public health internationally, often referred to as "the new public health" (World Health Organization [WHO], 1986). However, nursing and nursing education envisaged a different opportunity. Nursing and nursing education, particularly in Canada, recognized that connecting health promotion with caring could elevate Caring Science curricula and advance nursing's Caring Science agenda (Hills et al., 1994; Hills, 1998, 2002). This was a significant serendipitous moment because it placed a *Caring Science Curriculum* in a sociopolitical context. The Ottawa Charter (WHO, 1986) was a highly politicized attempt to move public health and coincidentally healthcare systems into a preventative health promoting context; its consequences were felt globally. Some nursing programs re-envisioned health promotion as an opportunity to reorient nursing from a biomedical orientation to a health promoting ideology. Some nursing education programs recognized the opportunity to partner caring and health promotion as a way to promote both ideologies and to give nursing an expanded language through health promotion to give nurses a way to further articulate caring theoretical perspective (Hills & Lindsey, 1994). Health promotion and caring share a similar goal—to shift from a biomedical emphasis from which to teach nurses to a caring and health promoting stance, which embraces health rather than medicine within nursing's domain of practice. "Nursing's disciplinary focus on the relationship of caring to health and healing differentiates it from other disciplines that relate caring to the unique concerns of their domain" (Watson & Smith, 2002, p. 456).

While we embrace The Ottawa Charter for Health Promotion's (WHO, 1986) definition of health promotion as "the process of enabling people to increase control over, and to improve their health," we also draw upon the expanded definition in the updated *Health Promotion*

Glossary, where the "how" and "why" *ideology* is linked to the "what" of the *determinants of health* (WHO, 1998). We believe this is crucial, because if health promotion is about anything, it is about *action* taken across the broad spectrum of health determinants, particularly directed towards the social, environmental, and economic conditions that support health (Carroll & Hills, 2015, p. 4). As the *Glossary* (WHO, 1998) definition describes,

> Health promotion represents a comprehensive social and political process, it not only embraces actions directed at strengthening the skills and capabilities of individuals, but also action directed towards changing social, environmental and economic conditions so as to alleviate their impact on public and individual health. Health promotion is the process of enabling people to increase control over *the determinants of health* and thereby improve their health [emphasis added]. (pp. 1–2)

The *Glossary* also emphasizes that "participation is essential to sustain health promotion action" and includes the three *Ottawa Charter* strategies for health promotion: "*advocacy* for health to create the essential conditions for health indicated above; *enabling* all people to achieve their full health potential; and *mediating* between the different interests in society in the pursuit of health" (WHO, 1986, p. 2).

These strategies are supported by five priority action areas as outlined in *The Ottawa Charter*:

1. Build healthy public policy
2. Create supportive environments for health
3. Strengthen community action for health
4. Develop personal skills
5. Reorient health services

These action strategies provide direction to those creating a Caring Science curriculum. For example, a Caring Science curriculum introduces senior undergraduate students to policy and its impact on nursing and healthcare systems as part of their professional growth. Reorienting health services guides us to provide practice experiences in primary healthcare, while strengthening community action encourages us to provide multiple practice experiences in diverse community settings. In a Caring Science curriculum, students have experiences in hospitals and institutions and community settings in every semester throughout the program.

The primary concept of health promotion that is so useful in a Caring Science curriculum is its focus on people and empowering them to have control over their determinants of health. This concept recognizes people's participation in decisions about their care. Historically, nurses have been taught to control the patient care experiences. Embracing health and a health promotion perspective aligns with Caring Science in placing people in the centre of their care. From this caring health promotion perspective, the WHO states:

> To reach a state of complete physical, mental and social well-being, an individual or group must be able to identify and to realize aspirations, to satisfy needs, and to change or cope with the environment. Health is, therefore, seen as a resource for everyday life, not the objective of living. Health is a positive concept emphasizing social and personal resources, as well as physical capacities. Therefore, health promotion is not just the responsibility of the health sector, but goes beyond healthy life-styles to well-being. (WHO, 1986, p. 1)

In fact, Caring Science and health promotion share several assumptions such as:

- People are holistic beings and cannot be broken down into component parts.
- People are able.
- People are always situated.
- Power and control are major influential factors in health.
- Diversity and intersectionality are valued.
- Health is individually defined and best understood by the person experiencing it.
- Health promotion and caring strategies seek to empower and emancipate.
- Health and illness coexist and are not points on a continuum.
- Social justice and equity are in nursing's domain of practice.

Nurses are in a unique position to lead change needed in healthcare systems (Hills, 2016). Nurses who are educated from a caring health promotion perspective do practice nursing from this perspective in acute-care settings (Hills, 1998; Hills, 2001). Examination of students' practice journals revealed three overall themes and several subthemes that were consistent with caring and health promotion (see Figure 4.1).

Many years ago, the United Kingdom, Royal College of Nursing, declared:

> The nursing workforce remains very much a sleeping giant. Its huge size means that nurses have enormous potential as agents of social [influence] in promoting health and well-being. It does not take too much to imagine what the impact might be if over half a million people (plus many more nurses in the world) became empowered, assertive and articulate agents of change for better health promotion. (Royal College of Nursing, 1998, p. 12)

Unfortunately, nursing remains a sleeping giant for health promotion. While we have made some gains, nursing has not yet realized its full potential to lead in this critical area. As Hills (2016) explains:

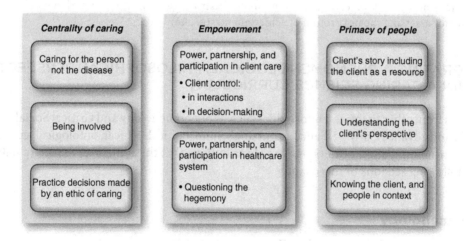

FIGURE 4.1 Themes and subthemes consistent with caring and health promotion.

Source: From Hills, M. (1998). Student experiences of nursing health promotion practice in hospital settings. *Nursing Inquiry, 5,* 164–173. https://doi.org/10.1046/j.1440-1800.1998.530164.x

> When nursing focuses on health and health promotion from a Caring Science perspective, there is an integration of several concepts that work in collaboration with one another. For example, concepts of wholeness and connection are reinforced by concepts of caring and health promotion working together in a synergistic alliance. (p. 305)

This insight provides the moment of opportunity for nurses to recognize the synergy that health promotion provides for nurses to lead teams to actually practice in collaborative, caring, intersectoral, multidisciplinary ways.

In nursing, health promotion is often seen as being limited to public health or community health and almost always focuses, in a limited way, uniquely on lifestyle behavioral change. For nursing to reach its full potential as a leader of health promotion, a Caring Science curriculum explicates health promotion as a "way of being" in all nursing settings including acute-care hospital settings. Introducing students to health promotion and the social determinants of health helps nurses to understand the context within which people live, work, and play.

The social determinants of health (Marmot, 2009), a legacy of the Ottawa Charter (1986) although often taught as relevant only to public health nursing, are actually extremely relevant in hospital institutions as they assist nurses in these settings to understand that patients do not live in hospitals (usually) but rather they live in families and in communities. The context of people's lives do determine their health. The social determinants of health are the conditions in which people are born, grow, live, work and age. These circumstances are shaped by the distribution of money, power, and resources at global, national, and local levels (Marmot, 2009). So, for example, being born in poverty determines your health status. The WHO acknowledged other health determinants as the prerequisites for health: "The fundamental conditions and resources for health are: peace, shelter, education, food, income, a stable ecosystem, sustainable resources, social justice, and equity. Improvement in health requires a secure foundation in these basic prerequisites" (WHO, 1986, p. 1). Thirty years later, the Ottawa Charter continues to be relevant, particularly for nursing. As Potvin and Jones (2011) explain:

> the significance of the Ottawa Charter lies in its longevity. . . . It continues to confirm a vision, orient action, and underpin the values that comprise health promotion today. Building capacity of the workforce, organizations and infrastructure for health promotion will be the crux for assessing the next round of achievements. (p. 246)

INTEGRATING A PHENOMENOLOGICAL/PHILOSOPHICAL PERSPECTIVE WITHIN A CARING SCIENCE CURRICULUM

Concepts from other theories/philosophies such as phenomenology and Critical Social Theory support and advance Caring Science as nursing's philosophical, ethical, ontological, epistemic, and practical foundation of nursing. The contributions that these theories make are outlined in the following sections of this chapter.

Phenomenology

Phenomenology is closely related to Caring Science and, from a nursing education perspective, it adds particular concepts that validate and expand Caring Science curriculum development and pedagogical practices. Phenomenology is a philosophical movement originating in the early 20th century and is usually attributed to the work of Husserl (1970). The primary aim of phenomenology was to directly understand and investigate human beings' experiences and the meaning they make of those experiences.

Just as Caring Science was created to ground our discipline in a nursing rather than medical perspective, phenomenology was created to overcome a strict adherence to rationalism/empiricism. Many scientists found the reductionistic procedures of the natural scientific approach to be unsatisfactory for understanding human beings, and so they were searching for alternatives (Giorgi, 1970, 2005). Phenomenology is one such alternative. As Reason (1994) explains,

> At the heart of the critique about orthodox inquiry is that the methods are neither adequate nor appropriate for the study of persons because persons are to a significant degree self determining. Orthodox social science inquiry methods, as part of their rationale, exclude human subjects from all the thinking and decision-making that generates, designs, manages and draws conclusions from the research. Such exclusions treats the subject as less than self determining persons, alienates them from the inquiry process and from the knowledge that is its outcome, and thus invalidates any claim the methods have to a science of persons. (p. 325)

To provide evidence for practice that involves people, those people themselves must be involved in deciding what the appropriate methods are for collecting evidence and how the evidence can be interpreted. "To generate knowledge about persons without their full participation in deciding how to generate it, is to misrepresent their personhood and to abuse by neglect their capacity for autonomous intentionally. It is fundamentally unethical" (Heron, 1996, p. 21).

This means that in a Caring Science curriculum, there needs to be a serious consideration and study of what it means to be human. How do I interact with people (patients) that honors their individuality and humanness regardless of their diagnosis? How do I learn about this particular person's experience of health and healing challenges?

Phenomenology is usually attributed to Husserl at the beginning of the 20th century (Giorgi, 2005; Giorgi & Giorgi, 2003). Phenomenology has evolved over the years to become an accepted and useful philosophy embraced by many nurse educators and academics to better understand people and their "lived experiences" and facilitate their students to learn this perspective. In addition, its research methods have also been used extensively in nursing research (e.g., Benner, 1984; Cara, 1997; Cara et al., 2017; Hills, 1998, 2002; Morse et al., 1994; Ray, 2019; Watson, 2012). Although we acknowledge that nursing research also embraces phenomenology as a useful research method, it is the philosophical and theoretical concepts embedded in phenomenology that are of interest in the evolution of our Caring Science curriculum including its pedagogical framework. In particular, we claim the following philosophical concepts as being necessary to design a Caring Science curriculum: the primacy of people's lived experiences, understanding the meaning people attribute to their health and healing experiences, and situatedness (context).

Primacy of People's Lived Experiences

For example, as nurse educators, we can use these concepts of people's experiences to design curriculum based on people's experiences of health and people's experiences of healing. We can level or scaffold people's experiences across the length of the program with a different emphasis in each semester (see Chapters 11 and 12), for example, focusing on people's experiences with health including students' self-understanding of their health, while in another semester concentrating on other people's experiences with chronic health challenges, and yet in another semester focusing on people's experiences of episodic health challenges. For example, people living with diabetes, a chronic health challenge, have their own unique experience of that disease. Or just like women who are pregnant, an episodic health challenge, have their own unique perspective of this lived experience. The significance of this type of structure is that it helps design curriculum with an understanding that no two people experience the same disease processes in the same way. We assert that every person has their own experience and their own story to tell. Every person who suffers from an illness is someone's sister or brother, someone's mother or father, or someone's daughter or son. Every patient is a person first. So a Caring Science curriculum development process needs to have a phenomenological philosophy that includes a science of people and understanding of their own and others' experiences of health and healing. The world can be known only as it is experienced and lived.

Furthermore, we can develop phenomenological pedagogical practices such as facilitating nursing students' learning of people's experiences by encouraging them to learn their patient's story from the person rather than the patient's chart. We can also develop evaluation strategies that are consistent with these concepts that encourage students to provide evidence of their ability to practice from this phenomenological perspective.

MEANING PEOPLE ATTRIBUTE TO THEIR HEALTH AND HEALING EXPERIENCES

In a Caring Science curriculum, it appears important that nurse educators support nursing students to understand how to acknowledge their patients' lived experience in order to assist them in finding meaning. For example, a textbook may report people's various reactions to a lower extremity amputation (e.g., depression, anger, frustrations, phantom pain, etc.). However, by inquiring about their patient's story, students will be able to grasp that their patient might perceive their lived experience of the amputation as being different (e.g., liberating, as the prosthesis will allow them to drive their vehicle again). Moreover, students need to acknowledge the uniqueness of their patients' lived experience in order to assist them in finding meaning in their health/healing experience. After learning her patient's story of living with Parkinson's disease, one student declared: "I feel good about this method of learning. No textbook could have told me this resident's personal story" (Hills, 1994, p. 8)

According to Giorgi (2005), "The meanings in the description also refer to the specific person's world, his or her hopes or ambitions and values and fears. . . . The key point is to appreciate that the meaning is not a third term between the act and the object, but the particular way that the object is experienced" (pp. 80–81, 82).

In other words, a patient's perspective is unique; so is the meaning attributed to it. Hence, phenomenology can bring an important perspective to a Caring Science curriculum.

As van Manen (2017) explains:

> The phenomenological gesture is to lift up and bring into focus with language any such raw moment of lived experience and orient to the living meanings that arise in the experience. Any and every possible human experience (event, happening, incident, occurrence, object, relation, situation, thought, feeling, etc.) may become a topic . . . Indeed, what makes phenomenology so fascinating is that any ordinary lived through experience tends to become quite extraordinary when we lift it up from our daily existence and hold it with our phenomenological gaze. (p. 812)

SITUATEDNESS (CONTEXT)

Phenomenology introduces us to the idea of being situated in time and place. As Mealeau-Ponty explains:

[S]pace always precedes itself. . . .. It is of the essence of space to be always "already constituted" . . . perceptual experience shows that they are presupposed in our primordial encounter with being, and that *being is synonymous with being situated* [emphasis added]. (Merleau-Ponty, 1962, p. 252)

This concept of "being situated" is very important in nursing and students need to learn how this concept of being in a particular context influences their actions. A Caring Curriculum supports this view and encourages students to develop contextual awareness so that they come to understand that as the context changes, so do their responses to situations. Nurse educators in a Caring Science curriculum ask probing questions such as: How is this situation similar or different than ones you have experienced before? How would you have handled this situation if this patient had been a woman instead of a man? How is this situation relevant to your other experiences in your life? They also, for example, may use case studies or different scenarios to facilitate the learning of this concept that one is always situated.

Furthermore, understanding situatedness supports students learning about "health/healing experiences" (rather than diseases) by encouraging and teaching them how to access their patients' unique stories and knowledge of their health challenge (condition/disease).

Integrating Concepts From Critical Social Theory Into a Caring Science Curriculum

The third theoretical perspective that is essential in a Caring Science curriculum development process is Critical Social Theory. There are several authors who claim to adhere to this perspective and central to our work in Caring Science curriculum is Paulo Freire's work (1972, 1993, 2009), who is generally considered the "inaugural philosopher" (Kincheloe, 2008, p. 70) of modern day Critical Pedagogy which is based on Critical Social Theory.

Critical Social Theory expands and advances Caring Science by bringing a specific focus on the ability to "critique" every situation, for example, to recognize patterns of behaviour that support advantage for some people and disadvantage for others, revealing systemic injustices and inequities within education and healthcare systems.

Again, our focus is to identify particular concepts, the building blocks of theory, that are particularly relevant when creating a Caring Science curriculum. Critical Social Theory provides this type of curriculum with several essential concepts including: understanding dialectical thinking, critical consciousness, social mandate, critical dialogue, reflective praxis, hegemony–counter hegemony, social justice, and inequity. These concepts are discussed in the context of the contribution that they make to a Caring Science curriculum.

Dialectical Thinking

Caring Science curriculum development reveals many examples that require teachers and students to deal with contradictions that need dialectical thinking. For example, teachers' ability to understand that they are both a teacher and learner in the same moment, and conversely for students, to realize that they too are teachers and learners in the same instance, is an essential component of a Caring Science curriculum. Another essential contradiction or "resolution of opposites" is that power in a teaching/learning situation has to be given and taken in the same moment in order to create "power with" relationships—a critical aspect of a Caring Science curriculum. Yet another example of this dialectical thinking is the ability to hold reflection and action as opposites that are reconciled through praxis—a dialectical relationship with each informing the other (see Chapter 8). In nursing education, theory is often taught as being separate from practice. In a Caring Science curriculum, theory is understood to also arise from practice and inform further theory development. In a Caring Science curriculum, students learn to think about their thinking (metacognition) and practice (act) differently based on new understanding. We call this "reflection-in-action" which is further explained in Chapter 8. In order to have this dialectical thinking, nurse educators need to have developed *critical consciousness* and they need to facilitate the development of this type of consciousness with their students.

CRITICAL CONSCIOUSNESS

Critical consciousness requires nurses to be aware of themselves, their circumstances, their social and political context, and that of others. This insight is developed in a Caring Science curriculum through a relational emancipatory pedagogy which encourages students to engage in collaborative caring relationships, critical dialogue, and reflective praxis (see Chapter 8). Students are seen as autonomous, capable, engaged learners who are responsible for their actions and their learning. Furthermore, they understand that health and education are inherently social and political in nature.

The development of critical consciousness involves a reflective awareness of the differences in power and privilege and the inequities that are embedded in social relationships—an act that Freire (1993) calls "reading the world"—and the fostering of a reorientation of perspective towards a commitment to social justice. The development of this type of consciousness, a process that Freire calls "conscientizacao," involves compassion, caring, critical thinking, and reflection and leads to engaged dialogue, collaborative problem-solving, and a "rehumanization" of human relationships (Freire, 1993) . Once students have developed this critical consciousness, they experience not only individual freedom and empowerment but also they feel compelled to be agents of change because they are aware of "privilege," inequities, and injustices embedded in society. They are driven to action; it is compelling and demanding. Critical consciousness is not a technique or a skill. It is a dialogical process that brings nursing students together to discuss issues in nursing (particularly practice). These issues are usually sociopolitical conditions within nursing practice and education. The students use a process of solution-seeking that results in new norms, rules, procedures, and policies. This emancipatory process transforms complex systems of interrelated realities and is not simply some change for a few individual nurses with the intention to reduce their individual negative consequences.

Nurse educators who do not have this critical consciousness are unable to see the contradictions so they are unable to embrace dialectical thinking. They tend to view teaching and learning in a more linear manner, as if one thing naturally follows another. For example, the nurse educator who claims to value students' thinking or opinions and yet never gives students opportunities to speak or engage in dialogue, struggles with dialectical thinking because they think it is their responsibility to teach the other; or the teacher who claims to believe in democratic decision-making and continues to make decisions in an authoritarian way. On the other hand, nurse educators who have developed critical consciousness have capacities to hold contradictory ideas, to reflect-in-action, and guide students to develop these capacities.

SOCIAL MANDATE

For nurses, this capacity to connect with one's position in one's life, in society, and in organizations is essential to commit to a Caring Science curriculum. Freire (1993) suggests that the thinking subject does not exist in isolation but, rather, in relationship to others in the world.

In fact, as Shor and Freire (1987) explain:

> Even when you individually feel yourself most free, if this feeling is not a social feeling, if you are not able to use your recent freedom to help others to be free...then you are only exercising an individualistic attitude towards empowerment and freedom. (p. 109)

In other words, although personal empowerment is acknowledged and important from a Critical Social Theory perspective, it is insufficient to bring about transformational changes.

So, whereas Caring Science and phenomenology focus primarily on individuals and their life world, Critical Social Theory adds an emphasis on the dimensions of group, community, and society to a Caring Science curriculum. This concept also integrates and reinforces nursing's social obligation and trust that is embedded in Caring Science.

CRITICAL DIALOGUE

The term "critical" is often misunderstood to be mean "criticism" or to have a negative connotation. In this context, from a Caring Science curriculum perspective, we want to be clear that we understand this term "critical" to mean *to critique*. The idea is that students are able to critique all perspectives, including the ones in which they believe deeply. This high-level capacity of being able to critique one's own strongly held beliefs, principles, and assumptions can be thought of as what Reason (1994) explains as *critical subjectivity*. So to be able to engage in critical dialogue and critical subjectivity, students need to have developed, or at least be in the process of developing, *critical consciousness*. Critical subjectivity is an individual capacity while critical consciousness is a social capacity.

So, although we support Shor and Freire's (1987) position, in a Caring Science curriculum, both individual empowerment and freedom as well as social empowerment and freedom are important, so we do acknowledge the need for individual emancipation, not just social emancipation. Also, like all concepts within a Critical Social Theory perspective, critical dialogue is political. As Shor and Freire (1987) explain:

> Dialogue does not exist in a political vacuum. . . . To achieve the goals of transformation, dialogue implies responsibility, directiveness, determination, discipline, objectives. . . . Nevertheless, a dialogical situation implies the absence of authoritarianism. (p. 102)

Critical dialogue is not merely facilitating discussion or getting students to speak, although these are important goals. It is about recognizing the important role that the teacher plays to direct the dialogue while at the same time remaining a colearner. This is another example of contradictions and the resolution of opposites (i.e., dialectical thinking).

This way of conceptualizing critical dialogue exposes another important principle that directs teachers' actions. That is that students can learn from one another. This powerful learning resource is often overlooked and hardly used in many nursing education programs. A Caring Science curriculum embraces this resource and designs learning activities that engage students in dialogical activities to activate this way of learning from each other. As one student nearing the end of a course so eloquently stated: "I wondered why you let us talk to each other so much; now I get it! We were learning from each other!"

A useful strategy to conceptualize critical dialogue is to imagine a spiral (see Figure 4.2). In the centre, you begin in the classroom asking students about a challenging experience that they might have had in their practice experience this week. Delve into an experience by asking

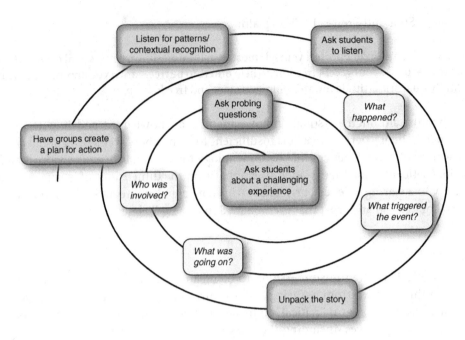

FIGURE 4.2 Critical dialogue: Teaching for change.

probing questions, such as: Who was involved? What was going on? What triggered the event? Then what happened? This facilitates the student to unpack the story. Listen and ask other students to listen. Listen for patterns and contextual recognition. Ask students what they are hearing. Add new information and theory. Ask students what they might do or say next. Have different students get into groups and take turns practicing how they might act or give each group an open-ended case study that allows them each to practice. Have groups create a plan for an action that they will try out in their next practice session. Begin your next class with students sharing their experiences in practice.

REFLECTIVE PRAXIS

There are at least two different types of reflective practices apparent in nursing education; *reflection-on practice* and *reflection-in-action*. These concepts are discussed fully in Chapter 8. However, within the context of this present chapter, the focus being on the contribution of Critical Social Theory to a Caring Science curriculum, it is important to articulate how these basic concepts are essential to *all* Caring Science curricula. Most nursing programs encourage *reflection-on practice*. For example, most nursing programs and nurse educators encourage preconference or briefing sessions and postconference or debriefing sessions with their students where they encourage this type of reflection: *reflection-on-action*. This type of reflection is important and significant for learning to occur, especially in a practice-based discipline like nursing.

However, the unique contribution of Critical Social Theory to advance a Caring Science curriculum is its conceptualization of *reflection-in-action*. This conceptualization of reflection is linked to critical consciousness and praxis. This perspective of reflection acknowledges the inextricable link between theory and practice (praxis) which views reflection as a dialectic.

So often in nursing education, we view theory as coming first, as if it is created in isolation. As Hills and Carroll (2017) explain:

> Theory is often talked about as if it belongs to the world of the academy; some form of abstraction that is separate from our day-to-day lives . . . It is our contention that theory is implicit in all human action and is critical in developing evidence for practice. (p. 124)

So, nurse educators tend to teach nursing theories and then require students to apply these theories in their practice. Also, these theories are often taught as definitive—this is the way nursing works: choose a theory that resonates with you and apply it to your practice.

A Caring Science curriculum does not see theory as something that is known and applied to practice, but rather as an "opposite" of practice. As Freire (1972) explains, this dialectical relationship of theory and practice acknowledges "the act of knowing involves a dialectical movement which goes from action to reflection and from reflection to action" (p. 31).

Reflective praxis is a "dialectical view of knowledge that supports the notion that theory and practice are inextricably linked to our understanding of the world and the actions we take in our daily lives" (Darder et al., 2009, p. 13).

Reflective praxis is one of the best examples of nurse educators living in the world of contradictions (paradoxes) comfortably. When nurse educators have developed dialectical thinking, they can theorize their practice and can draw from their experiences in practice back into their classroom courses and encourage students to do the same. In a Caring Science curriculum, learning activities are structured to engage students in situations that require them to draw from their practice experiences while in the classroom and theorize their practice during their practice experiences. In some Caring Science curriculum, each semester may have three or four courses in which they learn theoretical concepts and one practice course. Some nursing programs have called their practice course "praxis" to make sure that they draw the theory from the other courses in that semester into practice. For example, there might be three nursing courses, one support course (sociology or psychology) and one practice course (Praxis). Theory for all courses is integrated in the praxis experience and examples of praxis are shared in the classroom.

HEGEMONY—COUNTER HEGEMONY

Hegemony is political or cultural dominance over others. It is insidious and often invisible and shows up in unquestioned practices and actions. For nurses in acute care settings, it often is expressed in words such as "that is the way we do things here." It is prevalent in most practice and educational organizations. For example, when you walk into a classroom and the students are already sitting in chairs in rows facing the front of the room, they are following hegemonic practices. And when teachers walk in and stand in front of them and lecture, they reinforce that hegemony. Nurse educators who enter the classroom and see students sitting in rows and ask the students to help to put the chairs in a circle are disrupting the hegemony and creating a counter-hegemony. As McLaren (2009) explains:

> Hegemony refers to the maintenance of domination not by the sheer exercise of force *but primarily through consensual social practices, social forms, social structures produced in specific sites such as the church, the state, the school, the mass media, the political system, and the family* [emphasis added]. By social practices I refer to what people say and do. (p. 67)

Nurses are influenced by many of these forms in their daily lives. However, hegemony affects nurses in significant ways, often in ways that are invisible, in both their education experiences and their work life in practice. For this reason, this concept is taught and emphasized in a Caring Science curriculum. In fact, hegemony is so prevalent in practice that nursing students are expected to identify hegemony in their practice experiences (often referred to as "Praxis experiences") and identify ways that they can create a counter-hegemony.

For example, students write in their journals providing evidence that they are meeting predetermined quality indicators for that practice experience. As one student states:

> Another example of hegemony was last week while I was at coffee. Physiotherapy came and took my patient to the physio room. I was planning the morning so that I could give my patient's meds at 10:00. Physio usually comes at 10:30. They must know by now patients' medication times. I went to the physio room and suggested that I give them there. . .They did not seem too happy because it took 15 to 20 minutes but I thought, "the patient is the priority here." Maybe next time they will inform us if they need to come early. I have noticed with physio they seem to come when they decide to. I can sure see how important it is to critically question the hegemony of current nursing practice. (Hills, 2002, p. 236)

This student challenged the dominant institutional norms, taken-for-granted assumptions and procedures in hopes of changing those norms to improve patient care.

In another example, a student described a situation in which she tried to individualize nursing care to accommodate the patient's preferences. However, the patient was not sure how to respond to the idea that he could have some say in his care. As the student explains,

> I spent a great deal of time talking to him and giving him choices in his care. For example, when would he like to be washed up or when would he like to go for a walk. He would say to me "You're the one running the show, it doesn't matter what I want." I would reply, "Yes it does, you have a say in the care you receive." Here even the patient had accepted the hegemony! (Hills, 2002, p. 236)

A Caring Science curricula include hegemony as a critical concept to guide curriculum development and pedagogical practices.

All of these concepts embedded in Critical Social Theory inform a Caring Science curriculum and promote nurses to be graduates who understand the sociopolitical context within which they will work. That important learning enables them to be leaders advocating not just for their patients but also for caring and equitable healthcare systems. In other words, these emancipatory educational processes encourage graduates to develop their own voice, be the subject of their own world, and take their rightful leadership role in healthcare and other systems.

As nurse educators, we need to ask ourselves: *How do we participate in hegemonic practices?* And we need to encourage our students to do the same. In summary, hegemony in nursing, can be understood as:

- the domination of certain ideas and practices over others
- an insidious saturation of particular ideas into the consciousness of society
- becoming our perceived "only world"
- dictating what we learn as history and what we view as significant
- constituting "common sense"

- needing to recognize that a process of selection is operating which ensures that certain meanings are given credence and not others

SOCIAL JUSTICE AND EQUITY

Nursing has a long history of involvement in social justice. In fact, its origins can be traced back to Nightingale's "political efforts in social and economic issues" that are said to have 'kindled the light of justice' (Boykin & Dunphy, 2002, p. 14). Although some suggest that nursing's interest in social justice has waned (Boutain, 2005), others propose that there has been a resurgence of nursing interest in this concept. For example, Watson (2008) questioned "a world that is spending close to $600 billion for a war on terrorism and little or nothing to combat poverty and provide basic child healthcare for its citizens" (p. 54). She identified such things as poverty, mortality rates, disease, and suffering as the manifestations of social injustice. From a Critical Social Theory and health promotion perspective, we claim these health inequities and see them as linked to social injustices.

Social justice can be defined as "full participation in society and the balancing of benefits and burdens by all citizens, resulting in equitable living and a just ordering of society" (Buettner-Schmidt & Lobo, 2011, p. 948). They conclude that attributes of social justice include:

- fairness
- equity in the distribution of power, resources, and processes that affect the sufficiency of the social determinants of health
- just institutions, systems, structures, policies, and processes
- equity in human development, rights, and sustainability
- sufficiency of well-being

Nurses educators are particularly interested in conveying the impact of social justice to their students such as peace, freedom, emancipation, equity, acting on the social determinants of health, and obtaining health for all. This is especially true in acute-care settings where it is easy to forget that a patient is a "person" who usually lives with a family in a community and who is impacted by the social conditions of that community.

Providing international leadership, the World Health Organization (WHO) developed the Report on the Social Determinants of Health (2008), which determined that health inequities were impacted by political, social, and economic forces and recommended influencing the social determinants of health to improve health equity—closing the gap in a generation (Marmot, 2009). Achieving health equity to ensure social justice was described using the following terms: rights; distribution of power, income, goods and services; unequal distribution of health-damaging experiences; economic arrangements; politics; distribution of healthcare; society; social stratification; and living conditions (Marmot, 2009). Nurses are in a unique position to translate these concepts and perspectives into meaningful action strategies. As Kincheloe (2008) reminds us:

> Nothing is impossible when we work in solidarity with love, respect, and justice as our guiding lights. . .Freire always maintained that education [is] as much about a teachable heart as it [is] about the mind. Love is the basis of an education that seeks justice, equality, and genius. If critical pedagogy is not injected with a healthy dose of what Freire called "radical love," then it will operate only as a shadow of what it could be. (p. 3)

SUMMARY

In summary, a Caring Science curriculum endorses:

- a primary focus on people and their experiences
- a commitment to caring as the moral imperative of nursing—and the moral imperative to act ethically and justly
- a program philosophy that is informed by Caring Science, phenomenology, and Critical Social Theory
- an orientation that reflects a health/health promotion/healing, caring perspective
- content organized according to nursing rather than medical concepts and ideologies
- an orientation to teaching/learning that is interactive, challenging, and encourages the development of personal meaning and critical consciousness
- student/teacher relationships that are egalitarian, respectful, and caring
- a recognition of multiple ways of knowing such as intuitive, aesthetic, empirical, constructed
- courses and practice based on praxis
- the identification of hegemony

Caring Science curricula are devoted to instilling these perspectives within their programs and amplifying the voices of future nurses to echo these concepts proudly and loudly within their daily practices.

REFERENCES

Benner, P. (1984). *From novice to expert: Excellence and power in clinical nursing practice*. Addison-Wesley.

Benner, P., & Wrubel, J. (1989). *The primacy of caring*. Addison-Wesley.

Bevis, E. O., & Watson, J. (2000). *Toward a caring curriculum. A new pedagogy for nursing*. National League for Nursing Press. (Original work published in 1989).

Boutain, D. M. (2005). Social justice as a framework for professional nursing. *Journal of Nursing Education, 44*(9), 404–408. https://doi.org/10.3928/01484834-20050901-04

Boykin, A. (Ed.). (1994). *Living a caring-based program*. National League for Nursing Press.

Boykin, A., & Dunphy L. (2002). Justice-making: Nursing's call. *Policy, Politics, & Nursing Practice, 3*(1), 14–19. https://doi.org/10.1177/152715440200300103

Boykin, A., & Schoenhofer, S. O. (2001). *Nursing as caring: A model for transforming practice*. Jones and Bartlett Publishers & National League for Nursing. (Original work published 1993).

Boykin, A., & Schoenhofer, S. (2013a). Caring in nursing: Analysis of extant theory. In M. C. Smith, M. C. Turkel, & Z. Robinson Wolf (Eds.), *Caring in nursing classics. An essential resource* (pp. 33–42). Springer Publishing Company.

Boykin, A., & Schoenhofer, S. (2013b). Nursing as caring: A model for transforming practice. In M. C. Smith, M. C. Turkel, & Z. Robinson Wolf (Eds.), *Caring in nursing classics. An essential resource* (pp. 223–235). Springer Publishing Company.

Buettner-Schmidt, K., & Lobo, M., (2011). Social Justice: A concept analysis. *Journal of Advanced Nursing, 68*(4), 948–958. https://doi.org/10.1111/j.1365-2648.2011.05856.x

Cara, C. (1997). *Managers' subjugation and empowerment of caring practices: A relational caring inquiry with staff nurses* (Doctoral dissertation). Available from ProQuest Dissertations and Thesis Global. (UMI No. 9728055).

Cara, C., Gauvin-Lepage, J., Lefebvre, H., Létourneau, D., Alderson, M., Larue, C., . . . Mathieu, C. (2016). Le Modèle humaniste des soins infirmiers—UdeM: perspective novatrice et pragmatique. *Recherche en Soins Infirmiers, 125*, 20–31. https://doi.org/10.3917/rsi.125.0020

Cara, C., Hills, M., & Watson, J. (2021). *An educator's guide to humanizing nursing education: Grounded in caring science*. Springer Publishing Company.

Cara, C., O'Reilly, L., & Brousseau, S. (2017). Relational caring inquiry: The added value of caring ontology in nursing research. Dans S. Lee, P. Palmieri, & J. Watson (Eds). *Global advances in human caring literacy* (pp. 101–114). Springer Publishing Company.

Carroll, S., & Hills, M. (2015). Health promotion, health education and the public's health. In *Oxford Textbook of Public Health* (6th ed.). Oxford University Press.

Chinn, P. L., & Falk-Raphael, A. (2018). Embracing the focus of the discipline of nursing: Critical caring pedagogy. *Journal of Nursing Scholarship, 50*(6), 687–694. https://doi.org/10.1111/jnu.12426

Darder, A., Baltodano, M., & Torres, R. (2009). Critical pedagogy: An introduction. In A. Darder, M. Baltodano, & R. Torres (Eds.), *The critical pedagogy reader* (pp. 1–20). Routledge.

Duffy, J. R. (2018). *Quality caring in nursing and health systems* (3rd ed.). Springer Publishing Company.

Eriksson, K. (2013). Caring science in a new key. In M. C. Smith, M. C. Turkel & Z. R. Wolf (Eds.), *Caring in nursing classics. An essential resource* (pp. 193–200). Springer Publishing Company.

Forbes, M. O., & Hickey, M. T. (2009). Curriculum reform in baccalaureate nursing education: Review of the literature. *International Journal of Nursing Education Scholarship, 6*(1), 1–16. https://doi.org/10.2202/1548-923X.1797

Freire, P. (1972). *Pedagogy of the oppressed*. Penguin Books.

Freire, P. (1993). *Pedagogy of the oppressed: 20th anniversary edition*. Continuum.

Freire, P. (2009). From pedagogy of the oppressed. In A. Darder, M. Baltodano, & R. Torres (Eds.), *The critical pedagogy reader* (pp. 52–60). Routledge.

Giddens, J., & Brady, D. (2007). Rescuing nursing education from content saturation: The case for a concept-based curriculum. *Journal of Nursing Education, 46*(2), 65–69. https://doi.org/10.3928/01484834-20070201-05

Giorgi, A. (1970). *Psychology as a human science*. Harper & Row.

Giorgi, A. (2005). The phenomenological movement and research in human sciences. *Nursing Science Quarterly, 18*(1), 75–82. https://doi.org/10.1177/0894318404272112

Giorgi, A., & Giorgi, B. (2003). Phenomenology. In J. A. Smith (Ed.), *Qualitative psychology: A practical guide to research methods* (pp. 25–50). Sage Publications.

Goldin, M. (2016). Empathic and unselfish: Redefining nurse caring as love in action. In W. Rosa (Ed.), *Nurses as leaders: Evolutionary visions of leadership* (pp. 279–291). Springer Publishing Company.

Goldin, M. (2017). *Nursing as love: A hermeneutical phenomenological study of the creative thought within nursing* (Doctoral dissertation). Watson Caring Science Institute.

Goldin, M. (2019). Nursing as love: A hermeneutical phenomenological study of the creative thought within nursing. In W. Rosa, S. Horton-Deutsch, & J. Watson (Eds.), *A handbook for caring science: Expanding the paradigm* (pp. 433–446). Springer Publishing Company.

Halldorsdottir, S. (1991). Five basic modes of being with another. In D. A. Gaut & M. Leininger (Eds.), *Caring: The compassionate* (pp. 37–49). National League for Nursing Press.

Halldorsdottir, S. (2013). Five basic modes of being with another. In M. C. Smith, M. C. Turkel, & Z. R. Wolf (Eds.), *Caring in nursing classics. An essential resource* (pp. 201–210). Springer Publishing Company.

Heidegger, M. (1927/2011). *Being and time* (Macquarrie, J., Robinson, E., Trans.). Harper & Row.

Hendricks, S., & Wangener, V. (2017). Concept-based curriculum: Changing attitudes and overcoming barriers. *Nurse Educator, 42*(3), 138–142. https://doi.org/10.1097/NNE.0000000000000335

Herinckx, H., Paschall, M., Winter, E., & Tanner, C. (2014). A measure to evaluate classroom teaching practices in nursing. *Nursing Education Perspectives, 35*(1), 30–36. https://doi.org/10.5480/11-535.1

Heron, J. (1996). *Co-operative inquiry: Research into the human condition*. Sage Publications, Inc.

Hills, M. (1994). *Collaborative nursing program of BC: Development of caring science curriculum*. Report to the Ministry of Advanced Education. Centre for Curriculum Development and Professional Development.

Hills, M. (1998). Student experiences of nursing health promotion practice in hospital settings. *Nursing Inquiry, 5*, 164–173. https://doi.org/10.1046/j.1440-1800.1998.530164.x

Hills, M. (2001). Using co-operative inquiry to transform evaluation of nursing students' clinical practice. In P. Reason & H. Bradbur-Huangy (Eds.), *Handbook of action research, participatory inquiry and practice* (pp. 340–347). Sage Publications.

Hills, M. (2002). Perspectives on learning and practicing health promotion in hospitals: Nursing students stories. In L. Young & V. Hayes (Eds.) *Transforming health promotion practice: Concepts, issues and applications* (pp. 229–240). F. A. Davis.

Hills, M. (2016). Emancipation and collaborative: Leading from beside. In W. Rosa (Ed.). *Nurses as leaders: Evolutionary visions of leadership* (pp. 293–309). Springer Publishing Company.

Hills, M., & Cara, C. (2019). Curriculum development processes and pedagogical practices for advancing caring science literacy. In W. Rosa, S. Horton-Deutsch, & J. Watson (Eds.), *A handbook for caring science: Expanding the paradigm* (pp. 197–210). Springer Publishing Company.

Hills, M., & Carroll, S. (2017). Collaborative action research and evaluation: Relational inquiry for promoting caring science literacy. In D. S. Lee, P. Palmieri, & J. Watson (Eds). *Global advances in human caring literacy* (pp. 115–130). Springer Publishing Company.

Hills, M., & Lindsey, E. (1994). Health promotion: A viable curriculum framework for nursing education. *Nursing Outlook, 42*(4), 158–162. https://doi.org/10.1016/0029-6554(94)90003-5

Hills, M., Lindsey, E., Chisamore, M., Basset-Smith, J., Abbott, K., & Fournier-Chalmers, J. (1994). University-college collaboration: Rethinking curriculum development in nursing education. *The Journal of Nursing Education, 33*(5), 220–225.

Hills, M., & Watson, J. (2011). *Creating a Caring Science curriculum: An emancipatory pedagogy for nursing* (1st ed.). Springer Publishing Company.

Husserl, E. (1970). *The idea of phenomenology*. Nijhoff.

Josephsen, J. (2014). Critically reflexive theory: A proposal for nursing education. *Advances in Nursing, 2014*, 1–7. https://doi/10.1155/2014/594360

Kincheloe, J. (2008). *Critical pedagogy*. Peter Lang.

Leininger, M. (Ed.). (1981). *Caring: An essential human need*. Slack Inc.

Leininger, M. (2013). Caring—An essential human need: Proceeding of the three national caring conferences. In M. C. Smith, M. C. Turkel & Z. R. Wolf (dir.), *Caring in nursing classics. An essential resource* (pp. 127–141). Springer Publishing Company.

Marmot, M. (2009). Closing the health gap in a generation: The work of the Commission on Social Determinants of Health and its recommendations. *Global Health Promotion, 16*(1), 23–27. doi:10.1177/1757975909103742

McLaren, P. (2009). Critical pedagogy: A look at the major concepts. In A. Darder, M. Baltodano, & R. Torres (Eds.), *The critical pedagogy reader* (2nd ed., pp. 52–60). Routledge.

Merleau-Ponty, M. (1962). *Phenomenology of perception* (trans: Smith C). Kegan Paul.

Morse, J. M., Bottorff, J. L., & Hutchinson, S. (1994). The phenomenology of comfort. *Journal of Advanced Nursing, 20*, 189–195. doi:10.1046/j.1365-2648.1994.20010189.x

Newman, M. A., Sime, A. M., & Corcoran-Perry, S. A. (1991). The focus of the discipline of nursing. *Advances in Nursing Science, 14*(1), 1–6. doi:10.1097/00012272-199109000-00002

Newman, M. A., Smith, M. C., Pharris, M. D., & Jones, D. (2008). The focus of the discipline revisited. *Advances in Nursing Science, 31*(1), E16–E27. doi:10.1097/01.ANS.0000311533.65941.f1

Potvin, L., & Jones, C. (2011). Twenty-five years after the Ottawa Charter: The critical role of health promotion for public health. *Canadian Journal of Public Health, 102*(4), 244–248. doi:10.1007/BF03404041

Ray, M. A. (2010). *Transcultural caring dynamics in nursing and health care*. F.A. Davis Company.

Ray, M. A. (2019). Caring inquiry methodology: The aesthetic process in the way of compassion. In W. Rosa, S. Horton-Deutsch, & J. Watson (Eds.), *A handbook for caring science: Expanding the paradigm* (pp. 343–353). Springer Publishing Company.

Ray, M. A., & Turkel, M. C. (2019). Caring as emancipatory nursing praxis: The theory of relational-caring complexity. In W. Rosa, S. Horton-Deutsch, & J. Watson (Eds.), *A handbook for caring science: Expanding the paradigm* (pp. 53–72). Springer Publishing Company.

Reason, P. (Ed.) (1994). *Participation in human inquiry*. Sage Publications.

Roach, M. S. (2002). *Caring, the human mode of being: A blueprint for the health professions* (2nd ed.). CHA Press.

Roach, M. S. (2013). Caring: The human mode of being. In M. C. Smith, M. C. Turkel, & Z. R. Wolf (dir.), *Caring in nursing classics: An essential resource* (pp. 165–180). Springer Publishing Company.

Royal College of Nursing. (1998). *Imagine the future: Nursing in the new millenium*. Author.

Shor, I., & Freire, P. (1987). *A pedagogy for liberation: Dialogues on transforming education*. Bergin & Garvey.

Smith, M. C. (2013). Caring and the science of unitary human beings. In M. C. Smith, M. C. Turkel & Z. R. Wolf (dir.), *Caring in nursing classics. An essential resource* (pp. 43–57). Springer Publishing Company.

Smith, M. C. (2019). Advancing caring science through the missions of teaching, research/scholarship, practice, and service. In W. Rosa, S. Horton-Deutsch, & J. Watson, (Eds). *A handbook for caring science: Expanding the paradigm* (pp. 285–301). Springer Publishing Company.

Stickley, T., & Freshwater, D. (2002). The art of loving and the therapeutic relationship. *Nursing Inquiry, 9*(4), 250–256. doi:10.1046/j.1440-1800.2002.00155.x

Swanson, K. M. (2013). What is known about caring in nursing science: A literary meta-analysis. In M. C. Smith, M. C. Turkel & Z. R. Wolf (dir.), *Caring in nursing classics. An essential resource* (pp. 59–102). Springer Publishing Company.

Thorkildsen, K. M., Eriksson, K., & Raholm, M.-B. (2013). The substance of love when encountering suffering: An interpretive research synthesis with an abductive approach. *Scandinavian Journal of Caring Science, 27,* 449–459. doi/10.1111/j.1471-6712.2012.01038.x

Thorkildsen, K. M., Eriksson, K., & Raholm, M.-B. (2015). The core of love when caring for patients suffering from addiction. *Scandinavian Journal of Caring Science, 29,* 353–360. doi/10.1111/scs.12171

Tyler, R. W. (1949). *Basic principles of curriculum and instruction.* University of Chicago.

van Manen, M. (2014). *Phenomenology of practice.* Routledge Taylor and Francis Group.

van Manen, M. (2017). Phenomenology in its original sense. *Qualitative Health Research, 27*(6), 810–825. doi/10.1177/1049732317699381

Watson, J. (1979). *Nursing. The philosophy and science of caring.* Little Brown.

Watson, J. (1988). *Nursing: Human science and human care* (2nd ed.). National League for Nursing. (Original work published in 1985).

Watson, J. (2000). Transformative thinking and a caring curriculum. In E., Bevis, & J. Watson. *Toward a caring curriculum. A new pedagogy for nursing* (pp. 51–60). National League for Nursing Press.

Watson, J. (2005). *Caring science as sacred science.* F.A. Davis.

Watson, J. (2008). *Nursing. The philosophy and science of caring* (revised ed.). University Press of Colorado.

Watson, J. (2012). *Human caring science: A theory of nursing.* Jones & Bartlett learning.

Watson, J. (2017). Global Advances in human caring literacy. In S. M. Lee, P. A. Palmieri, & J. Watson, (Eds.), *Global Advances in human caring literacy* (pp. 3–11). Springer Publishing Company.

Watson, J. (2018a). Reflection on teaching and sustaining human caring. In D. D. Hunt (Ed.), *The new nurse educator: Mastering academe* (2nd ed., pp. 189–194). Springer Publishing Company.

Watson, J. (2018b). *Unitary caring science: The philosophy and praxis of nursing.* University Press of Colorado.

Watson, J., & Smith, M. C. (2002). Caring science and the science of unitary human beings: A trans-theoretical discourse for nursing knowledge development. *Journal of Advanced Nursing, 37*(5), 452–461. https://doi.org/10.1046/j.1365-2648.2002.02112.x

Watson, J., & Smith, M. C., & Cowling, W. R. (2019). Unitary caring science: Disciplinary evolution of nursing. In W. Rosa, S. Horton-Deutsch, & J. Watson, (Eds). *A handbook for caring science: Expanding the paradigm* (pp. 21–36). Springer Publishing Company.

Whelan, J. (2017). The caring science imperative: A hallmark in nursing education. In S. Lee, P. Palmieri, & J. Watson (Eds). *Global advances in human caring literacy* (pp. 33–42). Springer Publishing Company.

Wolf, Z. R., Giardino, E. R., Osborne, P. A., & Ambrose, M. S. (2013). Dimensions of nurse caring. In M. C. Smith, M. C. Turkel & Z. R. Wolf (Eds), *Caring in nursing classics. An essential resource* (pp. 347–356). Springer Publishing Company.

World Health Organization. (1986). *The Ottawa charter for health promotion.* Geneva. https://www.who.int/healthpromotion/conferences/previous/ottawa/en/

World Health Organization. (1998). *Health promotion glossary.* https://www.who.int/healthpromotion/about/HPR%20Glossary%201998.pdf?ua=1

A Relational Emancipatory Pedagogy for Caring Science Curricula

*If the [teacher] is indeed wise he does not bid you enter the house of his wisdom,
but rather leads you to the threshold of your own mind.*
—The Prophet, Khalil Gibran

In this unit, we present our relational emancipatory pedagogical framework for a Caring Science curriculum. This framework integrates four essential elements that when taken together create a dynamic relational inquiry process. These elements are described separately, but in reality they work synergistically to support the theory and philosophy of Caring Science. Pedagogy has become a central focus since Bevis (2000a) redefined nursing curriculum development as the interactions and transactions among teachers and students in order for learning to occur. With this redefinition comes an understanding that how we teach/facilitate learning becomes even more important or at least as important as what we teach. It places an emphasis on the need for nurse educators to understand how people learn.

Chapter 5 introduces the concept of pedagogy, identifies our conceptualization of pedagogy, and provides a rationale for why this type of pedagogy is required for a Caring Science curriculum. It describes our emancipatory pedagogy as relational inquiry, provides an overview of our relational emancipatory pedagogy, including a description of the four essential components of this pedagogical framework: creating collaborative, caring relationships; engaging in critical dialogue; reflection-in-action; and creating a culture of caring in nursing education. Also, this introductory chapter describes our conceptualization of knowledge and knowledge development as used in this pedagogy. Each subsequent chapter in this unit provides a detailed description of each of the essential components that constitute this pedagogy and gives examples of how to develop this component as part of a relational emancipatory pedagogy. The intention is that students can examine and critique this framework and develop their own relational emancipatory framework for a Caring Science curriculum.

Chapter 6 provides an overview of element one, creating collaborative caring relationships. Chapter 7 introduces the second element, engaging in critical dialogue. Chapter 8 describes the third element, reflection-in-action. Chapter 9 describes the final component, creating a culture of caring.

5

Emancipatory Pedagogy: The Transformation of Consciousness Through Relational Inquiry

The academy is not paradise. But learning is a place where paradise can be created. The classroom, with all its limitations, remains a location of possibility. In that field of possibility we have the opportunity to labor for freedom, to demand of ourselves and our comrades an openness of mind and heart that allows us to face reality even as we begin to move beyond boundaries, to transgress.—hooks, 1994, p. 207

INTRODUCTION

In this initial chapter of the unit, we begin by setting the context for our pedagogical framework. We describe some of the historical educational theories that have influenced the development of our current pedagogy. We continue by examining some definitions of pedagogy that are commonly used, and we describe our conception of them. Further, we explain why we claim our emancipatory pedagogy to be relational inquiry, and we describe our views of knowledge, various forms of inquiry, and knowledge development, all of which are inherent in our pedagogy. We end the chapter by introducing our relational emancipatory pedagogy and its essential components.

EDUCATIONAL THEORETICAL PERSPECTIVES: INFLUENCES ON THE DEVELOPMENT OF OUR EMANCIPATORY NURSING PEDAGOGY

Caring Science curricula can be considered in many ways; they are not dependent on a single theoretical perspective or view. There are many educational perspectives and nursing educational theories that are congruent with a Caring Science curriculum and we encourage you to explore them. Several of these educational views have influenced our current thinking about our relational emancipatory pedagogy. The four described in the following are important to us because they are congruent with a Caring Science curricula development process and its related pedagogies.

A Perceptual View

Combs (1982), in his historic education work in the United States, describes learning as a deeply personal experience that is always concerned with the discovery of personal meaning. His theory of teaching/learning is based on perceptual psychology. The theory postulates that an individual's behavior is understood to be the direct consequence of the total field of personal meanings existing at that instant. "These meanings extend far beyond sensory experience to include such perceptions as: beliefs, values, feelings, hopes, desires, and the personal ways in which people regard themselves and others" (p. 30).

Combs suggests that effective learning always consists of two aspects: the acquisition of new information or experience, and the individual's personal discovery of the meaning of the experience. As he explains, there are two faulty assumptions in education. One is: if I taught it, it was learned. The other is: if you don't understand the concept, what is needed is more information. As nurse educators, we know that we actually have no control over what students actually learn. Also, when students do not understand, often what they need is to discover the relevance of the information to their situation; their context. That is, they need to discover the *personal meaning* of the information to transform it into knowledge.

Combs suggests that teaching/learning has three components:

- *Creating a safe environment for learning.* From Combs's perspective, the teacher is responsible to create a learning environment that is free from threat and yet is challenging. He contends that, because learning is a deeply personal experience and thus requires self-exploration, people must put themselves in what they might perceive to be vulnerable positions in order to have significant learning experiences. The teacher must create an atmosphere that encourages daring and venturing forth. "Whatever narrows or hampers the exploration of ideas and the discovery of self must be rigorously eliminated from the teacher-education process" (p. 34).
- *Providing new information or experiences.* Most teachers concentrate considerable effort and energy on this aspect of teaching. Combs suggests that the way in which information or experience is delivered is of utmost importance. He contends that it is often assumed that learning is a simple process of presentation and absorption. "The genius of good teaching lies in the capacity to fire the imagination" (p. 51). Teachers need to feel passionate about their subject matter and their students and convey this passion in their facilitation of learning
- *Facilitating the discovery of personal meaning.* Combs believes that this aspect of teaching is often overlooked, yet it is the most critical. He suggests that learning is deeply personal and that, for information to be translated to knowledge, learners must be engaged in a process of discovering the meaning of information or experience for them personally. He states that "any information will affect a person's behavior only to the extent that he has discovered it's meaning for him" (p. 62). So, facilitating the discovery of personal meaning involves encouraging learners to struggle with ideas, share their thinking, make mistakes, experiment with new ideas and skills, and actively participate in all aspects of learning.

Combs (1982) cautions that teachers are often very good at the first two components but tend to ignore the final and most significant component—the discovery of personal meaning. Combs asserts that it is not the skills, knowledge, or methods of teachers that make them effective but rather the beliefs that they hold as outlined in Table 3.1 (see Chapter 3).

A Humanistic View

Rogers's (1969) views, based on his foundational work as an educator and therapist, are closely related to those of Combs. However, Rogers's humanistic psychological perspective brings a strong opinion about the role of teaching, contending that the teaching aspect of the educational process is "vastly unimportant and overrated." He suggests that to focus on teaching leads us to consider the wrong issues and ask the wrong questions.

> As soon as we focus on teaching, the question arises, what shall we teach? What, from our superior vantage point, does the other need to know? . . . What should the course cover? . . . this notion of coverage is based on the assumption that what is taught is what is learned. One does not need research to provide evidence that this is false. One needs only to talk to a few students. (p. 104)

Rogers contends that you cannot *teach* anyone anything and that we should place our emphasis in education on the facilitation of learning. In describing this possibility, he states:

> When I have been able to transform a group—and here I mean all the members of the group, myself included—into a community of learners, then the excitement has been almost beyond belief. To free curiosity; to permit individuals to go charging off in a new direction dictated by their own interest; to unleash the sense of inquiry; to open everything to questioning and exploration; to recognize that everything is in a process of change—here is the experience I can never forget. (p. 105)

Rogers contends that significant learning does not rely upon teaching skills, scholarly knowledge, curriculum planning, or a particular theoretical perspective. Rather, it is dependent upon certain attitudinal qualities that exist in the personal relationship between the facilitator and students. Rogers identifies three qualities that facilitate learning:

- *Realness in the facilitator of learning.* This means that the humanness, the personhood, of the facilitator is present in the relationship with students. The facilitator is aware of who they are and what they feel and relate to person-to-person in interactions with students. "There is no sterile facade. Here is a vital person, with convictions, with feelings . . . a transparent realness . . . that makes her an exciting facilitator of learning" (p. 107). We refer to this as *authenticity*.
- *Prizing, acceptance, and trust.* This attitude involves a nonpossessive caring about the learner and the acceptance of each individual as worthy and valuable in their own right. This attitude permits the facilitator to accept students' occasional apathy, anger, or disappointment in a learning situation. "What we are describing is a prizing of the learner as an imperfect human being with many feelings, many potentialities" (p. 109). It is an essential trust in the capacity of humankind. We think of this as unconditional *positive regard and respect*.
- *Empathic understanding.* "Being empathic is a complex, demanding and strong—yet subtle and gentle—way of being" (p. 142). Empathic understanding has several facets, including a deep, committed way of listening that momentarily suspends our prejudices so that we can truly hear the other's experiences; momentarily entering the perceptual world of the other; sensing what is present without it being spoken; and communicating our understanding in ways that honor the other's experience. "When the teacher has the ability to understand the student's reactions from the inside, has a sensitive awareness

of the way the process of education and learning seems to the student, then again the likelihood of significant learning is increased" (p. 111). We consider this to be empathic understanding and responding. We add the act of responding to emphasize the importance of the other person feeling and experiencing being understood.

An Emancipatory View

Freire (1972), a renowned education scholar and often referred to as "the inaugural philosopher of critical pedagogy" (McLaren, 2009), focuses on pedagogy in his discussions of teaching and learning. He describes a pedagogy for liberation by contrasting it to a traditional banking approach to education. Freire confirms the notions espoused by Combs, Rogers, and others by suggesting that, for education to be truly liberating, the student–teacher contradiction must be resolved. The resolution of this contradiction requires a transformation of the typical dichotomy of teacher as dominant and student as subservient to a partnership that recognizes that both parties are teachers and learners simultaneously.

Freire further suggests that education must focus on problem-posing rather than on problem-solving if we are to successfully engage students in a process of learning-to-learn rather than one of accumulating information. In other words, we must engage in emancipatory education rather than in a transfer-of-information pedagogy. "Liberating education consists of acts of cognition, not transferals of information" (p. 53).

The notion of power is a critical aspect of Freire's pedagogy. As he explains, "If teachers or students exercised the power to remake knowledge in the classroom, then they would be asserting their power to remake society" (p. 10). According to Freire, "the lecture-based, passive curriculum is not simply poor pedagogical practice. It is the teaching model most compatible with promoting the dominant authority in society and with disempowering students" (p. 10). Therefore, the touchstone of Freire's pedagogy for liberation is raising critical consciousness in order to transform society. Besides being an act of knowing, education is also a political act.

> That is why no pedagogy is neutral. They all have a form and a content that relate to power in society, that construct one kind of society or another, and they all have society relationships in the classroom that confirm or challenge domination. (p. 13)

A Nursing View

Bevis and Watson (1989/2000) in response to the curriculum revolution developed a transformative caring pedagogy for nursing education. Their emancipatory approach calls for encouragement of self-reflection wherein the educators can come in touch with their own humanity and encourage the release of the human spirit in teaching-learning-caring processes that must be considered in nursing education. Through this process, nurse educators seek to facilitate learning associated with human health and healing processes and expert human-caring practices.

Bevis (2000a) redefines curriculum to be "those transactions and interactions that take place between students and teachers and among students with the intent that learning take place" (p. 72). This requires that teachers provide opportunities for student engagement. Although Bevis and Watson (2000) describe education as an elusive concept, they call for a particular approach to education. Watson (2000a) suggests that this approach "appeals to freeing the human potential, an approach that allows one to develop not only rational and moral capacities, but emotional, expressive, intuitive, aesthetic, personal capacities and bring one's full self to bear with one's life work—in this instance, work of human caring" (p. 47). They further suggest that the teacher's main purpose is to provide the climate, the structure, and the dialogue that promotes praxis (Bevis & Watson, 1989/2000; Watson, 2000b).

Bevis (2000a) suggests that education should have as its goal "graduating students who are independent, self-directed and self motivated, and life-long learners with questing minds and a familiarity with inquiry approaches to learning" (p. 81).

These four theoretical educational perspectives have influenced our thinking about pedagogy and the development of our relational emancipatory pedagogy. Although we fully endorse these perspectives, it is our intention to expand and synthesize these conceptualizations of education to more fully embrace the most recent developments and understandings of pedagogies that are situated in a nursing Caring Science paradigm.

PEDAGOGY: WHAT IS IT?

The term "pedagogy" is given various definitions and interpretations. Merriam-Webster's dictionary defines pedagogy as the art and science of teaching (Merriam-Webster, n.d.). Historically, inspired by a feminist perspective, Chinn (1989) has described pedagogy as "the actions we take in the learning environment, the materials we use, how we use them, and the attitudes we convey" (p. 9). Similarly, Duffy (2018) indicates that "[p]edagogy refers to the art of teaching that encompasses specific methods, strategies, and instructional technology" (p. 258). Although the term pedagogy is often used synonymously with the process of teaching/learning, Ironside (2001) argues that pedagogy is more than teaching because it involves a way of thinking about and the comportment within education. More recently, Ironside (2015, p. 84) informed by several authors, suggests that:

> Narrative Pedagogy engages faculty in thinking about nursing education in ways that do not begin with selecting, sequencing, and covering content. Rather, it shifts the attention of teachers and students to interpreting their shared experiences in the process of learning nursing, challenging inherited perspectives, and envisioning ways that nursing education and practice can be improved (Brown et al., 2008; Diekelmann, 2005a, 2005b; Ironside & Cerbie, 2012).

Kenway and Modra (1992) also postulate that pedagogy includes what is taught, how it is learned, and the nature of knowledge and learning itself. Kenway and Modra (1992) encourage teachers to understand that pedagogy should recognize "that knowledge is produced, negotiated, transformed and realized in the *interaction* between the teacher, the learner, and the knowledge itself" (p. 140).

Smith (2019) argues that the common view of pedagogy is often seen as the art and science of teaching. As he suggests and we concur, viewing pedagogy in this way both fails to honor the historical experience, and to connect crucial areas of theory and practice. He suggests "that a good way of exploring pedagogy is as the process of accompanying learners; caring for and about them; and bringing learning into life" (Smith, 2019, para. 2). We support this view of pedagogy and advance it to further consider the need for an emancipatory perspective and the relevance of teacher–student relationships.

WHY DOES A CARING SCIENCE CURRICULUM REQUIRE A RELATIONAL PEDAGOGY?

Our current view is that pedagogy, especially an emancipatory pedagogy, is a relational inquiry process (explained in further detail in the following) that facilitates the transformation of consciousness (see Figures 5.1 and 5.2) through which learning and deeper insight occur. Transformation of consciousness within this context helps us realize that, ultimately, all knowledge becomes personal knowledge—it is the discovery of the personal meaning of information. This occurs when information is incorporated and integrated, with deep understanding and inner subjective knowing that connects with personal meaning. This process of insight and integration with a deeper connection of meaning for "personally knowing" results in transformation of consciousness.

While the earlier definitions of pedagogy, especially the latter two, capture much of what we believe to be relevant to a Caring Science, emancipatory pedagogy as a relational inquiry process, we believe that some critical aspects are often overlooked. From our broader perspective, important relationships and interactions reveal themselves. For example, Hills and Cara (2019) as well as Cara et al. (2021) emphasize the centrality of student–teacher relationships in nursing education. In this text, we also highlight the significance of the student-to-student relationships, acknowledging that students learn from each other and that teachers facilitate this type of learning by actively engaging students in group-learning activities.

It is our view that learning occurs at the juncture or intersection when the teacher and students are in a caring relationship and are cocreating knowledge. They are engaged in a process of transformational learning in which they cocreate knowledge through the complex caring

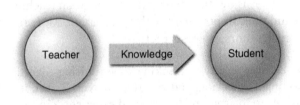

FIGURE 5.1 Banking conceptualization of teaching and learning.

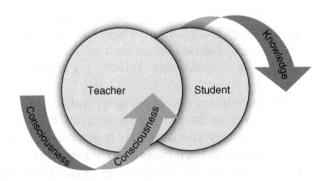

FIGURE 5.2 Emancipatory pedagogy as a relational inquiry process.

relational process: relation with subject matter; relation with one's own ideas and personal meaning; through relation with peers/classmates/social-political dynamics; and through caring student–teacher relationships among other relational dynamics of inner subjective experiences. Therefore, we believe that learning occurs in the intersection of the complexity of caring relationships that lead to new insights, new knowledge, and deeper understandings, resulting in the transformation of consciousness. Transformation of consciousness includes an evolution of consciousness, in that both student and teacher experience a higher dimension of integration from before, including a higher consciousness and repatterning of old into something new.

From our caring relational perspective, one aspect of the pedagogical process is not valued over another, and the teacher and student are engaged in a mutual inquiry process of learning—a relational inquiry process. In contrast to more traditional banking conceptualizations of teaching and learning in which the teacher is seen as the transmitter of information, this perspective does not permit the teacher to be viewed as an expert (see Figure 5.1) with knowledge to impart, the student to be a passive receipt of the knowledge, or the knowledge itself to be seen as merely information to be transmitted. This conceptualization of pedagogy highlights the complexity of the relational nature of the teaching/learning process and the teacher/learner relationship. Therefore, this perspective shows that emancipatory pedagogy is relational inquiry.

WHY DOES A CARING SCIENCE CURRICULUM REQUIRE A RELATIONAL EMANCIPATORY PEDAGOGY?

As we nursing educators begin to embrace Caring Science as a philosophical and theoretical foundation upon which to teach nursing, we must embrace a pedagogy that is congruent with this orientation. We argue that, in order to support Caring Science as the foundation of nursing, nurse educators need to develop pedagogical approaches that liberate, emancipate, and empower future nurses. As Bevis (2000b) explains:

> Without emancipation, education is an oppressive tool. It is an assembly line industry producing nurse-workers who on average follow the status quo. They may make waves, but they stay within the rules while living lives that are circumscribed by the inflexibility of large medical empire-bureaucracies and bear the inevitable stamp of banality and mediocrity. (pp. 162–163)

Hills and Watson (2011) expand this idea to suggest that "[e]mancipatory education encourages learners to ask the unaskable, confront injustices, inequities and oppression and be active agents in their lives and in their work" (p. 55).

As Bevis (2000b) claims, emancipatory education means "imbuing the spirit" with the following:

- The clarity to see things seen everyday but never really seen and to hear things heard everyday but never really heard before
- The energy to pursue an idea wherever it leads
- The vision to see beyond preconceptions and cultural conditioning and so enable departure from traditional bias
- A love of reflection and contemplation
- A trust of sensitivity and intuition

- An enthusiasm for insights and meanings that requires detecting the assumptions that underlie assumptions
- A fondness for strategizing
- A commitment to search for that elusive thing called truth
- A flexibility in generating and using options
- And last, to infuse the whole with the moral ideal of compassion and caring (p. 160)

Typically, in traditional pedagogies, teachers align themselves with the content to be taught. Combining a relational perspective with an emancipatory one aligns the teacher *with* the student and together they engage with the information to be learned. From this emancipatory perspective, it is not only the teacher who teaches. In fact, teachers often learn from their students. As Freire (1970/2000) explains, "through dialogue, the teacher-of-the-students and the students-of-the-teacher cease to exist and a new term emerges: teacher/student-with-student/ teachers. . .They become jointly responsible for a process in which all grow. . . Here no one teaches another, nor is anyone self-taught" (p. 80).

So, if we want to graduate nurses who embrace caring as their moral compass that guides all their actions and who are independent thinkers with confidence in their ability to make clinical judgments, we must educate them within a truly relational emancipatory pedagogy. We believe deeply and passionately that people are able, and that our responsibility as teachers is to create ambiguity, to challenge taken-for-granted assumptions, and to create an environment in which learners feel free to wrestle with ideas, challenge us and other learners, share half-baked ideas, and engage in critical dialogue about the issues at hand. A relational emancipatory pedagogy accomplishes this goal.

KNOWLEDGE DEVELOPMENT: FROM A RELATIONAL EMANCIPATORY PEDAGOGICAL PERSPECTIVE

Before describing our relational emancipatory pedagogy, we think it is important to mention our views on knowledge. Historically, there is so much that has been said about knowledge development and ways of knowing (Belinky et al., 1986; Carper, 1978) but, as these concepts are well developed elsewhere, we confine our comments to newer developments and aspects of knowledge development that are directly related to a relational emancipatory pedagogy.

Paradigm, Ontology, Epistemology, and Axiology

Our relational emancipatory pedagogy is based on a participatory paradigm (Heron & Reason, 1997) that includes a subjective–objective ontology as well as a relational subject-to-subject ontology; an extended epistemology and an axiology that values practical knowing and human flourishing. The meaning and importance of these terms in relation to knowledge development is described in this section of the chapter.

Participatory Paradigm

A paradigm is "a set of basic beliefs (or metaphysics) that deals with ultimates or first principles. It represents a worldview that defines, for its holder, the nature of the world, the individual's place in it, and the range of possible relationships to that world and its parts, as, for example, cosmologies and theologies do" (Guba & Lincoln, 1994, p. 105). A Caring Science curriculum and a relational emancipatory pedagogy is based in a participatory paradigm that rests on the belief that reality is an interplay between the given cosmos and the mind. The mind "creatively participates with [the cosmos] and can only know it in terms of its constructs, whether affective, imaginable, conceptual or practical" (Heron & Reason, 1997, p. 10). "Mind and the given cosmos are engaged in a creative dance, so that what emerges as reality is the fruit of an interaction of the given cosmos and the way the mind engages with it" (Heron & Reason, 1997, p. 279). As Skolimowski (1994) states, "we always partake of what we describe so our reality is a product of the dance between our individual and collective mind and 'what is there', the amorphous primordial giveness of the universe" (p. 20). That is a subjective–objective ontology which is relational.

In addition to this subjective–objective ontology, from a pedagogical perspective, this participatory paradigm also rests on a subject-to-subject ontology which is also relational. Teachers' and students' relationships are person-to-person with teachers sojourning with students which leads students to discover their own *selves*; their understandings, their meanings, their thinking, and their voices. This participatory worldview is at the heart of the relational emancipatory pedagogy that emphasizes participation as a core strategy.

Subjective–Objective Ontology

Watson (2018) states, "Ontology is the philosophical study of the nature of being, becoming (. . .) Indeed, ontology and the nature of our unitary being inform and guide moral caring/healing practices" (p. 12). Ontology also refers to the form and nature of reality and what can be known about it (Guba & Lincoln, 1994). In contrast to more orthodox pedagogies that are based on an objective ontology and that utilize traditional teaching methods to impart knowledge, a relational emancipatory pedagogy endorses a subjective–objective and an intersubjective relational ontology.

A subjective–objective ontology means that there is "underneath our literate abstraction, a deeply participatory relation to things, people and to the earth, a felt reciprocity" (Abram, 1996, p. 124). As Heron and Reason (1997) explain, this encounter is transactional and interactive.

> To touch, see, or hear something or someone does not tell us either about our *Self* all on its own or about a being out there all on its own. It tells us about a being in a state of interrelation and co-presence with us. Our subjectivity feels the participation of what is there and is illuminated by it. (p. 279)

So a relational emancipatory pedagogy is interested in the cocreation of knowledge as we together investigate our understandings and meanings as we experience them in the world.

An intersubjective relational ontology speaks to a *way of being* that recognizes that we are always in relationship. We are in relationship to our "self," others, communities, society, and the Earth. These relationships matter and are central to our experiences.

Extended Epistemology

Epistemology, the branch of philosophy that studies the nature of knowledge, deals with the nature of the relationship between the knower and what can be known. Often, the word "knowledge" conjures up a notion of factual information, facts, and theories that exist to explain phenomena. A relational emancipatory pedagogy embraces an extended epistemology that includes at least four types of knowledge and that endorses the primacy of practical knowing. Teachers and students participate in the "known" and generate knowledge in at least four interdependent ways—experiential, presentational, propositional, and practical (Heron & Reason, 1997).

EXPERIENTIAL KNOWING

Experiential knowing refers to direct encounters with persons, places, or things. "It is knowing through participatory, empathic resonance with a being, so that as the knower, I feel both attuned with it and distinct from it" (Heron & Reason, 1997, p. 281). Experiential knowing incorporates the participatory nature of perception as postulated by Husserl (1964) and Merleau-Ponty (1962/2005).

> Hardness and softness, roughness and smoothness, moonlight and sunlight, present themselves in our recollection not pre-eminently as sensory contents, but as certain kinds of symbiosis, certain ways the outside has of invading us and certain ways we have of meeting the invasion. (Merleau-Ponty, 1962/2005, p. 370)

Experiential knowing is the "lived experience of the mutual co-determination of person and world" (Heron, 1997, p. 164).

PRESENTATIONAL KNOWING

Presentational knowing is grounded in experiential knowing and is the way we represent our experiences through spatio-temporal images such as drawing, writing, dance, art, or stories. "These forms symbolize both our felt attunement with the world and the primary meaning embedded in our enactment of its appearing" (Polkinghorne, 1988; Reason, 1988, p. 281). This way of knowing is similar to Carper's aesthetic way of knowing (Carper, 1978; Chinn & Kramer, 2018).

PROPOSITIONAL KNOWING

Propositional knowing is factual knowledge: knowing about something conceptually. This type of knowledge is usually expressed in terms of statements, facts, or theories. This way of knowing, similar to Carper's (1978) empirics, is of utmost importance in more orthodox pedagogies. In a relational emancipatory pedagogy, propositional knowing is seen as interdependent with the other three ways of knowing.

PRACTICAL KNOWING

Practical knowing has primacy in a relational emancipatory pedagogy. Practical knowing is knowing how to do something—it is knowledge in action. "Practical knowledge, knowing how, is the consummation, the fulfillment, of the knowledge quest" (Heron, 1997, p. 34). This is similar to what Tanner (2006) refers to as "tacit knowing." This form of knowing synthesizes our conceptualizations and experiences into action (practice). It becomes a part of our being in the world.

Each form of knowing is, to some degree, autonomous and can be understood and can function on its own. However, of interest in this book is the interdependent nature of these four ways of knowing. Practical knowing, knowledge-in-action, is grounded in propositional, presentational, and experiential knowing (Heron, 1997). Intentional action or change is practical knowing. Consequently, change can be thought of as being based on evidence from all four ways of knowing. In relational emancipatory pedagogy, as nursing teachers and learners acquire knowledge through action and reflection, they build theory (propositional knowing) from practice about what constitutes good nursing practice. Teachers and students test these theories in the real world of their practice and reflect on their experiences in relation to propositional knowing. The more congruent their four ways of knowing are, the more valid the evidence for nursing practice. Another way of thinking about these ways of knowing that is relative to nursing as a practice-based discipline, is that practical knowing is primary. When we are "theorizing" our practice, we need to consider what theories or explanations are working in practice and which ones are not so that we can use different facts and theories to better understand our practice and vice-versa.

Several years ago, in nursing, Carper (1978) claimed that there were at least four ways of knowing. She described the pattern of *empirics* as the science of nursing; the *ethics* as the comportment of moral knowledge; *personal* knowing as knowledge of the self and others in relationship; and, the *aesthetics* as the art of nursing. This conceptualization of knowing was helpful at the time because it broadened the notion of knowledge in nursing beyond empirics. Adding to Carper's (1978) four ways of knowing, Chinn and Kramer (2018) have not only expanded the descriptions of these ways of knowing, but have advanced her work by carrying on with a fifth pattern of knowing, namely, *emancipatory knowing* which is pertinent to our request for nurse educators to develop a relational emancipatory pedagogy. Chinn and Kramer (2018) describe emancipatory knowing as:

> the human capacity to be aware of and critically reflect on the social, cultural and political status quo and to determine how and why it came to be that way. Emancipatory knowing calls forth action in ways that reduce or eliminate [inequity] and injustice. (p. 5)

In this text, we draw on Critical Social Theory and its inherent concepts of critical consciousness which requires self-awareness, insight, and metacognition; hegemony and creating counter-hegemony; power relations and praxis, which demands the integration of these multiple ways of knowing and reflection-in-action (see Chapter 4). Both emancipatory knowing and Critical Social Theory require actions to address inequities and injustices.

Before turning to a discussion of axiology, it is pertinent to further consider this relationship of theory to practice as it is critical to the development of knowledge, from a relational emancipatory pedagogical perspective. We refer to this relationship as "praxis."

PRAXIS—THE RELATIONSHIP OF THEORY TO PRACTICE IN KNOWLEDGE DEVELOPMENT

Theory is often talked about as if it belongs in the world of the academy—some form of abstraction that is separate from our day-to-day lives. But, simply put, theory is an explanation of phenomena, and it is our contention that theory is implicit in all human action and is critical in developing knowledge for nursing practice. "Only theory can give us access to the unexpected questions and ways of changing situations from within" (Schratz & Walker, 1995, p. 107). The relationship of theory to practice is key in a relational emancipatory pedagogy. As Lewin (1947) declared many years ago, "there is nothing so practical as a good theory and the best place to find a good theory is by investigating interesting problems in everyday life" (p. 149)—or nursing practice.

In contrast to more orthodox pedagogies, a relational emancipatory pedagogy does not see theory as something that is known and that "informs" practice. As van Manen (1990) suggests, "practice (or life) comes first and theory comes later as a result of reflection" (p. 15). In a relational emancipatory pedagogy, it is the cycling through the iterations of action and reflection, in which experiential knowing and propositional knowing are considered in relation to practical knowing that creates praxis and that generates new knowledge (and evidence) for future practice. This process grounds practice in theory rather than applying theory to practice. So often in nursing education, we teach nursing theory and then provide practice experience and encourage students to apply what they have learned in the classroom to the clinical practice setting. A relational emancipatory pedagogy recognizes the reflective nature of this learning process by drawing theory from practice, reflecting on it, and taking it back to practice.

This notion of praxis is a fundamental concept in Freire's (1972) work and is fundamental to a relational emancipatory pedagogy. Praxis does not involve a linear relationship between theory and practice wherein the former determines the latter; rather it is a reflexive relationship in which both action and reflection build on and inform each other. "The act of knowing involves a dialectical movement which goes from action to reflection and from reflection to new action" (Freire, 1972, p. 31). It is like a dance (see Exhibit 5.1). Through critical dialogue, people become "masters of their thinking by discussing the thinking and views of the world

EXHIBIT 5.1 The Dance of Praxis

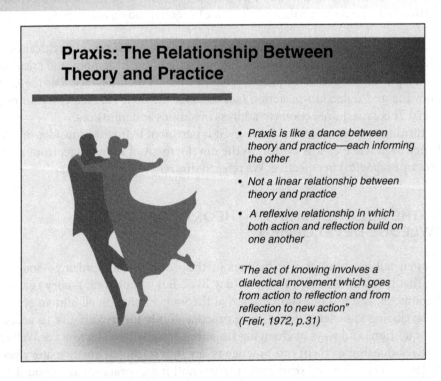

Praxis: The Relationship Between Theory and Practice

- *Praxis is like a dance between theory and practice—each informing the other*

- *Not a linear relationship between theory and practice*

- *A reflexive relationship in which both action and reflection build on one another*

"The act of knowing involves a dialectical movement which goes from action to reflection and from reflection to new action" (Freir, 1972, p.31)

explicitly or implicitly manifest in their own suggestions and those of their comrades" (Freire, 1970/2005, p. 124). Praxis, therefore, is constituted by both a theoretical and an experience component and is mediated by dialogue. As Wallerstein and Bernstein (1988) explain, "the goal of group dialogue is critical thinking by posing problems in such a way as to have participants uncover root causes of their place in society—the socio-economic, political, cultural, and historical contexts of people's lives" (p. 382). It is through this emancipatory dialogue that people are liberated to act in ways that enhance society by addressing inequities and injustices. Conceptualizing the relationship between theory and practice this way reorients our thinking about pedagogy from searching for understanding and explanation to ethical action toward societal good (Hills & Mullett, 2000). This conceptualization is clearly embraced by nursings' Caring Science theory and philosophy.

AXIOLOGY

Heron and Reason (1997) argue that any inquiry paradigm also must consider a fourth factor—axiology. This factor is often overlooked in other paradigms, but it is essential to the participatory paradigm.

Axiology deals with the nature of value and captures the value question of What is intrinsically worthwhile? The fourth defining characteristic of a relational emancipatory pedagogy, axiology, highlights the "values of 'being', about what human states are to be valued, simply because of what they are" (Heron & Reason, 1997, p. 287). The participatory paradigm addresses this axiological question in terms of human flourishing. Human flourishing is viewed as a "process of social participation in which there is a mutually enabling balance, within and between people, of autonomy, co-operation and hierarchy. It is conceived as interdependent with the flourishing of the planet ecosystem" (Heron & Reason, 1997, p. 11). Human flourishing is valued as intrinsically worthwhile and participatory decision-making and is seen as a means to an end "which enables people to be involved in the making of decisions, in every social context, which affect their flourishing in any way" (Heron, 1997, p. 11).

In this way, human flourishing is tied to practical knowing, knowing how to choose, how to be, and how to practice in ways that are not only personally fulfilling but that also enhance and transform the human condition. This concept of human flourishing is similar to Shor and Freire's (1987) notion of conscientization. As he explains, "Even when you individually feel yourself most free, if this is not a social feeling, if you are not able to use your freedom to help others to be free by transforming the totality of society, then you are only exercising an individualistic attitude towards empowerment and freedom" (p. 109). This valuing of human flourishing reconnects nurses to the human condition and recognizes the "truth" in our actions and practices. It means that in a relational emancipatory pedagogy, what is of interest is more than the usual educational outcomes. The utility of the educational outcome is judged based on the difference it makes to transforming the health and well-being of the society. Transforming students' consciousness and learning can assist nursing students to understand their societal obligations to humanity and Mother Earth.

Watson (2018), in her recent work, describes a call for a new science for nursing—a call for Unitary Caring Science that has "axiology as the starting point for science, [that means] we get to ask new questions of science as to where the moral values of caring, compassion, love, truth, beauty, unity of wholeness, and so on fit into a philosophy of science" (p. 9). Watson (2018) also explains that axiology "is associated with the ethics of science and moral imperatives, those ultimate intrinsic values essential for preserving humanity and human caring" (p. 9). Hence, a relational emancipatory pedagogy requires this inclusion of axiology to sustain the values embraced by a Caring Science curriculum.

RELATIONAL EMANCIPATORY PEDAGOGY: INTERLOCKING CIRCLES

In the previous sections of this chapter, we have presented the educational theories that have influenced our pedagogy, described our conceptualization of pedagogy, and explored knowledge development from a relational emancipatory pedagogy. Now, in this final section of the chapter, we synthesize those conceptualizations and understandings into our framework for a relational emancipatory pedagogy for Caring Science curricula and introduce and describe the four elements that compose our framework for a relational emancipatory pedagogy: Creating Collaborative Caring Relationships, Engaging in Critical Dialogue, Reflection-in-Action, and Creating a Culture of Caring.

We view the teaching–learning process as a relational inquiry because we believe that learning occurs in the relationship that is created by the teacher and learner and the knowledge that they cocreate together. Knowledge is not something that the teacher has that is somehow transmitted to the learner. Nor is it something that students discover by themselves, (although of course this can and does happen). We believe that learning actually occurs at the juncture of the authentic caring relationship that is created and lived by the teacher and students and the knowledge that they cocreate. Learning is a dynamic, lived, human experience.

A relational emancipatory pedagogy aims to create a relationship between teacher, learner, and knowledge that is based on a carefully edified thoughtfulness that attends to people's lived experiences and the meanings they create from those experiences. This notion of lived experience and its inherent concept of meaning–making are at the heart of understanding relational emancipatory pedagogies. As van Manen (1998, p. 36), explains, "lived experience is the breathing of meaning." He is inspired by the foundational work of Dilthey, who suggested that "lived experience is to the soul what breath is to the body" (see Chapter 4).

> Just as our body needs to breathe, our soul requires the fulfillment and expansion of its existence in the reverberations of emotional life . . . such lived experience is fully possessed only when it is brought into an inner relation with other lived experiences and its meaning is grasped thereby. (Dilthey, 1985, p. 59)

Transformational learning does not simply occur. In fact, we believe that four essential elements must be present and active for transformative learning to occur. They are: creating collaborative caring relationships, engaging in critical dialogue, reflecting-in-action, and creating a culture of caring. Each of these elements have underlying processes that drive the learning process. Each of the elements and their underlying processes are introduced here in this chapter and are described in detail in the chapters that constitute the remainder of this unit. Although we describe them separately, they work in synergy and, together, they represent our conceptualization of a relational emancipatory pedagogical framework.

Creating Collaborative Caring Relationships

The first essential component of a relational emancipatory pedagogy is *creating collaborative caring relationships*. In our own teaching, we are committed to fostering egalitarian teaching/

learning relationships based on trust, integrity, authenticity, caring, mutual respect, and shared power. We believe that, for learning to occur, all involved must feel safe, trust each other, and be committed to the process in which they are engaged. Creating collaborative caring relationships needs time to develop and usually requires several mutual experiences with positive outcomes to develop. Collaborative caring relationships usually result in a synergistic alliance of the participants, an alliance with one another, and with the knowledge that is cocreated. This element is described and discussed fully in Chapter 6.

Engaging in Critical Dialogue

For us, *critical dialogue* is the touchstone of a relational emancipatory pedagogy. When it is done well, it encourages critical thinking, critical reflection, the creation of new knowledge, and the discovery of personal meaning. It draws upon original thinking, unique personal interpretations, inner wisdom, and subjective life experiences. It is often the most difficult aspect of a teaching/learning experience because it requires that we challenge our own and others' assumptions, engage in healthy debate and dialogue, and be caring and respectful of each other, all at the same time. We believe deeply and passionately that people are able and that our responsibility as teachers/learners is to create and tolerate ambiguity, to challenge taken-for-granted assumptions, and to establish an environment in which learners feel free to wrestle with ideas, challenge us and other learners, share half-baked ideas, and engage in critical dialogue about the issues at hand (see also Chapter 4). During and after a critical dialogue, one should feel invigorated, thoughtful and, at times, exhausted. Feelings of pondering and exhilaration occur simultaneously. Most important, at the end of this kind of dialogue you should feel that your ideas were challenged but that your self-esteem and your caring relationship are intact!

The second component, engaging in critical dialogue, is explored in Chapter 7.

Reflection-In-Action

The third component of a relational emancipatory pedagogy is *reflection-in-action*. Reflection-in-action emphasizes the importance of having actual reflective, mindful experiences, integrated with knowledge development and learning. Reflection-in-action attends to the development of mindfulness, of catching oneself in the moment in learning, processing, of critiquing oneself. It is related to becoming a silent witness to your own feelings, thinking, and knowing. This process is related to how to mindfully take action and do something rather than merely being able to talk about how something should or could be done.

To be able to maximize reflection-in-action, we must be prepared to be self-aware in the moment: to be able to reflect in the midst of acting, being open to changes in thinking and practice, in our actions. Self-awareness, insight, and evolving consciousness of our own behavior in the moment is critical to our ability to be reflective and to develop insight. It involves self-correction on the spot in our actions, behaviors, and practices with ourselves and with others. This ability is generated from being intentional and conscious of both one's self and others—in the-moment. A critical caring environment within a relational emancipatory pedagogy reinforces safety of self-critique, and feedback allows one to examine our innermost concerns, doubts, questions, and queries, and, most importantly, express them. This process nurtures our development as learners and teachers; it fosters personal/professional growth and deepens our connection and abilities to further our own evolution and inner knowing. This third component is explored in Chapter 8.

Creating a Culture of Caring

The final component, *creating a culture of caring*, is covered in Chapter 9. This surrounds and encapsulates the other three elements of our relational emancipatory framework (Figure 5.3).

We must acknowledge our nursing culture—it exists. We have all experienced it in our workplaces or even when we meet other nurses in social situations. We have a way of talking, being with, and relating to one another and a shortcut way of engaging with each other because we share this culture, the culture of nursing. Our culture includes our values, taken-for-granted assumptions, traditions, our way of doing things, and our ways of relating to each other and others. It can be subtle or sometimes not, but it does exist.

As nurse educators working within a Caring Science curriculum, we need to include as part of our relational emancipatory pedagogy a deliberate effort to create a culture of caring in a way that transcends education and becomes a conscious, articulated way of practicing nursing. This requires more than simply creating a safe environment for learning. It means embracing a caring stance and being caring in our relationships with students and peers and colleagues so that we demonstrate how to enact our caring culture. Caring is not a soft and warm feeling; it is a moral obligation to act ethically and justly—it is a moral compass that guides our actions, our relationships and our decisions. In order to cultivate this caring way of being, nurse educators need to provide precedence for this caring culture over the more traditional biomedical/technocure/behaviorist culture that has been so dominant in nursing and nursing education. The precedence of this caring culture is the true reflection of the nature of nurse-client and teacher/student relationships, and it is within this context that nurses need to be educated if we are to fulfill our mandate to society. As Caring Science nurse educators we are obligated to attend to this development. This element is explored more fully in Chapter 9. The following diagram represents the interrelationship of the four key elements (Figure 5.3).

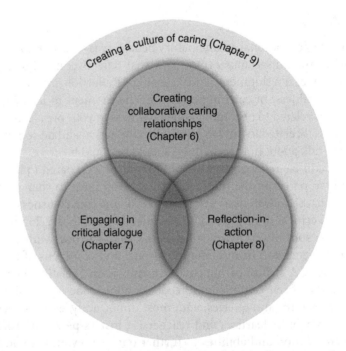

FIGURE 5.3 Interlocking circles of relational emancipatory pedagogy.

REFERENCES

Abram, D. (1996). *The spell of the sensuous: Perception and language in a more than human world*. Pantheon.

Belinky, M. Clinchy, B., Goldenberger, N., & Tarule, J. (1986). *Women's ways of knowing*. Perseus Books Group.

Bevis, E. O. (2000a). Nursing curriculum as professional education: Some underlying theoretical models. In E. O. Bevis & J. Watson (Eds.), *Toward a caring curriculum: A new pedagogy for nursing* (pp. 67–106). National League for Nursing.

Bevis, E. O. (2000b). Teaching and Learning: The key to education and professionalism. In E. O. Bevis & J. Watson (Eds.), *Toward a caring curriculum: A new pedagogy for nursing* (pp. 153–188). National League for Nursing.

Bevis, E. O., & Watson, J. (2000). *Toward a caring curriculum: A new pedagogy for nursing*. National League for Nursing. (Original work published 1989)

Brown, S. T., Kirkpatrick, M. K., Mangum, D., & Avery, J. (2008). A review of narrative pedagogy strategies to transform traditional nursing education. *Journal of Nursing Education, 47*(6), 283–286. https://doi.org/10.3928/01484834-20080601-01

Cara, C., Hills, M., & Watson, J. (2021). *An educator's guide to humanizing nursing education: Grounded in caring science*. Springer Publishing Company.

Carper, B. (1978). Fundamental patterns of knowing in nursing. *Advances in Nursing Science, 1*(1), 13–23. https://doi.org/10.1097/00012272-197810000-00004

Chinn, P. (1989). Feminist pedagogy in nursing education. In *Curriculum revolution: Reconceptualizing nursing education*. National League for Nursing.

Chinn, P., & Kramer, M. (2018). *Knowledge development in nursing*. Elsevier.

Combs, A. W. (1982). *A personal approach to teaching: Beliefs that make a difference*. Allyn & Bacon.

Diekelmann, N. L. (2005a). Engaging the students and the teacher: Co-creating substantive reform with narrative pedagogy. *Journal of Nursing Education, 44*, 249–252. https://doi.org/10.3928/01484834-20050601-02

Diekelmann, N. L. (2005b). Keeping current: On persistently questioning our teaching practice. *Journal of Nursing Education, 44*, 485–488. https://doi.org/10.3928/01484834-20051101-02

Dilthey, W. (1985). *Poetry and experiences*. Princeton University Press.

Duffy, J. (2018). *Quality caring in nursing and health professions: Implications for clinicians, educators, and leaders* (3rd ed). Springer Publishing Company.

Freire, P. (1972). *Pedagogy of the oppressed*. Continuum.

Freire, P. (1970/2000). *Pedagogy of the oppressed* (30th ed.). Continuum.

Guba, E., & Lincoln, Y. (1994). Competing paradigms in qualitative research. In N. K. Denzin & Y. S. Lincoln (Eds.), *Handbook of Qualitative Research* (pp. 105–117). Sage.

Heron, J. (1997). *Cooperative inquiry: Research into the human condition*. Sage.

Heron, J., & Reason, P. (1997). A participatory inquiry paradigm. *Qualitative Inquiry, 3*(3), 274–294. https://doi.org/10.1177/107780049700300302

Hills, M., & Cara, C. (2019). Curriculum development processes and pedagogical practices for advancing caring science literacy. In W. Rosa, S. Horton-Deutsch, & J. Watson (Eds.), *A handbook for caring science: Expanding the paradigm* (pp. 197–210). Springer Publishing Company.

Hills, M., & Mullett, J. (2000). Community-based research: Collaborative action for health and social change. In B. C. Victoria (Ed.), *Community health promotion coalition*. University of Victoria.

Hills, M., & Watson, J. (2011). *Creating a Caring Science curriculum: An emancipatory pedagogy for nursing* (1st ed.). Springer Publishing Company.

hooks, b. (1994). *Teaching to transgress: Education as the practice of freedom*. Routledge.

Husserl, E. (1964). *Field of consciousness*. Duquesne University Press.

Ironside, P. M. (2001). Creating a research base for nursing education: An interpretive review of conventional, critical, feminist, postmodern, and phenomenological pedagogies. *Advances in Nursing Science, 23*(3), 72–87. https://doi.org/10.1097/00012272-200103000-00007

Ironside, P. M. (2015). Narrative pedagogy: Transforming nursing education through 15 years of research in nursing education. *Nursing Education Perspective, 36*(2), 83–88. https://doi.org/10.5480/13-1102

Ironside, P. M., & Cerbie, E. (2012). Teaching strategies for quality and safety. In G. Sherwood & J. Barnsteiner (Eds.), *Quality and safety in nursing: A competency approach to improving outcomes* (pp. 211–225). Wiley-Blackwell.

Kenway, J., & Modra, H. (1992). Feminist pedagogy and emancipatory possibilities. In C. Luke & J. Gore (Eds.), *Feminisms and critical pedagogy* (pp. 138–167). Routledge.

Lewin, K. (1947). Frontiers in group dynamics: Concept method and reality in social science: Social equilibria and social change. *Human Relations, 1*(1), 5–41. https://doi.org/10.1177/001872674700100103

Merriam-Webster. (n.d.). Pedagogy. In *Merriam-Webster.com dictionary*. https://www.merriam-webster.com/dictionary/pedagogy

McLaren, P. (2009). Critical pedagogy: A look at the major concepts. In A. Darder, M. Baltodano, & R. Torres (Eds.), *The critical pedagogy reader* (pp. 52–60). Routledge.

Merleau-Ponty, M. (2005). *Phenomenology of perception*. Taylor & Francis. (Original work published 1962)

Polkinghorne, D. (1988). *Narrative knowing and the human sciences*. State University of New York.

Rogers, C. (1969). *Freedom to learn: A view of what education might become*. (1st ed.). Charles Merrill.

Reason, P. (1988). *Human inquiry in action*. Sage.

Schratz, M., & Walker, R. (1995). *Research as social change*. Sage.

Shor, I., & Freire, P. (1987). *A pedagogy for liberation: Dialogues on transforming education*. Bergin & Garvey.

Skolimowski, H. (1994). *The participatory mind: A new theory of knowledge and of the universe*. Penguin Books.

Smith, M. K. (2019). 'What is pedagogy?' *The encyclopedia of pedagogy and informal education*. https://infed.org/mobi/what-is-pedagogy

Tanner, C. A. (2006). Thinking like a nurse: A research-based model of clinical judgment in nursing. *Journal of Nursing Education, 45*(6), 204–211. https://doi.org/10.3928/01484834-20060601-04

van Manen, M. (1997). *Researching lived experience* (2nd ed.). Routledge.

Wallerstein, N., & Bernstein, E. (1988). Empowerment education: Freire's ideas adapted to health education. *Health Education & Behavior, 15*(4), 379–394. https://doi.org/10.1177/109019818801500402

Watson, J. (2000a). A new paradigm of curriculum development. In E. O. Bevis & J. Watson (Eds.), *Towards a caring curriculum: A new pedagogy for nursing* (pp. 37–49). Jones and Bartlett.

Watson, J. (2000b). Transformative thinking and a caring curriculum. In E. O. Bevis & J. Watson (Eds.), *Towards a caring curriculum: A new pedagogy for nursing* (pp. 51–60). Jones & Bartlett.

Watson, J. (2018). *Unitary caring science: The philosophy and praxis of nursing*. University Press of Colorado.

Creating Caring Relationships: Collaboration, Power, and Participation

A real humanist can be identified more by his trust in the people, which engages him in their struggle, than by a thousand actions in their favor without that trust.—Freire, 1970/2000, p. 60

INTRODUCTION

The purpose of this chapter is to explore the first component of a relational emancipatory pedagogy: creating caring relationships and to develop an understanding of how to create such relationships. This chapter examines the three elements involved in creating caring relationships: collaboration, power/empowerment, and participation. These elements are essential to the development of caring relationships (Figure 6.1).

STUDENT-TEACHER CARING RELATIONSHIPS: THE HEART OF A RELATIONAL EMANCIPATORY PEDAGOGY

Student-teacher caring relationships are the heart of a relational emancipatory pedagogy. It is the teacher's responsibility to create the space for these relationships to develop. It requires that teachers commit to and align first with their students. The teacher's deep first interest is with the students—*their* lived experiences, *their* understandings, *their* meanings, and *their* worldview. These student-teacher caring relationships emphasize the uniqueness of each individual student (Cara et al., 2021; Hills & Cara, 2019).

These relationships ground students and teachers in a mutual learning/teaching process that encourages students to realize that it is their understandings and experiences that are primary. The teacher enters the students' inner world and engages within their world without judgment, advice, or criticism. Teachers embrace the students' reality as "real" for them.

Such caring relationships are grounded on respect, commitment, equity, trust, safety, and authenticity (Cara et al., 2021). This respect, empathy, and nonjudgmental stance creates the conditions for the development of an authentic caring transpersonal relationship. As Watson (2012) explains, "[a] transpersonal caring relationship connotes... a connection/union with another person, a high regard for the whole person and their being-in-the-world" (p. 75). Accordingly, the aim of student/teacher transpersonal caring relationships would be to heighten and protect

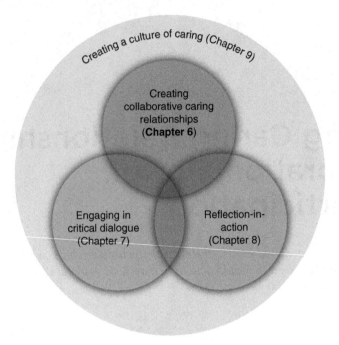

FIGURE 6.1 Interlocking circles of relational emancipatory pedagogy.

the students' human dignity as well as their learning (Cara et al., 2021). According to Watson (1988), "[h]uman care requires the nurse to possess specific intentions, a will, values, and a commitment to an ideal of intersubjective human-to-human care transaction that is directed toward the preservation of personhood and humanity of both nurse and patient" (p. 75). The same is true for the nurse educator-student relationships; both the nurse and the nursing teacher must also embrace caring as the moral imperative to act ethically and justly in nursing education.

It is now up to students to decide how they will engage with their teachers. This is a two-way street. It is important to note that these relationships still do not just happen. There is a lot of give and take at this stage of the development of this caring relationship. Generally speaking, when nurse educators engage in this humble and vulnerable way of being, it is reciprocated by students. In fact, reciprocity plays an important role in a caring relationship; both nurse educators and students join in a mutual search for meaning and wholeness as well as for the cocreation of knowledge within a trusting environment.

So, how do we develop these relationships? We suggest that there are three key elements to creating caring relationships: collaboration, negotiated power, and participation.

COLLABORATION: BEING-IN-RELATION

Building on earlier chapters, and our discussions of Caring Science as the ethical, philosophical, and theoretical foundation of nursing and therefore nursing education, we expand our discussion to include the necessary elements that must be present to create caring relationships: collaboration, negotiated power, and participation.

Throughout the literature and within scholarly debates about relational emancipatory pedagogies, there is agreement that, for significant learning to occur, the creation of collaborative, or what is often referred to as "egalitarian," relationships is essential. But the literature and debates too often lack discussion about how to create such relationships.

We live immersed in relationships of all sorts. We have our relationship to our *self*, to others (family members, colleagues, friends), and to society and the world. These relationships vary and have different characteristics, but we are always in relation even when we are alone. Further, we have a choice about how to be in those relationships, and we choose and change constantly in those relationships even though the dynamics within the relationship may try to keep it the same. It is also true that in nursing and nursing education, we choose how to be in relation to our patients/clients and our students. However, when you choose to embrace a Caring Science and relational emancipatory pedagogy, you are committing to developing a particular type of relationship with your patients and students. You are committing to developing a collaborative caring relationship.

What is Collaboration?

The notion of collaboration can mean different things to different people. So, what does it mean to collaborate?

Time Out for Reflection

In your journal, respond to the following questions:

What does it mean to collaborate?
What is the difference between cooperation and collaboration, partnerships?
How is power related to collaboration?
What needs to be present in order for you to feel that you are engaged in a collaboration?
What is your responsibility in contributing to this collaboration?

Collaboration has several definitions. In Merriam-Webster's dictionary, the first reads: "To work jointly with others or together especially in an intellectual endeavor" (Merriam-Webster, n.d.). Directly below this is a second definition: "To cooperate with or willingly assist an enemy of one's country and especially an occupying force" (Merriam-Webster, n.d.).

We believe this second definition captures a tension that can exist in collaborative relationships. When people who must work together (e.g., teachers and students; nurses and patients) view themselves as having different vested interests, each may feel like they have to protect their own "turf." We have all experienced situations in which we are trying to get someone to do something that we want to have happen, and they are not as invested in the same agenda and a certain tension results. The secret to overcoming this tension lies in finding a common vision: in cocreating what you each will work toward and how you will get there. This process for engagement needs to be transparent and agreed upon by teachers and students and/or nurses and patients. For us, the following definition, originating from Hills's (1994) work, best describes the collaborative caring relationship that we try to create within a relational emancipatory pedagogy.

> Collaboration is the creation of a synergistic alliance that honors and utilizes each person's contribution in order to create collective wisdom and collective action. Collaboration is not

synonymous with co-operation, partnership, participation or compromise. Those words do not convey the fundamental importance of being in a relationship nor the depth of caring and commitment that is needed to create the kind of reciprocity that is collaboration. Collaborators are committed to, care about and trust in each other. They recognize that, despite their differences, each has unique and valuable knowledge, perspectives and experiences to contribute to the collaboration. (Hills, 2016, p. 298)

Being Collaborative

Collaboration demands that teachers relate person-to-person with their students. It is not possible to develop a caring relationship with someone who hides behind a role or is not fully present in some way. So the key responsibility of the teacher is to show up! Being present in a relationship requires a teacher to relate in ways that communicate deep caring for the students and a recognition of the students as persons of worth, simply because they exist. As one faculty member who was attempting to shift from a behavioral evaluation method to one that embraced a Caring Science paradigm explains,

> our conversations and her journal allow me to see her [student] as a human being, a person seen in a holistic way; someone on a journey with her own way of knowing and understanding. The relationship with my past students was much more superficial; one based on a technical objective way of understanding . . . the old progress notes which constantly reflected the objectives seemed to keep us on task—the task of 'caring for people' who had a disease . . . Taking care tended to be doing something to someone rather than *being* with someone. (Hills, 2001, p. 340)

Time Out for Reflection

We invite you to write your reflections in your journal.

Review the key elements that you identified as being necessary for a collaborative relationship.
Note how they compare to those elements outlined in the previous definition.
Recall a time when you felt you were participating in a collaborative relationship within a teaching/learning situation.
What was it about the situation that made it collaborative?
List what you consider to be the key elements of a collaborative caring relationship.

LEARNING ACTIVITY: RELATIONSHIPS ARE PERSONAL

ENDS IN VIEW

The purpose of this learning activity is to examine the essential nature of a collaborative partnership as a personal commitment.

WRITE

In your journal, write five strategies that you could use to keep yourself in tune with how others perceive you. Reflect on the process you use to screen this information. How do you know the feedback someone gives you is "accurate"? How do you decide which information to act on? What strategies do you use to care for yourself? List five.

Share your responses to the above questions with a classmate or a colleague.

REFLECT

Do you have any concerns about relating in a personal way to students? In your journal, reflect on any such concerns. Set two goals that you can work on during this course that will assist you in developing this aspect of creating collaborative caring relationships.

Developing your "Self," becoming all you can be, is one of the greatest gifts teachers can give to their students. Buscaglia (1985), a famous psychologist who taught free classes on *Love* at the University of Southern California and became known as the "love" doctor, argues that only through actualizing your *self* as a person do you have something to give to others. In short, you cannot give what you do not have. "The most wondrous part of developing your *'Self'* is that you can give it away and you don't lose anything by giving your *Self* to others" (Buscaglia, 1985, p.49). Buscaglia encourages teachers to develop their uniqueness so that they can celebrate their humanness and have more to share with others:

> It all starts with you . . . If I grow and grow, I can give you more of me. I learn so that I can teach you more. I strive for wisdom so that I can encourage your truth. I become more aware and sensitive so that I can better accept your sensitivity and awareness. And I struggle to understand my humanness so that I can understand you when you reveal to me that you are only human too. And I live in continual wonder of life, so that I can allow you too to celebrate your life. What I do for me, I do for you. (Buscaglia, 1985, p. 50)

Similarly, Chinn and Kramer (2018) describe this process as "personal knowing" and suggest that it is: "an inner experience of becoming whole, aware, genuine Self . . . in relation to others" (p. 8). Being authentic and having integrity are also key ingredients to developing one's self. As Cara et al. (2021) suggest, nurse educators are invited to become role models for students to learn about the importance of integrity and imputability as future nurses caring for patients and families. Another action that is evident of one's growth of self is finding one's voice. In order for this to happen, nurse educators must be confident to speak with their "voice" in order to encourage students to find their voices.

If students do not *experience* these caring collaborative relationships with their teachers, it is not possible for them to create them with their patients. This requires *practical knowing*. It cannot be learned solely from propositional (theoretical) knowing (see Chapter 5).

PARTNERS IN LEARNING AND TEACHING

In creating caring relationships as part of a relational emancipatory pedagogy, teachers and students must be partners in the learning process. A "promotion" of learner-to-partner status is not the same as self-directed or student-centered learning. Self-directed and student-centered learning places the majority of the effort or work of learning on the learner. In relational emancipatory pedagogy, based on Caring Science, the work of learning is shared between teachers and learners. This idea may seem self-evident, but it is fundamental to the pedagogy that you develop. Teaching/learning practice looks very different within the different approaches. A relational emancipatory pedagogy is fundamentally a situation where the teachers and students both have to be learners, and both have to be cognitive-caring participants, in spite of them being different. For us, the first principle of a relational emancipatory pedagogy is for teachers and students to be critical agents in the act of knowing. As you are a teacher, so too, are you a learner. Every time you enter a situation with another for the purpose of engaging in an educational encounter, you simultaneously learn and teach. We are not suggesting that "teaching" is neutral or that how we are as teachers does not impact the learning experiences. Instead, we are trying to honor the importance of the cocreation of knowledge, when teachers and learners fully engage as passionate soul mates in their quest for deeper understandings, for wisdom. We believe this to be true no matter what the setting—classroom or practice setting. So, for example, when you enter a learning situation with clients, as a nurse you would approach the situation not as much to "teach" clients about some aspect of their health but to engage with them in a caring relationship in which you both cocreate mutually understood meanings about the client's situation; about their health and healing experience. All too often we hear teachers in teaching/learning situations say, "Well I gave them the information. I don't know what the problem is."

Combs (1982), a classic reference in education, states that there are two faulty assumptions about teaching/learning against which we must constantly guard. The first is "If I taught it, it was learned"; the second is "We are not learning unless we are getting new information" (Combs, 1982, p. 45). But we know that learning has more to do with the meaning we make of the information than the actual transmission of that information. Information is not knowledge. So in situations with nurses and clients, as with nurse educators and students, it is imperative that we ascertain the meaning that is being made of the information that we are sharing. We do that by being-in-relationship and having a collaboration within the learning/teaching process. Further, as Bevis (2000) explains, "Teachers of nurses have a special responsibility as do nurses who practice in settings where students learn. These nurses can be instrumental in being the students' mirror, revealing to the students things about themselves that will nurture the ethical ideal or destroy it" (p. 184).

LEARNING ACTIVITY

WRITE

In your journal, write about a teaching/learning situation in which you felt that you were a partner in the learning process. Consider and answer the following questions:

- What was it about the situation that made it a partnership? How was the partnership established?
- How did the relationship, being a partnership, affect you and the teaching/learning process?

DIALOGUE

Share your experiences with your learning partners or study group. Discuss how your experiences are similar to or different from each other.

REFLECT

In your journal, describe what you consider to be the essential characteristics of developing partnerships in teaching/learning situations.

POWER AND EMPOWERMENT

In this section, we explore the issue of power and discuss strategies for negotiating power while creating collaborative relationships. In addition, we discuss the concept of empowerment and its impact on the teaching/learning partnership.

The Pressure of Power

From a relational emancipatory pedagogy perspective, it is not possible to talk about pedagogy without talking about power. In fact, some pedagogies within this relational emancipatory perspective suggest that power is the key element upon which to focus (Freire, 1972, 1970/2000; hooks, 1994). Others recognize power as important but tend not to deal as directly with it.

Because of the influence of Freire (1972, 1970/2000), hooks (1994) and other Critical Social theorists (Darder et al., 2009) and Feminist theorists (Chinn, 2013, 2018; Chinn & Falk-Raphael, 2015; Lather, 2012, 2013) on our work, we view power as one of the most critical and pivotal concepts in any teaching/learning situation. Freire (1972) contends that if teachers and learners seized the power available to them in the classroom, they could remake society.

Power dynamics exist in all teaching/learning situations and, with each situation, there is a choice to be made about how power will be negotiated. You can choose to have power over others or you can choose to have power with others. Empowering relationships are characterized by power *with* partnerships that encourage full participation by all participants. Power lies at the centre of empowerment and "the empowering act exists only as a relational act of power taken and given in the same instance" (Labonte, 1990, p. 49). From a Caring Science perspective,

> there is no room for dominant–passive power relationships. Power relations need to be discussed and negotiated. It may not be possible to eradicate all power-over situations in nursing education, but it is possible to discuss them with students, which raises their consciousness and moves them to a state of greater awareness. (Cara et al., 2021, p. 52)

TIME OUT FOR REFLECTION

Think about a time when you were in a teaching/learning situation that felt empowering. In your journal, identify what the key factors were that made you feel you had control.

- Was there a power differential in this situation?
- How was power negotiated in this situation?
- What strategies were used to encourage "power sharing"?
- What strategies will you use to encourage students to share power?

In many situations it is not possible to have equal power. For example, in a formal teaching/learning situation such as in a nursing course in a nursing program, the teacher has responsibility to grade the students' assignments. Imagine that we are teaching you in such a course. We are automatically given power over students, but we can decide how to use that power. We can negotiate power but, in all of our years of teaching, we have not found a system that allows an equal distribution of power around this issue of grading. However, we can and should be transparent about the process, negotiate the criteria, and include peer and self-critique in the assessment of your work. An exemplar of such an approach is discussed in Chapter 18, contract grading. You always have the choice to offer alternatives and to negotiate other options. As Labonte (1997), a famous Canadian sociologist and health promotion expert states, "At its simplest, power is about choice" (p. 50).

Nurses often face issues of power when talking about other people's health issues. Nurses are familiar with labeling others' problems with medical terminology and reporting on others' progress using nursing or medical jargon, so it is sometimes difficult to let clients tell their story without similarly labeling their issue. Similarly with students, they are much more likely to describe any concern they might have in relation to learning as a *lived experience* rather than labelling it as a problem. Naming our own experiences is powerful in and of itself. "Our first claim to power—power being defined as the capacity to create or resist change—is naming our experiences and having that naming heard and respected" (Labonte, 1997, p. 31). In order to create collaborative relationships that are empowering, clients or students must name and describe the (health) issue or experience. As Beck (2019, p. 260) explains, students must learn to tell their own stories in order to be entirely present and "bear witness" to patients' stories. When students share their stories with each other, they learn from each other's stories. "As stories are communally witnessed and explored from multiple perspectives, even early students begin to identify shared concerns, assumptions, and ways their past experiences inform the learning they are now doing in nursing" (Ironside, 2015, p. 85).

One teaching strategy that was used in a Caring Science curriculum (Hills, 1998; Hills, 2002; Hills & Watson, 2011) was to teach students to learn about patients' health and healing experiences by learning about the patients' stories. One student, reflecting on her experience, states:

> My client is a good teacher. She openly explained the physiological factors of Parkinson's disease, her past history with the disease, and what her experiences had been like for herself, and how it has affected various members of her family. So far, I haven't been in a position to teach my client much. I've basically been learning from her. I feel good about this method of learning—no textbook could have told me this resident's personal story. (Hills & Watson, 2011, p. 77)

Nursing has been reluctant to trust people to act in their own best interests; "on the whole, professionals simply do not trust ordinary people, seeing them as lacking knowledge, living inappropriate lifestyles, absconding with resources, and generally not doing what they should to keep themselves healthy" (Raeburn & Rootman, 1998, p. 19). If we want to change this undermining of people/clients, nurse educators must develop teaching strategies that are empowering of students so that they in turn can empower their clients. Students cannot empower others, if they do not experience empowerment themselves. The following learning activity provides typical nursing situations that provide opportunities to practice empowering responses.

LEARNING ACTIVITY: NAMING HEALTH PROBLEMS

ENDS IN VIEW

In this learning activity, you will examine power in relation to naming health issues and concerns. When working with clients in teaching/learning situations, encouraging individuals or groups to name their health issue is one of the fundamental principles of creating a caring relationship.

CONSIDER THE FOLLOWING SCENARIOS

Scenario 1: You are a public health nurse doing a follow-up antenatal visit with a first-time mother. There were no complications with the birth, and you are expecting a routine visit. When you enter the home, you are greeted by a tired mother, who reports she has been up half the night and feels like she hasn't slept in days. She tells you that she feels like shaking the baby to make him stop fussing and asks you what you know about colic.

Scenario 2: You are a hospital nurse and you have been caring for Johnny (10 years old), who has been admitted for the third time in 6 months with asthma. You have been doing discharge teaching with his mother, who is divorced and on social assistance. You have had several discussions with her about the importance of keeping the home as dust-free as possible and of Johnny avoiding smoke or other pollutants. On the day before Johnny is to be discharged, his mother approaches you and says that she needs to speak to you about something important. You find a quiet place to sit, and she begins the conversation by telling you that she smokes.

WRITE

In your journal, write two responses to each of these scenarios. In the first, describe a way of responding that is not empowering, in which you, as the nurse, name what is happening. In the second, describe how you might respond in a way that is empowering and that encourages the client to name her health issue.

DIALOGUE

With your group, take turns sharing and critiquing each other's responses. Discuss how it might feel to be the recipient of the different responses (the client/learner). Did the empowering responses feel different than when the nurse was naming the health issue?

REFLECT

In your journal, identify strategies you could use to encourage clients to name their health issue or concern. How can you encourage clients to share their health experiences and stories?

PARTICIPATION

The third element, essential to creating collaborative caring relationships, is participation. Having full participation in a teaching/learning situation is not always easy. Students and teachers enter classrooms or clinical areas already consumed by daily life. Bevis (personal communication) used to comment that when you arrive somewhere different or new, you need to give your soul time to catch up to your body. This type of centering or preparing to be *present* is critical for participation to occur within a relational emancipatory pedagogy. In this section, we describe participation and suggest strategies for encouraging participation.

Participation Versus Involvement

Without participation, there can be no partnership or relationship. Participation is a slippery concept and is often confused with the notion of involvement. In the realm of community development, Labonte (1997) has conceptualized some interesting distinctions between these two terms. We have adapted his conceptualization for our relational emancipatory pedagogy. In this context, the following distinctions are important:

CHARACTERISTICS OF PARTICIPATION

- negotiated, formalized relationships
- open frame of "problem-naming"
- shared decision-making authority
- teacher/learner fully recognized as partners in learning
- shared responsibility and accountability for learning/teaching
- negotiated power

CHARACTERISTICS OF INVOLVEMENT

- learners are asked opinions that may or may not be used
- some sharing of power but ultimate authority rests with teacher
- decision-making rests with teacher
- power remains with teacher; students asked to contribute ideas

Considering the distinctions just presented, we can see that participation is very different than merely being involved. Participation requires commitment. It is a conscious decision to devote time, energy, and resources to teaching/learning. Participation demands engagement.

Recent literature (Hurlbert & Gupta, 2015) suggests that participation is critical in solving complex health, social, and environmental issues and describes an increased explosion of literature on this topic particularly in relation to Arnstein's (1969, cited in Hurlbert & Gupta, 2015) ladder of participation. Hurlbert and Gupta recommend a split ladder that addresses and links participation with learning, trust, governance (Figure 6.2). They provide four ideal typical circumstances and explain the nature of stakeholder participation for each circumstance. This split ladder can be used as a diagnostic or an evaluation framework to examine participation.

LEARNING ACTIVITY: PARTICIPATION OR INVOLVEMENT: WHAT SHALL IT BE?

The purpose of this learning activity is to examine your experiences of participation and involvement so that you can discover strategies for participation.

WRITE

Describe a teaching/learning situation in which you felt that participation was present. Use the previous criteria to list the critical elements that made it a situation of participation rather than one of involvement.

How do you see these two terms? How are they related to each other?

Think about strategies you can use to ensure you have participation in teaching/learning situations.

REFLECT

In your journal, list five strategies you can use to ensure participation. Describe any concerns you have about encouraging participation. Write down three of your strengths that will assist you to encourage participation.

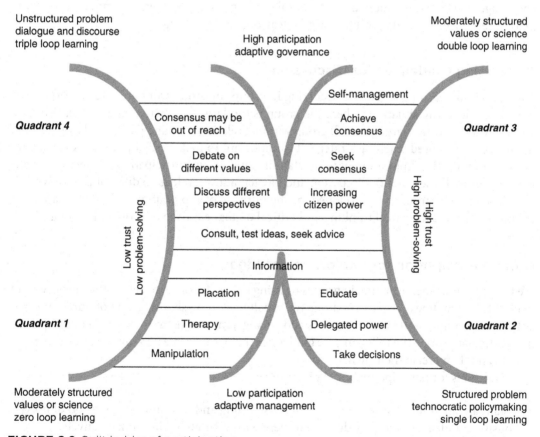

FIGURE 6.2 Split ladder of participation.

Source: Reprinted from Hurlbert, M., & Gupta, J. (2015). The split ladder of participation: A diagnostic, strategic, and evaluation tool to assess when participation is necessary. *Environmental Science & Policy*, *50*, 100–113. https://doi.org/10.1016/j.envsci.2015.01.011, Copyright 2015, with permission from Elsevier.

In her book, *Peace and Power*, Chinn (2013, 2018) describes several strategies for creating full group participation that rely on power with relationships: strategies that she refers to as "peace" processes. Chinn (2013) suggests the following guidelines for encouraging participation:

- Give every perspective a full voice.
- Demystify all processes and structures.
- Fully respect different points of view.
- Pay attention to the process itself so that how you do things is just as important as what you do.
- Rotate and share leadership according to ability and willingness.
- Value learning new skills so that the opportunity is accessible to all.
- Share responsibility for the processes of the group equally among everyone present.

As teachers, we each need to find our own ways to foster participation. There is no golden rule that works for everyone in every situation. However, following the guidelines just presented will create opportunities for participation that might not otherwise exist.

One way of implementing Chinn's recommendations for encouraging participation is to develop group guidelines for discussion. This not only demystifies the group process and encourages participation but it also creates solidarity between teachers and students resulting in joint responsibility and accountability for learning and teaching.

Developing Guidelines for Discussion

Many teaching/learning situations occurring in groups or group work are often incorporated in teaching/learning situations where the group is too large to function as a whole. Whether you are working with a large or small group within a relational emancipatory pedagogy group, discussion is a favored teaching strategy. It is important to make a distinction between group participation for the exploration of understanding and group participation for decision-making. Confusing these types of discussion and participation can lead to difficult group dynamics. Most learning groups are developed for the purpose of exploration. That is, they are used to engage students in critical thinking and critical dialogue for the purpose of learning.

Group Participation for Exploration of Ideas

We find it useful, when teaching in groups or using group dialogue, to clarify the purposes and to establish guidelines for participation. We usually begin by sharing some of our own, such as those that follow, and having students add, change, modify them to make them unique for this particular group. The following are guidelines that we have created that we ask students to discuss and then create their own.

Guidelines for participation for exploration:

- Maintain an attitude of searching for understanding and meaning. Try to let go of previously held ideas so that they do not interfere with your ability to think creatively.
- Share your "half-baked" ideas. They are often more interesting than what you already know.
- Stay in a state of not knowing. It is only when you do not know something that you can learn. If you already know something, there is no need to explore it.
- Cultivate the art of empathic listening. Try to synthesize or summarize what others have said before you make your contribution.

- Stay with the group. Follow the trend of the discussion and introduce new topics when old ones are complete.
- Talk briefly. Saying too much may cause others' minds to wander and then they may miss what you wish to express.
- When you disagree, be respectful. You can be challenging without being confrontational.

In addition to the guidelines just described, it is often helpful to ask groups to establish their own guidelines by asking: "What needs to happen for you to feel safe to explore your ideas?" Students and teachers can then together cocreate their ground rules for participation in the learning/teaching environment.

Time Out for Reflection

Think of different strategies you could use to establish patterns of working together in groups that enhance participation. How would you deal with students who are silent in the group? How will you deal with students who talk too much in the group? How will you ensure that the ground rules are honored? Who is responsible for maintaining collaborative relationships?

REFLECT

In your journal, list two strategies you could use for establishing group norms that are consistent with the ones just outlined. How will you ensure that the cocreated group norms will be honored in your relational emancipatory pedagogy?

In any teaching/learning situation, it is imperative to make the process for discussion and decision-making transparent. Using a learning activity, such as the one you just completed, is one way of ensuring that this process occurs. There are many other ways to accomplish this goal. You need to discover what will work best for you. In situations involving individuals, the same process needs to occur, but it is usually done through one-on-one dialogue rather than a learning activity.

LEARNING ACTIVITY: CHECKING IN AND CHECKING OUT

ENDS IN VIEW

The purpose of this learning activity is to provide opportunities for you to experiment with two strategies for encouraging ongoing collaborative partnerships.

CONNECTING AS A GROUP

"Checking In" and "Checking out" (Chinn, 2013, 2018) are useful strategies for continuously reminding the students of the collaborative nature of the group. These strategies help participants "clear" issues that might have happened before coming to the group and truly be fully present in the group. These strategies also ensure that you hear from each group member, at least twice during a learning session. The most powerful aspect of these strategies is that it reminds learning groups of our individual humanity and humanness. When well facilitated, these strategies develop group cohesion and a sense of belonging.

WRITE

You have probably had experiences using these two strategies in other courses you have taken in your nursing program. In your journal, write about times when you used these strategies and they really seemed to work well.

- What occurred to make them work well?
- You probably have had experiences with these strategies that were not positive.
- What was it that did not work?
- Describe your experiences. What needs to be in place for these strategies to work for you?

REFLECT

In your journal, write about how you will take responsibility for ensuring that, if you use these strategies, they are working for people.

LEARNING ACTIVITY: COLLABORATIVE DECISION-MAKING

In this learning activity, you will have opportunities to develop strategies for collaborative decision-making.

GROUP DECISION-MAKING

There may be times in a group when it is necessary to make decisions. How this process is handled must be congruent with the principles established for group process. For example, decisions may need to be made about negotiating for more time in a teaching/learning session, about a specific task that the group decides to take on, or about some point of controversy that the group stumbles upon. The point is that the decision-making process must support and be congruent with the group discussion process if you want to have collaborative relationships.

Groups often having difficulty coming to consensus on issues, resorting to voting as a way of being democratic. This strategy in fact can be coercive, and there are probably many other strategies that are more democratic. We have found the following strategy useful in our work with students. When we need to make a decision, we first have a full discussion so that everyone has an opportunity to share their views. A group member then states the issue and asks every member to give one of three responses: "I agree," "I disagree," or "I can live with it." If even one group member disagrees with the issue, further discussion is necessary.

WRITE

In your journal, write down five things that are important to you in group decision-making.

DIALOGUE

Decide how you will make decisions collaboratively. Be sure to get full agreement from each member of the class about the process to be used. Each time you meet, clearly identify times when you need to make decisions and use the agreed-upon process to do so.

REFLECT

In your journal, write down the collaborative decision-making process. Does it address the five issues that you wrote down earlier in your journal? If not, be sure to raise these issues at your next class for further discussion.

REFERENCES

Beck, M. D. (2019). Fostering metamorphosis through caring literacy in an RN-to-BSN program. In W. Rosa, S. Horton-Deutsch, & J. Watson (Eds.), *A handbook for caring science: Expanding the paradigm* (pp. 257–275). Springer Publishing Company.

Bevis, E. O. (2000). Teaching and learning: The key to education and professionalism. In E. O. Bevis & J. Watson (Eds.), *Toward a caring curriculum. A new pedagogy for nursing* (2nd ed., pp. 153–188). Jones & Bartlett.

Buscaglia, L. (1985). *Love.* Ballentine.

Cara, C., Hills, M., & Watson, J. (2021). *An educator's guide to humanizing nursing education: Grounded in caring science.* Springer Publishing Company.

Chinn, P. L. (2013). *Peace & power: New directions for building community* (8th ed.). Jones & Bartlett.

Chinn, P. L. (2018). *Peace and power handbook.* https://peaceandpowerblog.org

Chinn, P. L., & Falk-Rafael, A. R. (2015). Peace and power: A theory of emancipatory group process. *Journal of Nursing Scholarship, 47*(1), 62–69. https://doi.org/10.1111/jnu.12101

Chinn, P., & Kramer, M. (2018). *Knowledge development in nursing.* Elsevier.

Combs, A. W. (1982). *A personal approach to teaching: Beliefs that make a difference.* Allyn & Bacon.

Darder, A., Baltoodano, M., & Torres, R. (Eds.). (2009). *The critical pedagogy reader* (2nd ed.). Routledge.

Freire, P. (1972). *Pedagogy of the oppressed.* Penguin Books.

Freire, P. (2000). *Pedagogy of the oppressed* (30th ed.). Continuum. (Original work published 1970)

Hills, M. (1994). *Collaborative nursing program of BC: Development of caring science curriculum.* Report to the Ministry of Advanced Education. Centre for Curriculum Development and Professional Development.

Hills, M. (1998). Student experiences of nursing health promotion practice in hospital settings. *Nursing Inquiry, 5*(3), 164–173. https://doi.org/10.1046/j.1440-1800.1998.530164.x

Hills, M. (2001). Using co-operative inquiry to transform evaluation of nursing students' clinical practice. In P. Reason & H. Bradbury (Eds.), *A handbook action research* (pp. 340–347). Sage.

Hills, M. (2002). Perspectives on learning and practicing health promotion in hospitals: Students' Stories. In L. Young & V. Hayes (Eds.), *Transforming health promotion practice: Concepts, issues and applications* (pp. 229–240). F. A. Davis.

Hills, M. (2016). Emancipation and collaboration: Leading from beside. In W. Rosa (Ed.), *Nurses as leaders: Evolutionary visions of leadership* (pp. 293–309). Springer Publishing Company.

Hills, M., & Cara, C. (2019). Curriculum development processes and pedagogical practices for advancing caring science literacy. In W. Rosa, S. Horton-Deutsch, & J. Watson, (Eds.), *A handbook for caring science: Expanding the paradigm* (pp. 197–210). Springer Publishing Company.

Hills, M., & Watson, J. (2011). *Creating a Caring Science curriculum: An emancipatory pedagogy for nursing* (1st ed.). Springer Publishing Company.

hooks, b. (1994). *Teaching to transgress: Education as the practice of freedom.* Routledge.

Hurlbert, M., & Gupta, J. (2015). The split ladder of participation: A diagnostic, strategic, and evaluation tool to assess when participation is necessary. *Environmental Science & Policy, 50,* 100–113. https://doi.org/10.1016/j.envsci.2015.01.011

Ironside, P. M. (2015). Narrative pedagogy: Transforming nursing education through 15 years of research in nursing education. *Nursing Education Perspective, 36*(2), 83–88. https://doi.org/10.5480/13-1102

Labonte, R. (1990). *Empowerment practices for health professionals.* Participation.

Labonte, R. (1997). *Power, partnerships and participation in health promotion practice.* Australia Press.

Lather, P. (2012). "Becoming feminist": An untimely meditation on football. *Cultural Studies/Critical Methodology, 12*(4), 357–360. https://doi.org/10.1177/1532708612446438

Lather, P. (2013). Methodology-21: What do we do in the afterward? *International Journal of Qualitative Research in Education, 26*(6), 634–645. https://doi.org/10.1080/09518398.2013.788753

Merriam-Webster. (n.d.). Collaborate. In *Merriam-Webster.com dictionary.* https://www.merriam-webster.com/dictionary/collaboration

Raeburn, J., & Rootman, I. (1998). *People-centred health promotion.* John Wiley & Sons.

Watson, J. (1988). *Nursing: Human science and human care.* National League for Nursing.

Watson, J. (2012). *Human caring science: A theory of nursing.* Jones & Bartlett.

Engaging in Critical Caring Dialogue: Listening, Critical Questioning, and Critical Thinking

Education should have as one of its main tasks to invite people to believe in themselves. It should invite people to believe they have the knowledge.
—Freire, 1972, p. 80

INTRODUCTION

In this chapter, we present the second component of our relational emancipatory pedagogical framework: engaging in critical dialogue. The purpose of this chapter is to provide opportunities for you to examine the impact of engaging in critical dialogue as a fundamental element of relational emancipatory pedagogy (Figure 7.1). Critical dialogue consists of three essential interwoven processes and elements: listening, critical questioning, and critical thinking. We explore them in this chapter.

Critical dialogue, an essential component of Critical Social Theory (see Chapter 4), is the backbone of a relational emancipatory pedagogy. It provides the answer to the question: *How do we engage in a relational emancipatory pedagogy?* Dialogue might be considered simply a discussion, but critical dialogue is well planned, somewhat structured, and always purposive. The main purpose of critical dialogue is to create opportunities for critical thinking and critical reflection that result in the creation of new understandings (knowledge). Always transformative, critical dialogue aims to put teachers and students in situations where they encounter preconceived notions and ideas in ways that encourage them to question their assumptions. Without this type of encounter, they may be engaged in a discussion, but it would not be a critical dialogue.

LISTENING: THE HEART OF CRITICAL DIALOGUE

Listening is the most important process in critical caring dialogue, and it is the heart of a relational emancipatory pedagogy. Without effective listening, dialogue is reduced to mere words. We can begin to engage in the critical caring dialogue only through understanding another's meaning. As Watson (2018b) suggests, the nurse must "authentically *listen* to another person's

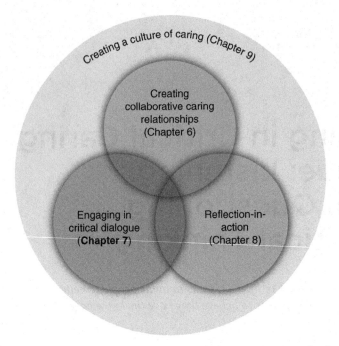

FIGURE 7.1 Interlocking circles of relational emancipatory pedagogy.

story without interrupting or trying to 'fix' anything, knowing that this moment of listening is a healing gift for both of you" (p. 84).

The Chinese characters that represent the verb "to listen" reveal the complexity of listening (Figure 7.2). Listening involves seeing, hearing, and your heart.

There is magic in listening. Being able to hear another's issues and concerns with deep understanding is a rare gift. Effective listening requires a depth of caring about the other that is characterized by warmth, genuineness, and mutual respect. Listening requires an ability to put aside, at least momentarily, our own thoughts and prejudices so that we can be open to the world of the other, so that we can be truly present with the other. Listening gives us access to the meanings that others are making in a given situation. Having this understanding of others permits us to respond in ways that are empathic and caring. In his early work, Moustakas (1977) eloquently describes this process:

> Listening is a magnetic and strange thing, a creative force. . .The friends that listen to us are the ones that we move toward, and we want to sit in their radius as though it did us good, like ultraviolet rays. . . . When we are listened to, it creates us, makes us unfold and expand. Ideas actually begin to grow in us and come to life. . .It makes people happy and free when they are

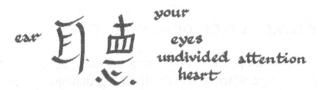

FIGURE 7.2 Chinese characters for listening.

listened to. . .When we listen to people, there is an alternating current, and that recharges us so that we never get tired of each other. We are constantly being recreated. (p. 32)

One of the most exciting things about this kind of listening, empathic listening, is that it can be learned. It is not easy to listen well—it takes concentration, willingness and practice. For those who persist, the rewards are truly astounding.

In order to truly listen to another, we need to prepare ourselves to be *present. Being present* has both physical and psychological characteristics. Being physically present, means orienting your body to the other: facing them, making eye contact, and having relaxed but attentive facial expressions. Being physically present also creates a psychological presence. It conveys to the student that you care about them and that you want to understand their situation, their perspective, the way that they are experiencing it. To enter this psychological space, we need to free ourselves from our preconceived notions, our beliefs, our tendency to prescribe, give advice, or make judgements.

Moustakas (1995) describes this psychological presence as "*Being In*" (being-in-the-world of the other) and suggests that "In the '*Being In*' I want only to encourage and support the other's communication of what is in the world and how that is, how it came to be, where it is going, just as it is offered" (p. 101).

Empathic listening requires not only that we hear what is being said by students but that we also can read the context and world-life of the student, what is being said between the words and the feelings that are being expressed nonverbally. Simply listening is not enough. We need to respond in ways that demonstrate that we understood students' experiences and meanings. The acid test for empathic listening is not whether *we* think we have demonstrated this understanding but whether *those being listened to*, students, feel that their meanings and experiences have been understood. Well-intentioned responses can often be misinterpreted as lack of understanding. This may be because, in general, *we tend to judge ourselves by our intentions and others by their actions*. For example, I might make what I intend to be a humorous comment; you might interpret that comment as sarcastic. I might say, "I was just trying to be funny!" but your interpretation can only be based on your observation and my action, not my intention. Others cannot access our thinking, so the only way they can interpret what we say or do is by our action, our response. That is how they will interpret how well we have understood them. So, it is the entire transaction that matters, not a single response and not just sitting silently in response to someone.

There are many different perspectives on the role of listening in teaching/learning. What Freire (1972) describes as listening for interests, Rogers (1979) and Combs (1982) describe as empathic listening. Regardless of its description, there is no dispute about the significance of the role that listening plays in the teaching/learning process within a relational emancipatory pedagogy.

For us, the main difference between these conceptualizations of listening is not in how they are labeled but in the way that these theorists have viewed listening throughout their study of the teaching/learning process. For example, Rogers (1979) suggests that listening, coupled with respect and genuineness, is sufficient to bring about change. Combs (1982) suggests that it is the beliefs that people hold that determine their actions. Freire (1972) argues that listening is important because it helps to identify the generative themes that need to be discussed through engagement in critical dialogue in order to move to action. All three may be accurate? What are your thoughts? How does listening fit into your relational emancipatory pedagogical model?

LEARNING ACTIVITY: LISTENING AND DEMONSTRATING UNDERSTANDING

ENDS IN VIEW

This learning activity engages you in a role-play to illuminate critical aspects of empathic listening.

DIALOGUE

Part A

Have a discussion with your learning partner to decide on an issue about which you both feel strongly but upon which you disagree. This role-play will be most effective if you discover an issue about which you really care. If more than two people are involved, take turns in a one-on-one situation. Take a few minutes to quietly think about the issue. Think about the last time you discussed the issue with someone. Recall your feelings. When you are ready, each of you take 5 minutes to try to convince the other of the merits of your side of the issue. After your turn, take a few minutes to talk about how it felt to be involved in this type of discussion. Did you feel you were understood?

Part B

Find a token that you can easily pass between you (a pen or piece of paper). Continue your discussion, but this time with one difference: only the person holding the token can state their opinion. The other must earn the token by demonstrating that they have understood the other's perspective by responding empathically. Once you have earned the token, you may state your opinion, and the other person will try to earn it back by listening and responding empathically.

If you are the person with the token, do not give it up easily. The token must be earned by having your feelings understood. Remember not to confuse agreement with empathy. The purpose of this activity is to experience truly being heard even when the one who is hearing you does not agree with you.

Part C

Discuss your reaction to the role-play experience. How did the second experience differ from the first? In the second experience, did you experience feeling understood? If not, what would have made a difference?

REFLECT

Write about your reactions to the exercise. How did it feel to try to listen to someone with whom you disagreed? Describe your experience of listening empathically.

The following poem (anonymous) highlights the complexity and importance of listening for understanding in a way that demonstrates caring. Sometimes, when we try to be understanding, we unknowingly can be very unhelpful by giving advice, trying to solve the problem, telling people what they should do or feel, or negating their feelings. This poem identifies some of the ways we are tempted to respond when all that is desired by the other is to be heard and to feel cared for.

Listen

When I ask you to listen to me and you start giving me advice,
you have not done what I have asked.

When I ask you to listen to me
and you begin to tell me why I shouldn't feel that way,
you are trampling on my feelings

When I ask you to listen to me
and you feel that you have to do something to solve my problem,
you have failed me; strange as that may seem.

Listen! All I ask is that you listen,
not talk or do—just hear me.
Advice is cheap—10 cents will get you both Dear Abby
and Billy Graham in the same newspaper.

And I can do for myself; I'm not helpless
Maybe discouraged and faltering. But, not helpless.

When you do something for me that I can and need to do
for myself, you contribute to my fear and weakness.

But, when you accept as a simple fact that I do feel what I feel,
no matter how irrational,
then I can quit trying to convince you
and I can get about the business of understanding what's behind
this irrational feeling.

And when that's clear, the answers are obvious
and I don't need advice.
irrational feelings make sense when we understand.

Perhaps, that is why prayer works, sometimes, for some people,
because God is mute and he doesn't give you advice or try to fix things.
"They" just listen and let you work it out for yourself.

So, please, listen and just hear me.
And, if you want to talk, wait a minute for your turn;
and I'll listen to you.

—Anonymous

This poem addresses the first component of listening, *hearing the other,* without interrupting, judging, or advising. But, empathic listening does demand a response—a particular type of response that acknowledges the other's feelings and perspective while being totally *present* with the other. This response needs to be respectful, authentic, and caring.

When you choose to teach from a relational emancipatory pedagogy, you enter a unique and special caring relationship. Teachers working within this pedagogy join the students in "genuine encounters of caring and being cared for" (Noddings, 2013, p. 175). As Noddings (2013) explains, no enterprise or special function (e.g., the role of a teacher) can relieve teachers from their responsibility as the one caring. In professions where encounter is frequent (as in teaching/learning situations) and where the ethical ideal of the other (student) is necessarily involved, "I am first and foremost one caring and, second, enactor of specialized functions. As a teacher, I am, first, the one caring" (Noddings, 2013, p. 177). This means that as a teacher, learning to listen with all your being and responding empathically is the key to being in relation in a relational emancipatory pedagogy.

Watson explains that nurse educators must, inspire, invite, and create safe space to listen, to ask questions, to disagree, and to evolve together. Be open to hear what students (and patients) have to teach you. You as the *faculty* become *expert learners* along with your students (Watson, 2018a, p. 189).

CRITICAL QUESTIONING

In this section of the chapter, we describe Freire's conceptualization of problem posing as a strategy for critical dialogue, and we present a variety of other ways to use critical questioning to engage in critical dialogue.

PROBLEM POSING

Freire's (1972; 1970/2000) model of empowerment education describes a three-stage methodology consisting of listening, which we discussed in the previous section; participatory dialogue, which we explore in this section; and action, which we will discuss in Chapter 8.

Freire (1972; 1970/2000) proposes that the main strategy of empowerment (emancipatory) education, namely critical dialogue, requires us to engage, as a group, in a process of problem-posing rather than a process of problem-solving. Problem-posing is different from problem-solving because it does not seek immediate solutions to problems. Rather, generative themes arising from the listening phase are "codified" and posed as problematics to raise group consciousness about specific issues. Wallerstein et al. (2018) contend that this process recognizes the complexity and the time needed to create effective solutions to societal issues. For a code to be effective it must reveal multiple sides of the issue that are familiar to the participants (Wallerstein et al., 2018). Freire describes these as generative themes because they generate energy that motivates people to act.

Freire contends that, through a process of dialogue that reflects on the generative themes raised through listening, people become "masters of their thinking by discussing the thinking and views of the world explicitly or implicitly manifest in their own suggestions and those of their comrades" (1972, p. 95). As Wallerstein et al. (2018) explain, using group dialogue with its critical questioning creates critical thinking by posing issues in order to have participants discover root causes of their position in society.

Freire (1972) cautions that "the liberating educator has to be very aware that transformation is not just a question of methods and techniques" (p. 35). If that were the case, we could simply substitute one set of methods for another. "The question is in a different relationship to knowledge and to society" (Freire, 1972, p. 35).

Critical thinking about generative themes identified in the listening phase does not occur spontaneously. The teacher is responsible for guiding this critical dialogue process by using a five-step questioning strategy that moves discussion from the personal to the social analysis and to the action level. People are asked (a) to describe what they see and feel, (b) as a group, to define the many levels of the issue, (c) to share similar experiences from their lives, (d) to question why this problem exists, and (e) to develop action plans to address the problem. Wallerstein et al. (2018), a Freirian scholar, created a questioning process for critical dialogue. She begins by using "triggers" to initiate dialogue. A trigger is a concrete, physical representation of a critical issue, generative theme, or obstacle that has arisen in the listening phase of empowerment education. For example, you might use a videotape, a role-play, a poem, or a story. In their description of developing learning activities, Bevis (2000) calls this notion "using a *hook*." A hook serves the same purpose. It grabs the student's interest and attention. It orients the student to the issue to be explored.

Wallerstein et al. (2018) uses the acronym SHOWED to represent the different stages of this teaching/learning process, which is built on a questioning cycle of What? Why? So what? Now what?

S See—What do I see here? How do we name this issue?

H Happening—What is happening? What is really happening to this person, group, or community? (These first two questions are the description stage during which the participants/students name the issue.)

O Our—How does this issue relate to our lives? How is my experience similar or different? How do I feel about the issue?

W Why—Why does this issue occur? What are the social, cultural, economic, and political influences that contribute to this problem?

E Empowered—How can we become empowered to deal with this issue?

D Do—What can we do? What action steps can we take to act on the problem? (These last two questions deal with the action-planning phase of the process.)

In a nursing education context, a trigger should

- be based on a generative theme that you have listened for in a teaching/learning situation;
- portray the theme as a familiar issue, immediately recognizable by the participants/students;
- focus on one concern but contain historical, cultural, and social connections.

TIME OUT FOR REFLECTION

Think about a teaching/learning situation for which you have to prepare. Consider the following questions:

What might you use as a trigger to engage learners?
How did SHOWED method of guiding critical reflection fit with your Caring Science pedagogy?

USING CRITICAL QUESTIONS TO PROMPT CRITICAL DIALOGUE

Learning to ask critical questions is the key strategy to facilitating effective dialogue. A dialogue method "systematically invites students or audiences to think critically, to co-develop the session with the expert or teacher, and to construct peer relations instead of authority-dependent relations" (Freire, 1972, p. 41). Using a dialogical learning process encourages teachers to move beyond the traditional lecture method to a dialectical process of interaction. This shift from lecture to dialogic teaching/learning transfers the responsibility from teachers being solely responsible for creating learning experiences to shared responsibility for learning that promotes the creation of new knowledge and self-actualization for teachers and students.

Learners also must develop the strategy of asking critical questions. As Bevis (2000) suggests, "Teaching, in its true form, is helping students learn new ways of approaching ideas and examining things by helping them learn to ask the appropriate questions" (p. 242). They learn to do so by experiencing positive caring, yet critical questioning, in their own learning.

People who want to use a dialogue method often struggle with the issue of how to incorporate information-giving into this process. Indeed, there are some who feel that lecturing has no place in a dialogue method of teaching/learning. "Regardless of its strengths, lecturing is an oppressive teaching strategy. It is oppressive because, among other reasons, learners must listen to information filtered through someone else's perspective and value system" (Bevis, 2000, p. 240). One strategy that works within a relational emancipatory pedagogy is to ask students if they want to hear your (the teacher's) conceptualization or the way you have synthesized the knowledge from the literature. Lecturing can be engaging, but it is very dependent on the teacher's charisma. If lecturing seems warranted, be sure that students are included in the process. Combining "mini" lectures with discussion also assists in reducing "teacher talk." The more you move away from lecturing toward dialogic teaching strategies the more you are situated in a relational emancipatory pedagogy. In general, *ask* rather than *tell*.

Bevis (2000) identified a passive-to-active continuum and recommended several methods that assist in active learning. Their description of a learning episode is reminiscent of Freire's (1972) three-stage method described earlier. A "learning episode is a natural grouping of events in which students engage in the process of acquiring insights, seeing patterns, finding meanings and significance, seeking balance and wholeness and making judgments or developing skills" (Bevis, 2000, p. 223). Bevis suggests that, for learning to occur, three stages—operation, information, and validation—must occur, although they can occur in any order.

Operation Phase

According to Bevis (2000), the operation phase is an issue or a problem that is used to "hook" the students' interest. The teacher's ability to invoke reality in an imaginative way and to raise real and relevant questions that stimulate students' interest and motivation is the key ingredient of this aspect of the learning episode. The operational aspect of the learning episode is most effective when students are provided with structure regarding how much time to spend, what questions are to be answered, and then are left to wrestle with their ideas in small groups.

Information Phase

The information phase is more passive and consists of the student acquiring data related to the issue or problem that was raised or will be raised in the operation phase depending on the sequencing of the phases. It is essential that the information that the students are seeking is needed to "solve" the issue raised. "Active learning requires that the students be engaged with an issue or with problems that require them to need information in order to solve the problem" (Bevis, 2000, p. 225). If the students do not need the information, and the lack of information flows over into the dialogue that is typical of the operation phase, students will pool their ignorance, not their knowledge. The most common way to gain information is by reading, watching, or listening. Teachers need to use their imaginations to devise strategies for engagement that motivate students to want information. Some examples include watching a video clip, listening to a tape, reading an article, going on a scavenger hunt, or engaging in some other type of activity.

Validation Phase

For Bevis (2000), the final phase of the learning episode, validation, is the testing aspect and it occurs in reality—the daily life of the nursing student. In nursing, the validation phase often occurs in the practice area. Validation allows students to see what they can do. This phase develops students' confidence. Simulations can help build competence but confidence comes only with reality validation.

As Bevis (2000) states, "If all three aspects have occurred, something will be learned, although it may not be what the teacher thinks will be learned" (p. 223).

LEARNING ACTIVITY: ASKING CRITICAL QUESTIONS

ENDS IN VIEW

There are many ways to engage in critical dialogue. In this learning activity, you will explore the use of critical questioning as a way to encourage critical dialogue.

READ

Review, in this text, the SHOWED framework, Bevis's description of the learning episode, and Freire's three-stage method for learning.

WRITE

In your journal, do a comparative analysis of Bevis's description of active learning, including the learning episode, and Wallerstein et al.'s SHOWED method. Identify the conceptual similarities and differences of these two models.

Does one model fit better than the other within your framework/model for teaching/learning practice?

Are there certain aspects of each that you would like to incorporate into your framework/model?

DIALOGUE

With your learning partners or study group, discuss your analysis of the two models. Discuss some of the scholarly modalities and educational heuristics identified by Bevis. Which of these will be helpful in developing your framework/model for teaching/learning practice?

REFLECT

In your journal, revisit your framework/model for teaching/learning practice. Have you considered what methodology you will use in it? Revise your framework in ways that may now seem appropriate. Describe how your methodology is congruent with other aspects of it.

So, if lecturing is perceived as a strategy that creates passive students, how can the teacher's information and knowledge be conveyed to learners? We suggest that there is no problem with teachers sharing their ideas and concerns. On the contrary, it is irresponsible not to share. In fact, as just described earlier, sharing information when it is needed is an excellent way to share information. The critical consideration is how teachers should share their ideas. There are two key points involved here: timing and process. As Shor and Freire (1987) explain, the critical question is not about lecturing or not lecturing. The point is whether you are lecturing or using a dialogical approach, "does it critically reorient students to society? Does it animate their critical thinking or not?" (p. 40).

If teachers begin sessions with lectures, there is an unstated assumption that what you have to say is more important than what students think about the topic or issue. This difficulty is related to the issue of power that was discussed in the previous chapters. Turning this process around by posing questions first and then sharing your ideas helps to reduce the power differential inherent in most teaching/learning situations. It must be stressed that it is the type of questions that you ask that is so important. Asking questions that require students to respond with memorized answers or "teacher knows the answer and you have to guess" is no different than lecturing. Asking questions that provoke learners to think in new and as yet undiscovered ways leads to insight and stimulates knowledge creation.

There are times when it is appropriate for teachers to share their synthesis of information. You might think of these as "mini raps" or "mini lectures." It is also important to remember that you, as teacher, have equal rights and responsibilities to be a full participant in the critical dialogue—sharing your views and learning from others. We have found the following strategies to be helpful when engaging in critical dialogue as a teacher.

- Share your ideas as opinions, not truths.
- Ask permission or ask for interest in hearing about what you know from the literature about the topic.
- Start a teaching/learning session by posing critical questions.
- Encourage students to work on issues in partnerships or small groups. Most students feel more comfortable testing out their ideas in a small group before sharing with a larger group.
- Create innovative ways of accessing students' understandings from their group work (other than reporting back). One strategy is to ask learners to come up with one question that still remains unanswered for them that they would like the large group to consider.
- Watch for teachable moments. Teachable moments are spontaneous occasions when students ask a question or pose an issue in such a way as to signify a readiness to learn that is urgent. These moments are basically enactments of the famous saying "When a child stands in awe and mystery of a falling rose petal, then it's time to teach the law of gravity."
- Learn to create and live with ambiguity. Being comfortable in a place of unknowing is a critical skill for a teacher who wants to practice from a relational emancipatory

pedagogy. Students need space and time to struggle in that place of not knowing and teachers need to support their struggle without providing their answer to the issue or struggle.

It is a magical moment in a teaching/learning situation when you see students living in that moment of uncertainty, of not knowing, on the brink of discovery—of learning. We talk about creating this moment of *confusion* as essential for teachers to create for students so they can enter that space of not *knowing*. We claim that it is only when you are in a state of *not knowing*—of *ambiguity*—that you are in a space to learn.

CRITICAL THINKING

In this section of the chapter, we examine the role of critical thinking within a relational emancipatory pedagogy. Opportunities are provided for you to examine your critical thinking development and abilities.

WHAT IS CRITICAL THINKING?

Critical thinking is a process that requires that we continuously and critically question the assumptions that underlie our customary, habitual ways of acting and thinking. It involves much more than analytical, rational processing of information or analyzing information for logical fallacies. At its core, critical thinking requires that we question our assumptions as they are enacted in our daily lives. Meizerow (1997) states that this can be very demanding because:

> Admitting that our assumptions might be distorted, wrong, or contextually relative implies that the fabric of our personal and political existence might rest upon faulty foundations. Even considering this possibility is profoundly threatening. If our past lives have been lived within faulty assumptive worlds, we are faced with the question of whether we have to jettison our current relationships, work, and political commitments in favor of some more authentic ways of living, whatever they may be? (p. 192)

Critical thinking is a productive and positive activity. Critical thinkers are totally engaged in and passionate about life circumstances. They see themselves as creators of life experiences and they exude a sense of vitality and hope. They are optimistic and see the potential that being "critical" offers. They are passionate and committed yet open and flexible.

In his early writing, Brookfield (1993) identifies five characteristics of critical thinking. Although we are using his headings here to describe critical thinkers, we have taken considerable poetic license in describing the attributes of critical thinkers.

CRITICAL THINKING IS A PROCESS, NOT AN OUTCOME

Critical thinkers are constantly in a state of becoming. They are consistently engaged in a process of wondering or of questioning assumptions. They are skeptical not only of universal truths but of simplistic explanations of any phenomena. Regardless of their own biases, they can always raise doubts about the way a situation is being viewed. "Central to the interpretation of critical thinking is a realization that critical thinking is not a method to be learned, but rather a process, an orientation of the mind, and includes both the cognitive and affective domains of reasoning" (Simpson & Courtney, 2002, p. 98).

Manifestations of critical thinking vary according to the contexts in which they occur; there is no formula or right or wrong way to be a critical thinker. Critical thinkers vary enormously in terms of how they appear in everyday life. Sometimes they are more apparent to us because of the way they process information. It is easier to recognize the critical thinking abilities of those who externalize their thinking than it is to recognize those whose thinking is internal.

CRITICAL THINKING IS TRIGGERED BY POSITIVE AS WELL AS NEGATIVE EVENTS

Much of the literature describes critical thinking as being triggered by only negative events (Dobrzykowski, 1994). These negative events apparently cause people to question previously held assumptions about the way the world and the people in it work and relate to each other and this questioning prompts careful scrutiny of what were previously unquestioned views. However, it is just as reasonable to think that critical thinking can arise from joyous occasions in which our previously held assumptions are called into question.

CRITICAL THINKING IS EMOTIVE AS WELL AS RATIONAL

At times, critical thinking is presented as if it were removed from emotions and feelings. But emotions are in fact central to critical thinking. Questioning our unquestioned assumptions, our taken-for-granted values, and the way in which we live our lives touches on the core of our emotions and requires that we tune into our feelings.

TIME OUT FOR REFLECTION

In your journal, draw a line down the middle of a page. On the left-hand side of the page, list the five characteristics of critical thinkers. On the right-hand side, next to each characteristic, write at least two behaviors that you exhibit that you feel demonstrate this characteristic in the way you engage in teaching/learning situations. Would others recognize these characteristics in you?

List five strategies you could use to help others to develop critical-thinking characteristics.

Write about what seems new to you regarding the way you now view critical thinking. What stands out for you as being important or needing attention?

ESSENTIAL COMPONENTS OF CRITICAL THINKING

Brookfield (originally in 1993 and more recently in 2012) identifies four essential components for critical thinking. Again, we use his headings and our experiences in nursing education to describe these components in order to make them relevant to nursing.

- *Identifying and challenging assumptions*—For us, the questions How do you know that?, Who told you that that is true?, and Why does that have to be the case? all challenge our taken-for-granted assumptions. So often, we wander through nursing practice and education accepting what seems, for us, to be the natural order of events. It is by asking, Why must this be so? that we begin to uncover what is usually and naturally assumed to be so. Challenging assumptions is often difficult because many nurses and students would prefer that you not upset their equilibrium.

- *Challenging the influence of context*—Critical-thinking nurse educators and students are aware that practices, structures, and actions are never context-free. They are able to see the influence of the context on a particular situation and understand the dynamics that occur because of this context. It is as though they are tuned into the nuances of a situation. Because they understand the complexity of context, particularly in healthcare systems, they can respond instantaneously to a given situation even though they may have never previously been in such a situation.

- *Imagining and exploring alternatives*—Nurse educators and students who are critical thinkers are aware of many different ways of operating other than the one that seems most apparent. Although they understand that the context of a situation makes something appear to be the most obvious way of doing something, they also realize that, if the context were to shift slightly, something else could appear to be the most obvious thing to do.

- *Reflective skepticism*—Nurse educators and students who are critical thinkers have a healthy optimism about being skeptical. They know that the best way of understanding a situation is to be critical and to raise questions about it. They are wary of quick-fix solutions. They are able to question practices that have existed for a long time because they recognize that, just because they have worked in the past, they may not be appropriate now. And, just because everyone else agrees with them, that does not make them right!

LEARNING ACTIVITY: COMPONENTS OF CRITICAL THINKING

ENDS IN VIEW

This learning activity is designed to have you examine your ability to think critically.

WRITE

In your journal, write the four components of critical thinking. Take a few minutes to think about yourself in a teaching/learning situation. Beside each component, describe one experience that you have had in which you either experienced yourself or experienced someone else struggling with this component of critical thinking.

DIALOGUE

Describe these experiences you have written about in your journal to your learning partners or study group. Discuss how you felt as you struggled with these issues. Describe some of the main things you learned about critical thinking as a result of these experiences.

DEVELOPING CRITICAL THINKING

Many authors have described and theorized about the development of critical thinking. Brookfield (2012) has summarized others' thinking about it and suggests that the pattern of the development of critical thinking involves five phases.

Phase 1: Trigger Event

Some unexpected event occurs that results in inner feelings of discomfort or perplexity. Many theorists suggest that these events are often negative. We like to conceptualize this occurrence as creating ambiguity or confusion. We often tell students that part of our jobs as teachers is to create this ambiguity or confusion. For us, this is related to the issue that we raised earlier. We believe that you cannot learn—or maybe we should say think critically—if you are in a state of knowing. Significant learning occurs when you are in a state of dis-ease, or confusion. The brain is a wondrous organ for it will not allow you to stay in this state of dis-ease. It will keep mulling around the confusion until you sort it out.

Phase 2: Appraisal

This is the period of self-scrutiny—the mulling around the issue—we described. During this phase, the issues and concerns are identified and clarified.

Phase 3: Exploration

Having seen discrepancies or anomalies, new ways of explaining them begin to be explored in order to decrease the discomfort that is experienced. During this phase, new ways of thinking or acting are tested out that seem more congruent with the perceptions of what is happening in our practice and our learning. During this phase, we search for new ways of doing things, new answers, new ways of organizing one's worldview. For us, it is a time of possibility; a time for creating new ways of being-in-the world; a time for developing our caring capacities.

Phase 4: Developing Alternative Perspectives

From these explorations come new ways of thinking that begin to make sense for our current situations. This is a transitional phase during which the old is left behind and new ways are embraced. New knowledge and skills are developed for the way you now wish to be.

Phase 5: Integration

Once you have decided on the worth, accuracy, and validity of your new ways of thinking and living, you begin to weave these into the fabric of your life. At this stage, you achieve some level of integration of the previously conflicting feelings or ideas. Meizerow (1997) describes this process as "perspective transformation" suggesting that this is the point at which students experience having learned, or having come to a satisfactory point of closure, in relation to an issue.

TIME OUT FOR REFLECTION

Write in your journal about a time when you felt that you experienced the development of critical thinking as just described. Think about a problem you had to solve or a decision you had to make. Try to be specific in describing your experience in relation to the stages suggested by Brookfield (2012).

Respond to the following questions:

- Did you experience all of these stages?
- Did some of the stages seem more important than others?
- Recall your assumptions and how they might have changed during the process.
- What alternatives did you consider?
- How did you evaluate the effectiveness of your choice of alternatives?

REFERENCES

Bevis, E. (2000). Teaching and learning: A practical commentary. In E. Bevis & J. Watson (Eds.), *Toward a caring curriculum: A new pedagogy for nursing* (pp. 217–259). National League for Nursing.

Brookfield, S. (1993). On impostorship, cultural suicide, and other dangers: How nurses learn critical thinking. *The Journal of Continuing Education in Nursing, 24*(5), 197–205. https://doi.org/10.3928/0022-0124-19930901-04

Brookfield, S. (2012). *Developing critical thinkers.* Jossey-Bass.

Combs, A. W. (1982). *Personal approach to teaching: Beliefs that make a difference.* Allyn & Bacon.

Dobrzykowski, T. (1994). Teaching strategies to promote critical thinking skills in nursing staff. *The Journal of Continuing Education in Nursing, 25*(6), 272–276. PMID: 7868746.

Freire, P. (1972). *Pedagogy of the oppressed.* Penguin Books.

Freire, P. (/2000). *Pedagogy of the oppressed* (30th ed.). Continuum. (Original work published 1970)

Meizerow, J. (1997). *Fostering critical reflection in adulthood.* Jossey-Bass.

Moustakas, C. (1977). *Creative life.* Van Nostrand Reinhold.

Moustakas, C. (1995). *Being-in, being-for, being-with.* Rowman & Littlefield.

Noddings, N. (2013). *Caring: A feminine approach to ethics and moral education* (2nd edition, updated). University of California Press.

Rogers, C. R. (1979). *Freedom to learn.* C.E. Merrill Pub. Co.

Shor, I., & Freire, R. (1987). *A pedagogy for liberation: Dialogues on transforming education.* Bergin & Garvey.

Simpson, E., & Courtney, M., (2002). Critical thinking in nursing education: Literature review. *International Journal of Nursing Practice, 8*, 89–98. https://doi.org/10.1046/j.1440-172x.2002.00340.x

Wallerstein, N., Duran, B., Oetzel, J., & Minkler, M. (2018). *Community-based participatory research for health: Advancing social and health equity* (3rd ed.). Jossey-Bass.

Watson, J. (2018a). Reflection on teaching and sustaining human caring. In D. D. Hunt (Ed.), *The new nurse educator: Mastering academe* (2nd ed., pp. 189–194). Springer Publishing Company.

Watson, J. (2018b). *Unitary caring science: The philosophy and praxis of nursing.* University Press of Colorado.

Critical Reflection-In-Action (Praxis): Emancipatory Action

Even when you individually feel yourself most free, if this feeling is not a social feeling, if you are not able to use your recent freedom to help others to be free by transforming the totality of society, then you are exercising only an individualistic attitude towards empowerment and freedom . . . While individual empowerment, the feeling of being changed, is not enough concerning the transformation of the whole of society, it is absolutely necessary for the process of social transformation.—Shor & Freire, 1987, p. 109

INTRODUCTION

Critical reflection-in-action is the third element of our relational emancipatory pedagogical framework. We assert that, in order to create transformational learning, students must be provided with actual experience in which they can discover reflecting and acting in the moment. We refer to this practice and integration of knowledge from experience as *praxis*. We reach that goal at the end of the chapter. Beforehand, we explore the relationships between experience, reflection, and action. This process of reflection is recognized as an important aspect of all learning. We examine the complexities of reflection by presenting different perspectives that help to distinguish reflection as an internal process and reflection as dialectic. It is reflection as a dialectic—*reflection-in-action*—that we argue is the key to transformational learning. Reflection *on* action can lead to change; reflection-in-action always leads to change (Figure 8.1).

REFLECTION-ON-ACTION

Reflection is sometimes referred to as a process that occurs internally and in isolation. Boud et al. (2013a) state that "reflection in the context of learning is a generic term for those intellectual and affective activities in which individuals engage to explore their experiences in order to lead to new understandings and appreciations" (p. 19). Reflection is often linked to experience and can be thought of as the process of internally examining an issue of concern, triggered by an experience, that creates and clarifies meaning in terms of self, and that also results in a changed conceptual perspective. Nurse educators use this type of reflection often, for example in pre- and postconference sessions or teaching moments in practice settings. It is straightforward to trigger this type of reflection by asking questions such as What just happened in

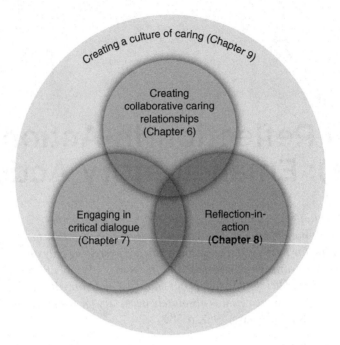

FIGURE 8.1 Interlocking circles of relational emancipatory pedagogy.

that situation? or Think about what happened when . . .? These types of questions quite easily trigger *reflection-on-action*. According to Sherwood and Horton-Deutsch (2017), "*reflection-on-action* is a retrospective process; it's the thinking that occurs after an incident. The goal is to make sense of what happened and process the outcomes to rethink future actions" (p. 12).

REFLECTION AS A THREE-STAGE PROCESS

Boud et al. (2013a) describe a three-stage process of reflection. They suggest that, in any learning experience, there are three stages—preparation, engagement, and processing—each of which requires a different type of reflection. In the *preparatory phase*, students deal with the anticipation of the experience, reflecting perhaps on what might be expected of them and what contribution they might make. In the *engagement phase*, the actual experience, students' reflections usually include recognition of the disparity between what they learned in the classroom and what they experience in the field. The final *processing phase* occurs after the field experience and involves retrospectively reflecting on the experience to make sense of it.

ASSUMPTIONS UNDERLYING REFLECTION IN LEARNING

Boud et al. (2013b) also detailed three key assumptions regarding reflection in learning:

- Only students themselves can learn and only they can reflect on their own experiences. Although, by a variety of methods, facilitators can access students' thoughts at a basic level, students have complete control in a teaching/learning situation by choosing what they are willing to share.

- Reflection is pursued with intent. It is a purposive activity directed toward a goal.
- Reflection is a complex process in which both feelings and cognition are closely interrelated and interactive.

LEARNING ACTIVITY: REFLECTION ON OWN EXPERIENCES

ENDS IN VIEW

In this learning activity, we invite you to reflect on your own experiences and thoughts about reflection in learning.

WRITE

In your journal, write about a recent experience in which you felt that your learning was significant and meaningful. Address the following questions:

What role did experience play in this situation?
How was reflection involved? Try to describe your process of reflection as concretely as possible.
What was the relationship between experience and reflection?

DIALOGUE

With your study group, discuss your responses to the questions just asked. Also, consider and discuss the following questions. How does reflection occur? What conditions influence one's ability to reflect? How does one know that reflection has occurred?

REFLECT

Review your journal entries in response to learning activities and/or time out for reflection activities that you have completed throughout this book. Pay particular attention to the notes that you have written for each reflection component of your numerous learning activities. Note any themes that seem to emerge. What characteristics of reflection seem evident?

COMPONENTS OF REFLECTION IN LEARNING

Boud and his colleagues' (2013a) model for reflection in learning consists of two components: the experience and the reflective activity. They define experience as the total response of people to a situation or event: what they "think, feel, do and conclude at the time and immediately thereafter" (p. 18). They contend that the experience is followed by a processing phase of reflection. Reflection is "an important human activity in which people recapture their experience, think about it, mull it over and evaluate it" (Boud et al., 2013a, p. 19). In their view, one of the most important ways to enhance learning is to strengthen the link between experience and the reflective activity that follows it. It is recommended that teachers plan consciously for the reflective phase as it is often overlooked and undervalued. Although this may be true in education in general, it seems that nursing education has fully embraced the importance of reflection and continues to praise its significance in nursing to this day (Josephsen, 2014;

Nelson, 2012). As Sherwood and Horton-Deutsch (2017) explain: "deep learning can only be made known as it comes to the surface . . . Reflection enables that process through the ability to construct, deconstruct and reconstruct" (p. 14).

Three elements were identified as being central to this reflective process (Boud et al., 2013b) and we have adapted them with nursing students:

1. *Returning to the experience*—This element involves recollecting the salient aspects of the experience. It is descriptive in nature and requires that the nursing students recall what actually occurred in practice as accurately as possible. The simple recollection of an event can develop insight. As we witness the events again, they become available to us to reconsider and examine afresh; we realize "what we were feeling and what responses prompted us to act as we did" (Boud et al., 2013a, p. 27). Boud et al. (2013a) recommends that the description itself be as free from judgments and interpretations as possible.

2. *Attending to feelings*—This element involves the nursing students consciously recalling positive and negative feelings that they may have encountered during the experience. Nursing students are encouraged to use their own positive feelings to assist them in pursuing what otherwise might be a very challenging situation (Boud et al., 2013a).

3. *Reevaluating the experience*—During this element, the experience is reexamined in light of the nursing students' intent, while associating new knowledge with what was already known and integrating this new knowledge into the students' conceptual framework. Four aspects have been identified within this element of reevaluation (Boud et al., 2013a):

    a. *Association*—Association is the connecting of the ideas and feelings that were a part of the original experience with those that have occurred during reflection. Through this process students may come to realize that their previous attitudes are no longer consistent with their new understandings.

    b. *Integration*—During this aspect of reevaluating the experience, the process of discrimination assists nursing students in sorting out what is meaningful to them. Two processes are involved in this aspect: searching for the nature of relationships that have been observed in the association aspect and drawing conclusions while arriving at insights. The nursing students experience a coming together or creative synthesis of the information previously taken in and the formation of a new solution or change in the self—what might be called a new *gestalt*.

    c. *Validation*—In this aspect, nursing students begin to test their new understandings for consistency with their existing knowledge and beliefs. If discrepancies appear, the situation needs to be reassessed in order to decide on what basis to proceed. Rehearsal is a useful strategy to use in the validation aspect.

    d. *Appropriation*—This aspect does not occur in all instances of reevaluating the experience. This aspect involves the nursing students owning the new information in a personal way. Strong emotions are involved in this process and nursing students often are deeply affected by the learning. The inclusion of the emotional quality to information radically alters the way that information is treated by the nursing students' consciousness as they experience the personal meaning of the experience.

REFLECTION-IN-ACTION

Some theorists make a distinction between reflection-on action and reflection-in-action. Both of these concepts are important for nurses and nurse educators because of the practice-based nature of their work. Much of the first section of this chapter dealt with reflection-on-action/experience and provided insight into how some of the ways of engaging in this type of retrospective reflection assist learning. In this section of the chapter, we examine three different ways of reflecting-in-action: practical knowledge-in-action, skill acquisition, and praxis and the prerequisites for this type of reflection. This type of reflection, reflection-in-action, is intrinsically linked to critical consciousness.

Critical Consciousness

To be able to reflect in this way, in-action, nurses must have critical consciousness. Critical consciousness from a Freirean perspective, means,

> [T]he ability of individuals to take perspective on their immediate cultural, social, and political environment, to engage in critical dialogue with it, bringing to bear fundamental moral commitments including concerns for justice and equity, and to define their own place with respect to surrounding reality. (Mustakova-Possardt, 1998, p. 13)

Critical consciousness requires nursing students to develop self-awareness, insight, and critical subjectivity. In most nursing schools, we have courses that assist students to develop self-awareness. Insight and critical subjectivity are more difficult to teach because they require the students themselves to engage in self-development and critical reflection; in metacognition. They have to be able and want to engage in thinking about their thinking. It requires that students have a heightened awareness of their immediate *and* their socio-political context.

"Insight" and "critical subjectivity" are similar but different. *Insight* is an instance of apprehending the true nature of something, especially through intuitive understanding, or it can be thought of as discernment; being able to see the inner character or underlying truth. *Critical subjectivity* is an awareness of the explanations that explain one's actions in the world and to see the extent to which their experiences are congruent with these ideas or theories. In this way, both theory and practice are developed. This developed form of consciousness is called "critical subjectivity" (Reason, 1994). This type of awareness allows nursing students to increase their consciousness and as a consequence, they are able to change their practices.

Critical consciousness can be thought of as operating on three levels of awareness. At the lowest level of consciousness, nurses, nurse educators, or students can be unaware of their surrounding context. They simply go about their daily practices without paying any attention or having any awareness of the political or cultural context within which they are working. On the next level, nurses are aware of their political and cultural context but they choose not to act. They like to think of themselves as being *neutral* but in reality there is no position of neutrality. As Freire (1985) eloquently claims: "Washing one's hands of the conflict between the powerful and the powerless means to side with the powerful, not to be neutral" (p. 122). The final level of critical consciousness requires a wide-awakeness to the political, cultural, and hegemonic practices that require action. At this level of consciousness, it is not possible to not act. We are driven to action because of our insights, our understanding of the context, our being-wide-awake-in-the-world. We are compelled to act.

For example, one of the authors had the experience of being in an emergency waiting room with her friend and colleague when they were travelling for their research. An Indigenous woman entered the emergency room and approached the triage nurse. The nurse barely acknowledged her, took some information from her. She passed the patient a wastepaper basket when she indicated that she was nauseous. The woman was obviously weak and distressed and asked if she could lie down. Without looking up, the triage nurse said that there was a gurney around the corner and the patient could lie down there if she wanted. The author got up and went to the patient, introduced herself and noted that she was a nurse, and asked if she could help the woman get to the gurney. The woman thanked the nurse and the nurse took her arm and led her to the gurney that was out of site for the triage nurse. The gurney was raised and there would have been no way that the woman would have been able to get on the gurney. The nurse observer lowered the gurney and assisted the woman onto it. The nurse observer told the woman where she was going to sit in the waiting room, and explained that she would be able to keep an eye on her from where she would be sitting. Later, the woman's family came and after seeing their mother, they came into the waiting room looking for the person that had helped their mother. The point here is that there was no choice in this action. The nurse (author) observing this scenario did not have to think about what to do. She was compelled to act. And so it is with many of us. When you have this level of critical consciousness, the right thing to do—the caring way of being—guides us to act justly. It is a moral imperative!

Nurses need to be able to think about their thinking; that means being able to engage in metacognition " to think about one's own thoughts and emotions, link the present to the past, to provide a view for the future and construct meaning of events" (Josephsen, 2014, p.2). This level of consciousness needs to be developed over time in nursing education programs. Jemel suggests that "being around others, especially those in roles of authority, with higher levels of critical consciousness may be the source of support for [critical consciousness] development" (Jemal, 2017, p. 614). So, nurse educators and nurses who supervise students must have this critical consciousness so that they can assist in its development for students. By the time nursing students graduate, they need to be able to face the challenges of increasingly complex and rapidly changing healthcare systems and have this level of critical consciousness.

Tacit Knowing-In-Practice

Schön (2016) contends that this type of reflection—reflection-in-action—is often overlooked completely, and yet is of paramount importance to practitioners such as nurses. This type of reflection is important in most aspects of nursing education because of the practice-based nature of our discipline. However, this type of reflection is critically important in teaching/learning situations that require the acquisition of skills. It is this type of knowing-in-action that Benner and Wrubel (1982) describe in their foundational research that illuminates nursing practice. Schön (2016) supports their position and claims that reflection is an intuitive, creative, artistic process, much more than a cognitive/affective process of analysis. Reflection-in-action means that practitioners respond instantaneously to unfamiliar situations in appropriate and skillful ways. As Schön (2016) explains:

> When we go about the spontaneous, intuitive performance of the actions of everyday life, we show ourselves to be knowledgeable in a special way. Often we cannot say what it is that we know. When we try to describe it we find ourselves at a loss, or we produce descriptions that are obviously inappropriate. Our knowing is ordinarily tacit, implicit in our pattern of action and in our feel for the stuff with which we are dealing. It seems right to say that our knowing is in our action. (pp. 49–50)

Sherwood and Horton-Deutsch (2017) defined *tacit knowledge* as: "implied and difficult to articulate objectively but may be shared through interactive conversation or narrative. It is the integration of knowledge with experience for new understanding and operating related to specific situations in practice" (p. 10; see also Chapter 5).

As with nursing practice, much of teaching practice is chaotic and unpredictable. No matter how much you prepare, you cannot prepare for the unexpected. So much of teaching requires that you be able to think on your feet, read the situation, and recognize teachable moments. In other terms, we must be able to think about doing what we are doing while we are doing it.

LEARNING ACTIVITY: KNOWING AND DOING

ENDS IN VIEW

In this learning activity, you will explore experiences of knowing-in-action.

WRITE

In your journal, consider and respond in writing to the following statements and questions.

- Think of a time in your nursing experience when you had to respond to an unexpected situation.
- Describe what happened.
- Who was involved?
- Think about how you knew what to do.
- Try to recall your thinking about the situation. Did you systematically analyze the situation?
- Did you act and then think?

DIALOGUE

Discuss the situation that you wrote about from your practice with a learning partner. Consider and discuss the following questions: How are your experiences similar or different? How do you account for being able to do something without being able to provide a rationale/analysis for why you did what you did?

REFLECT

Contemplate the following question: What is the relationship between knowing and knowing what to do (action)? Write a full description of this relationship in your journal.

Skill Acquisition: More Than Behavioral Performance

Part of a nurse's education involves learning particular skills. Also, nurses are often called upon to teach particular skills to clients or groups. Usually, nurses think of skillfulness as being able to do something such as a specific task, for example, being able to give an injection. Benner and Wrubel's (1982, 1989) and Benner's (1984, 2001) work on explicating nursing practice has contributed significantly to our understanding of this particular type of reflection-in-action in nursing. Their work and that of others (Dreyfus & Dreyfus, 1986) expand our understanding of skillfulness from its usual focus on behavior to include other equally important aspects. As they explain, there are at least three critical aspects of being skillful. Hills (1989) adds a fourth.

Perceptual awareness—This aspect refers to the ability to perceive the salient features of a given situation. Certain aspects of a situation stand out as being more important than others (Dreyfus & Dreyfus, 1986).

Behavioral performance—This aspect describes the ability to actually perform a certain task. There is a tendency to focus solely on this aspect of skillfulness (Dreyfus & Dreyfus, 1986).

Discretionary decision-making—This refers to the ability to make judgments about what is appropriate as a way to be or what to do in a given situation (Dreyfus & Dreyfus, 1986).

Confidence—This aspect refers to feelings in relation to capabilities. Benner and Wrubel (1989) did not identify this aspect of skillfulness in their original work. However, our work with learners acquiring skills revealed that confidence is also an important aspect of skillfulness (Hills, 1989).

Benner (2001) also uncovered the critical role of experience in developing skillfulness. Although she claims that there are some aspects of practical knowledge that can be learned only from practice (experience), she also asserts that this way of knowing is generally under-valued and not well understood. Benner (2001) explains that Western culture traditionally places a premium on abstract reason. As a result, we understand theoretical knowledge better and value it more than knowledge gained through practice or experience. This view is sup-ported by Reason's explanation of practical knowing substantiated earlier (see Chapter 5).

In her research examining knowledge embedded in nursing practice, Benner (1984, 2001) reveals that nurses display different characteristics in their performance depending on their level of development. She identifies five levels of competency: novice, advanced beginner, competent, proficient, and expert. What is of interest from a reflection-in-action perspective is the role that experience plays in acquiring skilled knowledge. Benner explains that experience is not mere passage of time or longevity; rather, it is the transformation of preconceived notions and expec-tations by means of encounters with actual practical situations; that is, reflection-in-action. This means that, for situations involving skill acquisition, learners require actual concrete experiences in order to become more proficient or expert nurses.

LEARNING ACTIVITY: SKILL ACQUISITION

ENDS IN VIEW

This learning activity provides opportunities for you to examine teaching/learning situ-ations that involve skill acquisition.

WRITE

In your journal, write about a recent experience in which you had to teach someone a skill or you had to learn a skill. Using the four aspects of skillfulness, describe how you paid attention to each aspect.

DIALOGUE

Share your experiences with your classmates or colleagues. Discuss the approaches you used to teach this skill. What aspects of skillfulness did you find most difficult to attend to?

Praxis: The Dialect of Reflection and Action

In this section of the chapter, we explore the concepts of reflection and action as a dialectic.

The notion of dialectic from Merriam-Webster's dictionary is based on the concept of the unity of opposites (thesis/antithesis) and their continual resolution (synthesis) (Merriam-Webster, n.d.). The unity of opposites is the recognition of the contradictory, mutually exclusive opposite tendencies in all phenomena and processes of nature (including mind and society).

Dialectical thought involves seeking a synthesis of two or more seemingly opposing viewpoints.

For our relational emancipatory pedagogy, this means understanding the opposing notions of action and reflection and to find synthesis through the process. As Kemmis (2013) explains, reflection is a dialectical process.

> It looks inward at our thoughts and thought processes and outward at the situation in which we find ourselves; when we consider the interaction of the internal and the external, our reflection orients us for further thought and action. Thus, reflection is meta thinking—thinking about thinking in which we consider the relationship between our thoughts and actions in a particular context. (p. 140)

Kemmis argues that reflection is action-oriented, social, and political. We tend to think of reflection as something that happens quietly and personally inside of us. But Kemmis (2013) suggests that to do so is "to ignore the very things that give reflection its character and significance: it splits thought from action" (p. 141).

The significance of understanding reflection and action as dialectic is that it frames our understanding in a historical and political context. We do not reflect without reason; we reflect because something has occurred to make us aware of ourselves. We understand that the way we act, to some degree, will impact future events for ourselves and possibly others. From a dialectic position, "reflection is a political act, which either hastens or defers the realization of a more rational, just and fulfilling society" (Kemmis, 2013, p. 140).

So, when people make decisions about their health practices, or learn new ways of being healthy, and by doing so realize that the healthy choices they are making not only improve their health but also the health of the society in which they live, they are engaged in a process of transformational change. These kinds of transformations in perspective are said to have been accomplished through a process of "conscientization" (Freire, 1972), "perspective transformation" (Mezirow, 1990), or "emancipatory learning" (Habermas, 1991). These terms are used to describe situations in which students make fundamental changes in the way that they view themselves, their communities, and their place in the world.

Mezirow (1990) contends that "the most significant learning experiences in adulthood involve critical self-reflection—reassessing the way we have posed problems and reassessing our own orientation to perceiving, knowing, believing, feeling, and acting" (p. 13).

> Perspective transformation is a three-stage process: becoming critically aware of how and why our presuppositions have come to constrain the way we perceive, understand, and feel about our world; reformulating these assumptions to permit a more inclusive, discriminating, permeable, and investigative perspective; and making decisions or otherwise acting upon these new understandings. (Mezirow, 1990, p. 14)

In a relational emancipatory pedagogy, teachers are constantly mindful of potential opportunities to create a situation in which this type of learning can occur. Learning that endures, that is, learning that is retained and easily transferred to other situations, is created through this type of process.

LEARNING ACTIVITY: ENHANCING SOCIETY THROUGH EMANCIPATORY ACTION

ENDS IN VIEW

In this learning activity, you will consider experiences you have had that are examples of transformative change.

READ

Read the following example of transformative change:

In 1990, I was a very keen jogger and was fairly conscious of what I ate because of my interest in running. One evening, I was talking to someone I had just met—she had recently published a book on vegetarian cooking—and we were discussing the merits of being vegetarian. I had had these types of conversations before and was quite happy with my decision to continue to eat meat. I recall when I was leaving she said light-heartedly, "Remember nothing with a face or a heart!" Later that evening, for some reason I began to view things differently. I became aware of myself acting in habitual ways—I ate meat because that was what I had always done. It was easy. I began to understand that not only did I not need to eat meat but, if I chose not to eat it, I could make a difference to society, to the environment, and to thousands of animals that could continue to live! When I awoke the next morning, I decided I would not eat anything with a face or a heart again.

WRITE

In your journal, write about a time when you had a similar type of transformative experience. Try to recall as many of the details as possible that will assist others in understanding your experience. Write about what it was that heightened your awareness or triggered your reflection. Try to recall your thinking about this situation as you were experiencing it.

DIALOGUE

Share your experiences with your classmates or colleagues. Discuss what characteristics your experiences seem to have in common and how they are different. Together, describe the critical aspects that are present in this type of transformative process.

REFLECT

In your journal, describe your understanding of this process of transformative change. What aspects seem most important to you? What strategies can you use to encourage this type of transformative change? What are the benefits of engaging in this type of learning?

Freire (1972, 1970/2000) considers reflection-in-action as praxis. The constituent elements of praxis are action and reflection, and their relationship is reflexive. Emancipatory action is informed by the dialectal movement from action to reflection and to new action. So, there is a theoretical component, an experience component, and a dialogue component that liberate people to act in ways that enhance society. This dialectal way of viewing reflection-in-action reorients our consideration of this concept from one of searching for understanding or explanation to one of ethical action toward societal good. This is similar to Mezirow's (1990) explanation that,

> conscientization is not merely speculative or theoretical interpretation of an experience, nor is it merely a new way of making sense of nonsensical and oppressive conditions. It is critical reflection—looking back on assumptions underlying our experience and redefining our own being not merely as knowers but as reflective doers. (p. 89)

Emancipatory action recognizes the dialectic of action and reflection—it is praxis. Emancipatory action has a different relationship to knowledge than other forms of reflection. From an emancipatory perspective, action flows from practical and theoretical reflection. Grundy (1987) explains that "it is action that seeks, through reflective praxis, to make meaning of the social situation in the light of authentic insights into the nature of the socially constructed world" (p. 135). If we can understand the world "as being socially constructed, we can understand how we can act in the world to change those social constructions toward a more emancipatory position. Emancipatory praxis is realized via the medium of critical self-reflection" (Grundy, 1987, p. 188). Viewed from this perspective,

> reflection is a power we choose to exercise in the analysis and transformation of the situations in which we find ourselves when we pause to reflect. It expresses our agency as the makers of history as well as the awareness that we have been made by it. (Kemmis, 2013, p. 139)

What is so compelling about understanding the dialectical nature of reflective praxis and its inextricable link to critical consciousness is that once you operate in this way of being, you have the capacity to choose how you will practice and how you will think; how you will be in-the-world. It is emancipatory!

REFERENCES

Benner, P. (1984). *From novice to expert: Excellence and power in clinical nursing practice.* Addison-Wesley.

Benner, P. (2001). *From novice to expert: Excellence and power in clinical nursing practice* (commemorative edition). Prentice Hall.

Benner, P., & Wrubel, J. (1982). Skilled clinical knowledge: The value of perceptual awareness. *Nurse Educator, 7*(3), 11–17. https://doi.org/10.1097/00006223-198205000-00003

Benner, P., & Wrubel, L. (1989). *The primacy of caring: Stress and coping in health and illness.* Addison Wesley.

Boud, D., Keogh, R., & Walker, D. (2013a). Promoting reflection in learning: A model. In D. Boud, R. Keogh, & D. Walker (Eds.), *Reflection: Turning experience into learning* (pp. 18–40). Kogan Page.

Boud, D., Keogh, R., & Walker, D. (Eds.). (2013b). *Reflection: Turning experience into learning.* Kogan Page.

Dreyfus, H. L., & Dreyfus, S. E. (1986). *Mind over machine: The power of human intuition and expertise in the age of the computer.* Blackwell Press.

Freire, P. (1972). *Pedagogy of the oppressed.* Herder & Herder.

Freire, P. (2000). *Pedagogy of the oppressed* (30th ed.). Continuum. (Original work published 1970)

Freire, P. (1985). *The politics of education: Culture, power and liberation.* Bergin & Garvey Publishers.

Grundy, S. (1987). *Curriculum: Product or praxis?* Falmer Press.

Habermas, J. (1991). *The theory of communicative action* (Vol. 1). (Trans. T. McCarthy). Polity Press.

Hills, M. (1989). The child and youth care worker as an emerging professional practitioner. *Journal of Child and Youth Care, 4*(1), 17–31.

Jemal, A. (2017). Critical consciousness: A critique and critical analysis of the literature. *Urban Review, 49*(4), 602–626. https://doi.org/10.1007/s11256-017-0411-3

Josephsen, J. (2014). Critically reflexive theory: A proposal for nursing education. *Advances in Nursing, 2014,* 1–7. https://doi.org/10.1155/2014/594360

Kemmis, S. (2013). Action research and the politics of reflection. In D. Boud, R. Keogh, & D. Walker (Eds.), *Reflection: Turning experience into learning* (pp. 139–163). Kogan Page.

Merriam-Webster. (n.d.). Dialectic. In *Merriam-Webster.com dictionary*. https://www.merriam-webster.com/dictionary/dialectic

Mezirow, J. (1990). *Fostering critical reflection in adulthood.* Jossey-Bass.

Mustakova-Possardt, E. (1998). Critical consciousness: An alternative pathway for positive personal and social development. *Journal of Adult Development, 5*(1), 13–30. https://doi.org/10.1023/A:1023064913072

Nelson, S. (2012). The lost path to emancipatory practice: Towards a history of reflective practice in nursing. *Nursing Philosophy, 13*(3), 202–213. https://doi.org/10.1111/j.1466-769X.2011.00535.x

Reason, P. (Ed.). (1994). *Participation in human inquiry.* Sage.

Schön, D. A. (1983/2016). *The reflective practitioner: How professionals think in action.* Temple Smith.

Sherwood, G. D., & Horton-Deutsch, S. (2017). Turning vision into action: Reflection to develop professional practice. In S. Horton-Deutsch, & G. D. Sherwood (Eds.), *Reflective practice: Transforming education and improving outcomes* (pp. 3–27). Sigma Theta Tau International Honor Society of Nursing.

Shor, I., & Freire, P. (1987). *A pedagogy for liberation: Dialogues on transforming education.* Bergin & Gavey Publishers.

Creating a Culture of Caring

Who am I being that you are not shining?—Lululemon Athletica Inc., personal communication, 2010

INTRODUCTION

One of the authors had the opportunity to attend a leadership-training session that was being facilitated by her daughter who was a culture corporate coach in the western United States for a successful corporate retailer. During this experience, it struck her that this business, which sold athletic clothing, was investing considerable effort and resources into educating leadership for managers and staff to create a culture of authenticity within the organization. All of their training programs were designed to give them access to what it means to be great in life. As Jenna, her daughter, explains, "The only way to truly be great is to be your true authentic self" (Hills, personal communication, 2010). As she reflected on this notion, she began to wonder about our culture of nursing. Why doesn't nursing proactively teach and nurture its culture of caring?

We believe that nursing, as a discipline and a profession, embraces a culture of caring, yet it is not often articulated nor do nurses deliberate about what it is or how to develop it. As we were developing this idea, it occurred to us that we need to openly recognize the culture aspect that permeates our relational emancipatory pedagogy. By making this *culture of caring* an explicit component of our pedagogy, we hope to highlight its importance within the education process and to provide nurses with language to express their practice in a way that counters the predominant, traditional, medically based nursing culture that tends to infiltrate our culture of caring.

In this chapter, we describe creating a *culture of caring*, the fourth and the final component of our relational emancipatory pedagogy that encapsulates the other three elements. Just as the embryonic sac surrounds and nurtures a developing embryo, so too does the caring culture surround, nurture, and nourish a student nurse developing within the discipline of nursing. Including this fourth component in our framework highlights the teacher's responsibility to include the component in their pedagogical framework (Figure 9.1).

Culture is all the values, perceptions, past associations, past learning, past experiences, and shared mind-sets of all the individuals in a system, many of which are hidden, often unknown, and latent. Our nursing culture includes our taken-for-granted assumptions, traditions, ways of doing things, and ways of relating to each other. It is sometimes subtle and sometimes not, but it is always there, forming the horizons of our being-in-the-world. We nurses have all experienced this culture in our workplaces or even when we meet our colleagues in social situations.

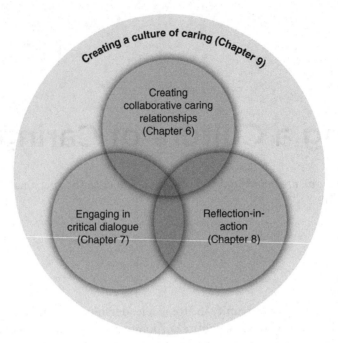

FIGURE 9.1 Interlocking circles of relational emancipatory pedagogy.

We have a way of talking, being with each other, relating to one another, and a shortcut way of engaging with each other because we share a culture, the culture of nursing. "The culture of nursing . . . has a vital social-scientific role in advancing, sustaining, and preserving human caring as a way of fulfilling its mission to society and broader humanity" (Watson, 2008, p. 18). "If one accepts the proposition that caring is the moral ideal of nursing . . . then teaching caring becomes the moral imperative of nursing educators" (Bevis, 2000, p. 183).

Nursing is a deeply moral activity requiring the performance of "the most difficult drudgery that human misery generates and some of the most sublime activities that one person ever has the opportunity to do for another" (Bevis, 2000, p. 183). Nursing is intensely intimate and touches people when they are most vulnerable: often in suffering, alone, afraid, and threatened.

> If we are to entrust society to [nurses'] hands, teachers must do all that is possible to engender the moral ideal of caring so that that caring will compel nurses to act in ways that are positive for these vulnerable individuals and families that are [in] their trust. (Bevis, 2000, p. 183)

Nurse educators must keep this moral ideal at the forefront of their minds as they plan curricula, develop courses and learning opportunities, and interact with students. As Whelan (2017) states, "[f]rom an educator's perspective, helping students develop caring literacies is a moral imperative because caring is the very essence of nursing. How we, as educators, instill and nurture caring among students is vital" (p. 40). The moral ideal of caring, nurses' societal mandate, must infiltrate every moment of everyday that teachers spend with students. "Such a moral imperative transcends nurse educators' usual teaching role, guiding their leadership . . . raising their awareness to foster nursing's larger social mandate" (Cara, Hills, & Watson, 2021, p. 43).

One strategy that assists students to develop a culture of caring is journaling. We have developed a particular strategy for journaling that includes students writing narratives as exemplars from their practice. They are provided with guidelines for developing a story and a framework consisting of domains of nursing practice and relevant quality indicators for critiquing the narrative (Hills, 2002). This process is described more fully later in the book.

For example, one student explained,

> I cannot believe I am in the last three weeks of my first year of nursing . . . it was frustrating at first not doing a lot of hands-on work . . . but when it comes down to it . . . the skills have been the easiest of the two to learn. You can *train* almost anyone to do skills but . . . when it comes down to it. . .becoming a part of the patient's healthcare team, to talk and listen to their needs, to understand and believe that patients have rights and beliefs about their own health; that has been the challenge of the first year . . . I feel that I have gained the confidence and education to successfully achieve what is asked of me as a first year nurse. I have achieved everything from doing a bed bath, to repositioning and turning, to vital signs, medications, enemas, commodes, assisting with feeding, understanding the administrative use of oxygen, and charting . . . and the list could go on . . . Yet, the most important thing that I have learned is that the hands-on skills are not the only thing that makes you a nurse . . . it has been exciting to see the pieces fall into place. As I look back to September, everything seemed to be in its own place: biology, health, professional growth, psychology. Now at the end of my first year as I look back, I realize that it is all becoming one—nursing: I am becoming a nurse! (Hills & Watson, 2011, p. 125)

The following excerpt fully illustrates that if students are taught from an ethic of caring and a moral obligation to act ethically and justly, nothing will stand in their way. This student is attempting to illustrate that nursing is primarily about people and their experiences of health and healing and not about the disease. She explains:

> A friend of mine died the other day. I didn't know her very well but in the short time that I knew her I learned a lot about myself. She was in hospital because of a bacterial infection, possibly tuberculosis, and I, as a nursing student, was asked if I wanted to be assigned to care for her. Usually, I am quite eager to get a chance to increase my knowledge about different disease processes and to help others understand their situation, but I found myself hesitating to take her as my patient. You see, she was HIV positive. I tried to sort out the different feelings that I was experiencing, the biggest one being fear.

> Fear immobilized me. I found that I couldn't think clearly but I was really hoping that I wouldn't have to be her nurse. At that point, I can honestly say that I cared more about myself than I did about her. I worried that somehow getting infected; I thought of what I might be bringing home to my children. I approached her bed with hesitant steps and introduced myself. She was very pleasant and very willing to have a student care for her. She told me that she was also a nurse and that she could remember what it was like being a student. Then, very efficiently, she explained to me about the equipment around her and what the doctors were attempting to do for her while she was in hospital. That day and the next, we spent some time getting to know each other.

> Over the next few weeks I chose her as my patient assignment. As my fear dissipated and my knowledge of her illness grew, I began to understand some of what she was going through. I also began to see how other nurses were caught up in their fear. When she would press her call bell, a nurse would answer over the intercom and avoid entering her room. When staff did enter her room, they would put gloves on, even if they were not doing an invasive procedure. No one touched her other than to do something with her equipment, and even then

they did not linger long at her bedside. I felt myself bristling at the injustice and unfairness, although I am ashamed to say that I didn't speak up for her when others would make assumptions about her. The world of a student is a double-edged sword. I was only there two days a week and I felt powerless to help her.

As her illness progressed, she experienced behavioral changes and would occasionally lash out at me. Although she was sometimes quite demanding about the way things were done, I was able to look beyond the behavior and appreciate her frustration because others had not taken the opportunity to get to know the person, they saw only the disease and labeled her accordingly.

This woman taught me that fear is natural and that you can get beyond it if we take the first step. When we learn about our fears we are able to look beyond them. I call her my friend because she did everything that friends do for one another, and I tried to do the same for her.

Sadly, though, she died in a hospital filled with people too afraid of illness to care for the person. She had hopes and dreams just as you and I do. Despite the struggle near the end of her life, no one stayed with her to face the inevitable, to calm her fears, to tell her that she would be missed. I wish I had thanked her for helping me to make the journey from ignorance to knowledge. I will miss her, but she will always be with me as will others that have taught me so much about caring. (Hills, 1998, p. 13)

This student is clearly practicing from a moral ethic of caring. Identifying and overcoming her own fear, being cognizant and observing how others were treating the patient, and developing insight into caring practices demonstrate the development of becoming a nurse who will practice from an ethic of caring. A *culture of caring* needs to embrace a moral stance of relational ethics.

ETHICS OF CARE: A RELATIONAL PERSPECTIVE

Typically, the ethics of care is considered to be a normative ethical theory; it is a theory about what makes actions right or wrong. It was one of several normative ethical theories that were developed by feminists in the second half of the 20th century. Carol Gilligan's (1993) work in moral psychology challenged "justice-based" approaches to moral discussions. As she describes,

> Women's construction of the moral problem as a problem of care and responsibility in relationships rather than as one of rights and rules ties the development of their moral thinking to changes in their understanding of responsibility and relationships, just as the conception of morality as justice ties development to the logic of equality and reciprocity. Thus the logic underlying an ethic of care is a psychological logic of relationships, which contrasts with the formal logic of fairness that informs the justice approach. (Gilligan, 1993, p. 73)

Beauchamp and Childress (2001), in describing Gilligan's perspective, explain that,

> Men *tend* to embrace an ethic of rights using quasilegal terminology and impartial principles, . . . whereas women *tend* to affirm an ethic of care that centers on responsiveness in an interconnected network of needs, care, and prevention of harm. The core notion involves caring for and taking care of others, and it is modelled on relationships. (p. 371)

Of course, there is nothing preventing men from adopting an ethic of care and we should be careful not to "essentialize" gender differences here, even if Gilligan's perspective is clearly a feminist one.

Ethics of care contrasts with more well-known ethical views, such as Kohlberg's development of moral judgment theory (Gilligan, 1993), utilitarianism, and deontology, or Kantian ethics (Beauchamp & Childress, 2001). This sort of outlook is what feminist critics call a "justice view" of morality. A morality of care rests on the understanding of relationships as a response to another, in their terms (Gilligan, 1993; Noddings, 2005). So, while the consequentialist and deontological ethical theories emphasize the importance of universal standards and applying them impartially, ethics of care perspectives emphasize the importance of relationships. "The care perspective is especially meaningful for roles such as parent, friend, physician, and nurse, in which contextual response, attentiveness to subtle clues, and deepening special relationships are likely to be more important morally than impartial treatment" (Beauchamp & Childress, 2001, p. 372). As a result, nurses need to become expert ethicists because they encounter, in a day, more complex moral and ethical dilemmas than most people do in a lifetime. The guidance they need to make decisions when faced with these complex moral issues cannot be found in any rule-bound objective ethical guideline. As Bevis (2000) declares,

> *no code of ethics, no list of injunctions, no fear of punishment or hope of reward, and no rules or logic decision tree will affect these tasks of moral education. Only a mentor / preceptor / teacher modeling a humanistically caring ethic and having dialogue with students that underscores constructed knowing and encourages them to be personally related to the ethical issues involved can facilitate and enhance students in their moral development for life and for nursing.* (Bevis, 2000, p. 184; italics by original author)

Nurse educators and nurses who work in practice settings where students learn, play a critical role in the students' moral development, and they must together nurture this culture of caring if students are to graduate as competent, caring nurses. This is not an easy task.

Hegemonic Power

One factor that makes it so difficult to engage in a culture of caring is the existence of hegemonic power. Labonte (1990) describes hegemonic power as:

> the ability of a dominant group to control the actions and behaviors of others . . . Hegemonic power is that form of "power-over" that is invisible, internalized and structured within the very nature of our day to day living so that we come to take it for granted. (p. 50)

Hegemonic power is difficult to deal with because it is insidious. Freire (1970/2000) contends that:

> Any situation in which "A" objectively exploits "B" or hinders his and her pursuit of self-affirmation as a responsible person is one of oppression. Such a situation in itself constitutes violence, even when sweetened by false generosity, because it interferes with the individual's ontological and historical vocation to be more fully human. (p. 55)

Freire (1970/2000) describes the phenomenon of horizontal violence and suggests that it is a primary characteristic of oppression. It is well documented that this type of oppression and resulting horizontal violence exists in nursing practice. In their study, Stanley et al. (2007) reported that "46% of the study participants reported lateral violence as a 'very serious' or 'somewhat serious' problem, and 65% reported frequently observing lateral violence behaviors among coworkers" (p. 1247).

> The existence of this internal battle within nursing is particularly important because it has allowed other groups to maintain control and not be challenged by nursing as a result of the inability of nurses to join together to support each other. (Roberts et al., 2009, p. 290)

Culture is the total sum of our inter- and innersubjective life-worlds, and it exists below the surface of our outer words, actions, and expressed intentions. This culture is intangible but nevertheless palpable; it has sustaining power that can detour the most elegant and highest ideals. This detouring of vision and dreams and highest ideals is grounded in insecurity, distrust, projection, lack of clear communication, and often fear. This sort of environment can be threatening; whereas, inviting people into a place of caring, of trust, and of meaningful and honest communication can be reassuring. As Cara et al. (2021) underline,

> Nurse educators can embody their valuing of human dignity in their classrooms by suggesting that everyone be open to each other's uniqueness and diversity in order for students to learn in a 'humanistic space.' . . . It is critical for students to learn in safety so that they can explore delicate or controversial issues. (p. 26)

They further mention, in a caring environment "both nurse educators and students join in a mutual search for meaning and wholeness as well as for the cocreation of knowledge within a safe environment" (Cara et al., 2021, p. 94).

This culture triggers one's inner relationship with self and other; the inner fears behind the scenes and in the silence of the person's private world that is subtly translated into overt but subtle behaviors. It can manifest through an energetic presence of negativity, of critical assessment internally and externally; it becomes threatening because it is facing self and other through self-disclosure. In the long run, the culture of a faculty, of a subgroup, or of the system will trump all the other aspects of a Caring Science curriculum and all the best efforts toward a relational emancipatory pedagogy. For this reason, it is critical for nurse educators to focus on creating a supportive culture that contrasts with often negative cultural surroundings that nurses experience in their everyday working lives.

One way to overcome this negativity and to live a culture of caring is to choose to be in *power with* relationships. Nurses have a choice about how to use their power. Power can be exerted over those who hold less power: that has been termed "power over." Power can be exerted against one's peers: that has been termed "horizontal violence." Where power is shared, either with those in peer positions or with those who have less of it, you are sharing *power with*. Having *power with* relationships is the only power situation wherein a culture of *caring* can flourish. We could easily make the logical assumption that power is a limited finite resource so that, in order to share power, we must give up some of our limited supply of power. With some forms of power, that might be the case. But, the power that leads us to our humanness is infinite. We have come to know that the more of this type of power we share, the more we have returned to us. As Hills and Cara (2019) explain,

> [t]o be informed by a Caring Science perspective, nurse educators must choose 'power with' strategies to create the emancipation necessary to cultivate a graduate who will be an

independent, self-reliant, and confident nurse who also demonstrates critical thinking and lifelong learning. (pp. 203–204)

LEARNING ACTIVITY: HORIZONTAL VIOLENCE

The purpose of this learning activity is to provide opportunities for you to examine the relationship between horizontal violence and teaching/learning.

The following parable was told to us by a former student.

Do you know the story of the crabs and the dolphins? Did you know that if you put a bunch of crabs in a pot, not a single crab will get out of the pot? They could escape if they were able to climb one on top of the other, but every time one tries, one of the other crabs pulls it down. At times, they even pull each other's legs off!! Not one of the crabs ever escapes!

In contrast, if you watch a school of dolphins, they display a very different type of behavior. When it becomes time to feed, one of the dolphins will swim in the middle and the others will swim around in a circle to protect it. The dolphin in the center will feed for as long as it wants and when it is finished, the dolphin will swim to the outer circle and another dolphin will swim into the center and feed for as long as it wants.

So often in nursing, crab behavior is evidenced in the horizontal violence that we display to one another. It is as if we don't know how to behave any differently. So the question then becomes: Do you want to be a crab or a dolphin?

WRITE

In your journal, recall a teaching/learning situation in which you experienced horizontal violence. Describe what would need to occur to transform these experiences into empowering teaching/learning situations.

REFLECT

In your journal, describe how you would promote a "dolphin culture" rather than a "crab culture."

Another way to overcome such latent underlying energetic cultural drains is to transform; to transmute human fears, apprehensive feelings, and concerns into higher order of love, of compassion and gentleness, of trust, safety, transparency, open and honest communication, and meaningful caring relationships. There must be a safe trusting space where nurses are given permission to be human, to be vulnerable, to experience their own healing, and to be accepted and honored with unique gifts as well as frailties. A caring culture has to permeate the consciousness, the intentionality, and the practices of each person within the environment. However, each individual has to be valued and affirmed for their contributions, unique reason for being where they are, their talents, and their diverse points of view.

Another successful intervention for cultural transformation is to invite individuals and the collective consciousness of a group into a vision of contributing to something greater than self, to appeal to their role in translating their own human gifts into compassionate human service through their teaching, their roles, whatever they may be: into assisting their colleague, a student, a community group; in offering up their heart and mind to that which inspires and inspirits them for this work that is shared by others and makes a difference; in letting others know they are important and making an important difference; and, in inviting nonconformity, creativity, inspired vision, and ideals beyond the norm.

At the same time, the program leader, the head person *holds the space* for self and others to live out this broader and deeper vision of Caring Science, of caring practices, of emancipatory pedagogies. The Caring Science container is large enough to hold the evolving cultural consciousness of the whole, while still sustaining a common vision, a common context, and container for liberation for the evolved consciousness of humanity alike, toward a moral community, a moral culture of caring, and liberation/emancipation.

There has to be room for safe disagreement of individual and group ideas without diminishing the individuals or the groups; allowing and creating open space for consensus building; for sharing common human-to-human caring processes and relationships that honor the whole.

Without such elevated vision to appeal to the higher senses of all; without leadership that invites the highest level of ideals and values and ethics into daily practices; without a vision of excellence that affirms the highest ethical caring values of each faculty, each student, each administrator, each employee and holds them in this consciousness, even if the individuals cannot see that for themselves in the moment, then any attempts at creating and sustaining a Caring Science curriculum and emancipatory pedagogies will be undermined and diluted, and ultimately destroy the program by default, not because of the design.

The very same principles for emancipatory pedagogy for faculty/student relations have to come alive and be lived out at all levels in the program, the curriculum, the classroom, the clinical area, the organizations: between and among faculty to faculty, faculty to student, administrators to administrators, administrators to faculty and students alike. In other words, the caring values and actions that compose the entire culture have to be lived out within the whole; the whole caring consciousness, the liberated thinking and consciousness of emancipation have to be lived out in "caring moments" across the entire organization, from the inside out.

> Such humanistic relationships . . . can contribute to the development of a sense of belonging within the nursing education workforce. Finally, embracing the Political Caring Literacy Model could prove itself to be significant to implement caring relationships that will hopefully contribute to enhance nurse educators' personal well-being, professional satisfaction, and meaningfulness in one's daily learning/teaching praxis. (Brousseau & Cara, 2021, p. 175)

As nurse educators in a Caring Science curriculum, we need to include as part of our relational emancipatory pedagogy a deliberate effort to create a culture of caring in a way that transcends education and becomes a conscious, articulated way of practicing nursing. In order to cultivate this caring way of being, nurse educators must provide precedence for this caring culture over the more traditional biomedical/technocure culture that has been so dominant in nursing and nursing education. The precedence of this caring culture is the true reflection of the nature of nurse/client and teacher/student relationships, and it is within this context that nurses must be educated if we are to fulfill our mandate to society. As nurse educators who embrace a Caring Science philosophy and theoretical perspective, we are obligated to attend to this development.

Ultimately, the culture of caring created by liberated nurse leaders will contribute to our ability to sustain human dignity, to sustain humanity for an evolved human consciousness of connectedness, of unitary views of human-environment, of unity of mind-body-spirit, returning us to the very roots, the very foundation of Caring Science theory, ethics, values, philosophical orientations toward humankind itself. It is only when we pause, when we are free to critique and find another way to serve our evolved self and others, in safe space, in a communion of caring, that we are truly educating for a moral society, a deeply human, caring culture that ultimately contributes to world healing and peace.

As Smith (2019) explains,

> Beliefs and values of the faculty create the culture of an organization. In a Caring Science-based program, Caring informs the ways of relating to self and others within the academic community. . . . Faculty and students are engaged in a reflective process of growing in Caring. They are invited to intentionally engage in the process of caring for self so critical to the ontological development of a nurse. (pp. 288–289)

Finally, with respect to caring culture and open honest communication regarding this book, we too can disclose our motivation, our deepest desire for this book: to offer a transformed vision for Caring Science; to bring forth the ideals and values of Caring Science, to help the evolution of humankind and nursing's ancient and noble contributions to humanity through new ways of understanding education, the liberated human in teaching and learning processes, structure, pedagogies, and informed practices; ultimately to contribute to the evolution of nursing as a discipline and profession that can help sustain human caring and healing for humankind.

REFERENCES

Beauchamp, T. L., & Childress, J. F. (2001). *Principles of biomedical ethics* (5th ed.). Oxford University Press.

Bevis, E. (2000). Teaching and learning: The key to education and professionalism. In E. Bevis & J. Watson (Eds.), *Toward a caring curriculum: A new pedagogy for nursing* (pp. 153–188). National League for Nursing.

Brousseau, S., & Cara, C. (2021). Nurse educators' political caring literacy and power to promote caring relationships in nursing education. In C. Cara, M. Hills, & J. Watson (Eds.), *An educator's guide to humanizing nursing education: Grounded in caring science* (pp. 161–182). Springer Publishing Company.

Cara, C., Hills, M., & Watson, J. (2021). *An educator's guide to humanizing nursing education: Grounded in caring science*. Springer Publishing Company.

Freire, P. (2000). *Pedagogy of the oppressed* (30th ed.). Continuum. (Original work published 1970)

Gilligan, C. (1993). *In a different voice: Psychological theory and women's development*. Harvard University Press.

Hills, M. (1998). Student experiences of nursing health promotion practice in hospital settings. *Nursing Inquiry*, 5(3), 164–173. https://doi.org/10.1046/j.1440-1800.1998.530164.x

Hills, M. (2002). Perspectives on learning and practicing health promotion in hospitals: Nursing students' stories. In L. Young & J. Hayes (Eds.), *Transforming health promotion practice: Concepts, issues and applications* (pp. 229–240). FA Davis.

Hills, M., & Cara, C. (2019). Curriculum development processes and pedagogical practices for advancing caring science literacy. In W. Rosa, S. Horton-Deutsch, & J. Watson (Eds.), *A handbook for caring science: Expanding the paradigm* (pp. 197–210). Springer Publishing Company.

Hills, M., & Watson, J. (2011). *Creating a Caring Science curriculum: An emancipatory pedagogy for nursing* (1st ed.). Springer Publishing Company.

Labonte, R. (1990). *Empowerment practices for health professionals*. Participation.

Noddings, N. (Ed.). (2005). *Educating citizens for global awareness*. Teachers College Press.

Roberts, S. J., Demarco, R., & Griffin, M. (2009). The effect of oppressed group behaviours on the culture of the nursing workplace: A review of the evidence and interventions for change. *Journal of Nursing Management*, 17, 288–293. https://doi.org/10.1111/j.1365-2834.2008.00959.x

Smith, M. (2019). Advancing caring science through the missions of teaching, research/scholarship, practice, and service. In W. Rosa, S. Horton-Deutsch, & J. Watson (Eds.), *A handbook for caring science: Expanding the paradigm* (pp. 285–301). Springer Publishing Company.

Stanley, K., Martin, M., Michel, Y., Welton, M., & Nemeth, S. (2007). Examining lateral violence in the nursing workplace. *Issues in Mental Health Nursing, 28*(11), 1247–1265. https://doi.org/10.1080/01612840701651470

Watson, J. (2008). *Nursing. The philosophy and science of caring* (Revised Updated ed.). University Press of Colorado.

Whelan, J. (2017). The caring science imperative: A hallmark in nursing education. In S. Lee, P. Palmieri, & J. Watson (Eds.), *Global advances in human caring literacy* (pp. 33–42). Springer Publishing Company.

UNIT III

Creating a Caring Science Curriculum

In this unit, we present the phases of the curriculum development process and provide seven exemplars of programs and courses that have used Caring Science as the philosophy and theory to develop a curriculum.

There are eight chapters in this unit. Chapter 10 describes the phases of the curriculum development process within a Caring Science curriculum. It provides a blueprint for transcending reductionistic curriculum development models. Chapter 11 presents a program that used this curriculum development process, this blueprint (see Chapter 10), which was based on Caring Science and Health Promotion—the Collaborative Nursing Program of British Columbia (CNPBC), the first in Canada. In Chapter 12, Rollison and Jung, contributors from Vancouver Island University, provide more details regarding how this blueprint (Chapter 10) can be used to develop courses within a Caring Science curriculum. This particular innovative course is offered in a conference format to assist students to transition to the workforce.

The remaining chapters in this unit are exemplars from contributing authors that illustrate practical examples of ways to develop and implement a Caring Science Curriculum. Chapter 13 is a contribution from Boykin, Touhy, and Smith that describes a Caring Science Nursing Program that was developed and implemented over 35 years ago at Florida Atlantic University. This program continues to be highly successful to this day. Chapter 14 is a contribution from Thrall, Lally, and Thate that describes the development of a Human Science Curriculum at Siena University in New York State. Chapter 15 is a contribution from Lally that describes a leadership course based in Caring Science that was created as one of the final courses in the Siena Baccalaureate Program. Chapter 16 is a contribution from Bourque Bearskin, Kennedy, Poitras Kelly, and Chakanyuka that emphasizes the importance of Indigenous caring ways of being and knowing in nursing education. It illustrates how much we have to learn from our Indigenous colleagues and Elders. The final chapter, Chapter 17, is a contribution from Christopher that addresses a leading edge issue in nursing education. It highlights simulation, narrative pedagogy, and Caring Fidelity™ as a new reality for the future.

Each of these exemplars is unique, demonstrating different perspectives of a Caring Science Curriculum. Together, they demonstrate exciting and innovative ways to create a Caring Science Curriculum.

Collaborative Caring Science Curriculum Structure and Design: Transcending Reductionistic Models

Over the years this adherence to strict behaviorism has made critical aspects of nursing. . .invisible. As nursing evolves its disciplinary foundation, it is time to stand in this base and claim those invisible aspects of nursing as core to our practice and therefore nursing education.—Hills, 2017

INTRODUCTION

In this chapter, we describe the processes, structures, and organizational frameworks for designing a Caring Science curriculum. In the previous chapters, we have concentrated mainly on the philosophical underpinnings of a Caring Science curriculum and the related transformative relational pedagogy. It is time now to turn our attention to the structure and design for a Caring Science curriculum. As you know, we cannot teach everything all at once, so we need organizational structures to assist us in this development process. This is an interesting dilemma because over the past 30 years, largely due to the "curriculum revolution" starting in the late '80s and early '90s (National League for Nursing, 1988, 2003), we have all but ignored the structural and design elements of curriculum development. Most of our attention has been focused on the development of innovative pedagogical approaches. However, we still need to figure out where to begin and how to proceed in a logical fashion so that the structure of our programs has coherence and some semblance of order.

Recent Conceptualizations of Curriculum Structure and Design

As discussed in previous chapters dedicated to this topic, relational emancipatory pedagogical practices, those that are consistent with a Caring Science curriculum, are a significant factor in implementing a caring curriculum. Indeed, many, including us, would argue that pedagogy is the primary influencing factor in curriculum development. That which actually occurs in the classroom/clinical area among teachers and students impacts learning the most. However, such components as the development of a program philosophy, the program goals and outcomes, the curriculum design, the way the courses are structured and sequenced, the teacher–student relationship, the learning environment, and the sociopolitical context within which the program is delivered are all significant contributing factors to successful curriculum development. It is not easy to develop a curriculum that captures the complexities of the discipline and that reflects the realities of nursing practice. Although their focus is not on Caring Science curricula per se, Jillings and O'Flynn-Magee (2007) offer a helpful framework for creating nursing curricula. As they explain,

> the nursing curriculum provides the infrastructure for organizing and delivering content and learning experiences, building cognitive, affective and psychomotor outcomes. The crucial interplay between forms of knowledge, ways of knowing, and the process of curriculum development cannot be understated; if the curriculum is to provide experiences that extend beyond mere content delivery and skill acquisition, it must reflect all dimensions of nursing and in addition, achieve a profound connection with the learner who must ultimately understand and enact the core concepts, theories, and competencies. (p. 384)

Further, they suggest that, currently, we seem to be returning to a more balanced perspective in nursing education where there is focus on the integrity of the curriculum, as well as on teaching/learning processes. They outline "six critical phases of curriculum design: contextual elements, philosophy and mission, program outcomes or goals, curriculum framework, curriculum design, and instructional design" (Jillings & O'Flynn-Magee, 2007, p. 395).

Iwasiw et al. (2018) also focus on the entire curriculum development process; however, they pay less attention to pedagogy. They recommend a 12-step process: determining need for change, gain support, organize for curriculum change, plan and implement faculty development, gather data about internal and external contextual factors, agree on philosophical approaches, determine curriculum directions and outcomes, formulate curriculum goals, design the curriculum, design courses, plan evaluation, and plan implementation.

Each of these authors offers valuable and complementary perspectives that are useful in creating a Caring Science curriculum. Both call attention to the contextual factors that can influence curriculum development; both promote the importance of the philosophical orientation as being critical to successful implementation; and, both include curricula design, instructional design, and evaluation in their curriculum development process. Iwasiw et al. (2018) add an interesting emphasis on early phases of curriculum development and note some of the particular challenges at the beginning of a curriculum development process. Also, they include, as recommended by Bevis and Watson (1989/2000), a particular focus on faculty development. Depending on the situation, this might be an important aspect early in the curriculum development process. However, none of these conceptualizations includes a Caring Science perspective that we consider essential to nursing and therefore nursing education and curriculum development.

CURRICULUM DESIGN AND STRUCTURE FOR DEVELOPING A CARING SCIENCE CURRICULUM

In this section, we incorporate some of these recent conceptualizations of nursing curriculum with processes that are recommended to develop a Caring Science curriculum. Even though these processes are described in a linear fashion, curriculum development is actually an iterative process in which each subsequent phase builds on the other while also creating new learning that may result in changing the phase just completed. It is difficult to describe the recursive nature of the curriculum development process because we can really describe only one thing at a time. However, we will attempt to point out typical places where the iterative process is most apparent.

The curriculum processes within a Caring Science curriculum are described in the next section and include the development of the philosophy, program purpose, and goals; the curriculum framework that describes the overall organizing framework; the curriculum design that demonstrates the sequencing and structuring courses; the instructional design that includes detailed course development with learning outcomes; a description of teaching methods to be used; and, finally, an evaluation plan that includes strategies for student evaluation, course evaluation, and an overall program evaluation plan. These curriculum development processes are built on the theoretical/philosophical framework described in Chapter 4.

Collaboration is Key

The most important single element in curriculum design, redesign, revision, or refresh is the relationship that the leader of the process, whether that be an outside consultant or an internal faculty member, needs to live in a facilitative position as a leader who leads from beside (Hills, 2016). This style of leadership and collaboration encourages shared responsibility and accountability and it empowers faculty members to own their work. This is key to the sustainability and integrity of any curriculum. When faculty members are engaged and committed, anything is possible.

In Hills's early work as the director of the Collaborative Nursing Program of British Columbia (BC) (see also Chapter 11), she created the following definition of collaboration and, to this day, continues to use it in all her work.

> Collaboration is the creation of a synergistic alliance that honours and utilizes each person's contribution in order to create collective wisdom and collective action. Collaboration is not synonymous with co-operation, partnership, participation or compromise. Those words do not convey the fundamental importance of being in relationship nor the depth of caring and commitment that is needed to create the kind of reciprocity that is collaboration. Collaborators are committed to, care about, and trust each other. They recognize that, despite their differences, each has unique and valuable knowledge, perspectives, and experiences to contribute to the collaboration. (Hills, 1992, p. 14)

This process begins as soon as the key stakeholders are identified and form a curriculum team. This initial time together involves establishing guidelines for engagement. These are group guidelines for discussion (deciding how the team will work together), group process development activities, learning individuals' perspectives, backgrounds, and preferences. Through these activities and processes, mutual ownership of the curriculum development process is created. It is critical that a trusting working relationship is established so that the team can complete their work together and feel safe to contribute ideas openly.

Standing on that foundation of true collaboration, the group enters into a series of meetings and interactions through which they both advance through the curriculum development process and engage in a series of iterative cycles of reflection and review to refine the curriculum evolution. As the new or revised curriculum develops, so too does faculty's learning.

In essence, the group:

- creates a collaborative working relationship;
- creates rules of engagement—to ensure that faculty members feel safe to express their ideas openly and to allow committee members to take shared responsibility for the process;
- establishes agenda of face-to-face meetings;

- concludes every meeting with clear goals, identified deliverables, and nominations of persons responsible before its next encounter;
- prearranges teleconferences or virtual conferences that will occur between meetings; and;
- establishes agendas for workshops that are interspersed throughout the process.

It is important to establish a mutually agreed upon meeting schedule in the initial phase of the curriculum process. Initially, we could anticipate that monthly meetings would be required for the first 6 months. These monthly meetings need to have mutually developed and agreed upon, clear, well-established goals, expectations, identified responsible personnel, and deliverables. The tasks for each month will be clearly articulated with persons assigned (point persons) to guide their completion. These point people will prepare a brief report that will be submitted to the chair of the curriculum committee and consultant (if they are not the same person). Each meeting should begin with a report from the curriculum chair and/or consultant.

Initially, the faculty and curriculum development will be done as a group involving all members of the curriculum team. Subsequently, the team will create task forces and theme teams that accomplish specific tasks. For example, the curriculum team might want to establish a program-evaluation subcommittee to monitor the curriculum alignment with accreditation standards and professional regulatory competencies. Eventually all members of the nursing department become involved.

Through the use of iterative review cycles, the team ensures that all phases of the curriculum development process are paradigmatically consistent. In addition, faculty members are taught and coached to use participatory evaluation strategies so that they can create evidence from practice throughout the curriculum development experience. This iterative process will create changes by reflecting on current practices in relation to an established curriculum framework. This process allows nurse educators to collect evidence while simultaneously implementing innovations.

Develop a Work Plan

The following describes the components of a systematic, evidence-informed, work plan to collaboratively create a state of the art Caring Science curriculum that anticipates how nursing will be practiced in 10 years. Holding this futuristic perspective assists faculty to let go of what they currently are doing and how they are being and imagine how nursing could be taught.

This work plan outlines four development phases—Assessing, Envisioning, Developing, and Evaluating—and includes the development processes to be used during each phase. Depending on the available time devoted to the curriculum development process, the work plan should reflect reasonably obtainable deadlines to keep the team motivated and to have a sense of accomplishment. The first 2 years will focus on the development of pedagogy, philosophy, program goals, curriculum framework, course development, and evaluation. In addition, during the initial phase, a task force should be established to oversee the curriculum development in relation to established professional standards and competencies for entry to practice with the final phase of the curriculum development process. The team will analyze and cross reference the developed curriculum with these standards of practice and competencies. It is imperative that the development process and the standards and evaluation processes be coordinated; however, these processes should not be allowed to drive the creative process of curriculum development.

PHASE 1: ASSESSING THE CURRENT SITUATION

Continuing to develop a collaborative relationship for the team includes understanding the current state of curriculum development and faculty members' perspectives, commitments, desires, and pedagogical practices. This initial phase involves reading existing materials available regarding the current curriculum, including the School of Nursing's strategic plan and its recent Accreditation Report. The team needs to familiarize themselves with state/provincial/local nursing standards, review any recommendations, and discuss a strategy for providing evidence that the revised curriculum will address these recommendations.

It is anticipated that members of the faculty will have differing views and perspectives as discussions and deliberations begin. So, it is important to establish a shared responsibility for critical dialogue so that all members feel a sense of responsibility for the success of the group's work. Several heuristics can be used to create this relationship. Some examples are provided in Chapter 11.

PHASE 2: ENVISIONING: CREATING A COMMON VISION

The team engages in a number of value-based activities to assist all faculty members to articulate their perspectives about their ideal nursing curriculum. One strategy that has proven to be very successful is using a phenomenological method and thematic analysis to explore faculty members' perspectives on what nurses will need to know, how they will need to be, and what they will need to be able to do to practice nursing 10 years from now. This orientation helps faculty members to imagine the discipline of nursing in the future. It also helps faculty members identify areas of agreement and points of difference so they can be discussed. Typically, this strategy is used in a workshop format with faculty members working in small groups to generate the "know" "be" "do's" on sticky notes. The facilitator places large newsprint paper on the wall throughout the room with "KNOW" "BE" or "DO" posted at the top of the page. Each of the groups posts their post-it notes on the large papers. The team visits each paper and groups concepts that seem to be related to each other. The team continues this process of grouping concepts that are similar to each other (thematic analysis), resulting in the creation of a vision that is mutually agreed upon. These themes are revisited during the curriculum design phase to identify and organize content themes (see the following).

This strategy can be repeated by gathering data through focus groups that include local nurse administrators, alumni, students, bedside and community-based nurses, and representatives of the Nursing Association and/or Union. This process combined with the faculty members' identified themes results in an understanding of many perspectives for the education of future nurses and a common vision held by all participants.

PHASE 3: DEVELOPING A UNIFIED PROGRAM PHILOSOPHY, PROGRAM GOALS, AND CURRICULUM FRAMEWORK

The third phase is the most substantial, extensive, and consuming of time, commitment, and resources. It involves the following seven steps, which will be explained in detail afterward:

Step A: Developing a philosophical statement
Step B: Developing program purpose and goals
Step C: Articulating pedagogical practices based on nursing and educational theories and philosophies
Step D: Embracing curriculum structure and design

Step E: Develop course blueprints and course descriptions
Step F: Developing learning activities
Step G: Establishing student classroom and clinical evaluation as authentication

Step A: Developing a Philosophical Statement

Once consensus is reached that the draft vision (Phase 2) is aligned with faculty members' perspectives (Phase 1), the vision is further articulated by developing a draft philosophical statement. The statement will outline the faculty members' views, positions, beliefs, and assumptions about caring, persons, health/health promotion, healthcare, nursing, and curriculum. It is important to consider the sociopolitical context of the program (e.g., Indigenous, health promotion, primary healthcare, and socio-ecological).

Whether you are developing a new program or revising an existing one, developing a philosophical statement is usually where most nurse educators begin. If the curriculum is to claim to be a Caring Science curriculum, it obviously needs to incorporate a philosophy that is consistent with Caring Science. We are not suggesting that there is only one theory or one philosophical perspective that is consistent with the Caring Science paradigm; in fact, there are many (see Chapter 4). The program's philosophical statement basically outlines the faculty members' views, positions, beliefs, and assumptions, and it needs to be alive and evolving. It guides every other decision you will make, so it is worth spending the time it takes to have it be congruent with all those involved in curriculum development.

This statement will remain alive and will continue to evolve during the curriculum development process; therefore, it will be necessary to develop it only to the point of reaching general consensus even though the statement might not be yet perfect. As you move forward with other aspects of the curriculum, an iterative process is created to revisit and review the philosophy so it continues to evolve as other aspects of the curriculum emerge. Although the philosophy may be a published document, its primary purpose is internal. It assists the faculty members to stay grounded in this nursing disciplinary philosophical foundation (see Chapter 4) and it unites the faculty members.

Step B: Developing Program Purpose and Goals

The program purpose and goals emerge directly from the philosophical statement and make that statement more concrete. Whereas the philosophical statement is an internal statement for faculty members, the program purpose and goals are developed as a public statement. They declare what the specific department of nursing stands for and the expectations they have for their graduates. This is a time when the process can be very iterative. Depending on the team's comfort with moving between two aspects of the curriculum process at the same time, the team can go back and forth between these first two phases, developing the philosophy and the program purpose and goals with relative ease.

The program purpose is a broad public statement that links the philosophy and essential concepts that are embedded in the program to the anticipated outcomes of the program. It describes, in a broad sense, the capacities, capabilities, and attitudes of the graduate. The program goals further articulate the program purpose by identifying more specifically how the student will "be" as a graduate.

Usually, the team reviews the existing program purpose and goals and critiques it. Often, some examples from other exemplary programs are reviewed to clarify precisely how this program will be unique. If the philosophy is clearly articulated (Step 2), it is reasonably straightforward to articulate the program purpose and goals (see Chapter 11).

Step C: Articulating Pedagogical Practices Based on Nursing and Educational Theories and Philosophies

This phase of curriculum development is often overlooked and yet, in our opinion, it is one of the most influential factors affecting students' learning. In 2000, Bevis and Watson redefined curriculum as something beyond simply curriculum structure and design; rather, to be those transactions and interactions that take place between teachers and students and among students, with the intention that learning occurs. The first nine chapters of this book expand this idea by describing pedagogy as both relational and emancipatory and present a pedagogical framework for Caring Science curriculum development. So, yes, structure and design are important but how we teach and how students learn is as important, if not more so.

So at this phase, the curriculum team engages in activities that lead to the development of a clear articulation of their pedagogical framework: how they will teach students in a way that is consistent with their vision, philosophy, and program goals. Several educational and nursing theories can be explored to ascertain how the faculty wishes to position itself.

Step D: Embracing Curriculum Structure and Design

This step involves the delineation of core concepts and conceptual maps to guide the curriculum design process. As many nurse theorists and educators argue, these concepts should come from nursing models, theories, and conceptual frameworks to ensure that the curriculum is grounded in nursing's disciplinary knowledge (see Chapter 4) and not education or medicine as has happened so often in the past. Nursing is now adequately developed to use its own knowledge base to inform curricula development to educate future nurses.

One strategy that is helpful in articulating the content to be taught is to engage nurse educators, sessional instructors, preceptors, and others involved in students' educational experiences in focus groups.

Based on our experiences, in order to keep the discussion futuristic and imaginative, we suggest asking the following three questions:

- How do nurses need to *be* to practice nursing 10 years from now?
- What do nurses need to *know* to practice nursing 10 years from now?
- What do nurses need to be able to *do* to practice nursing 10 years from now?

Working in small groups, participants write their ideas on post-it notes. The facilitator places large sheets of newsprint with different titles at the top of the page (BE; DO; KNOW) on the walls around the room. The facilitator reviews a previously prepared handout on how to do a thematic analysis, for example, using a phenomenological approach (van Manen, 2014). The participants post their ideas on the post notes on the appropriate newsprint page. Then the groups take turns reading all the post-it notes and grouping them and creating "themes" that emerge from the post-it notes. Then the whole group, led by the facilitator, engages in a dialogue further sorting the ideas/concepts within themes.

This strategy has been well tested several times with great success. It ensures that the content themes are contextualized within the local setting while maintaining a broader understanding of standards of practice. During this phase, in addition to identifying content themes, permeating variables (e.g., health promotion and indigenization) that would be incorporated in each semester, the team can identify critical concepts that would be integrated into each course (e.g., ways of knowing). See Chapter 11 for an example.

The result will be a draft curriculum structure. Usually this results in a logo or a drawing that pictorially represents the overall high-level curriculum.

Once the overall curriculum structure is designed (see example in Chapter 11), the team can explicate what courses will be developed, by whom, what content will be taught, what learning outcomes can be anticipated, and what teaching and evaluation strategies will be used. Faculty teams are created to develop course templates that include the aforementioned information and the recommended textbooks and other learning resources.

Step E: Developing Course Blueprints and Course Descriptions
This phase focuses on detailed course development including explicating which courses will be developed by whom, what content will be taught, what learning outcomes will be anticipated, and what teaching and evaluation strategies will be used. Also, it involves articulating how each course will support the program's purpose and goals and how theoretical/philosophical integrity will be achieved and maintained.

Each course usually has a course title, a course description, and a purpose. These essential elements are typically published in an institutional calendar or catalogue. Additional course materials are usually developed for students that include teaching strategies, expectations of students and teachers, and methods of evaluation. In a Caring Science curriculum, courses need to be designed to maximize student engagement, promote caring-teaching student relations, and have evaluation strategies that are emancipatory and caring.

Course design and development is another of those processes in curriculum development that is iterative. Courses inevitably change over time as faculty members receive feedback from students and revise the course. This keeps the curriculum alive and evolving.

Course blueprints are developed to provide more detailed guidance to identify the essence of what is expected for each faculty member who might teach this course. Academic freedom is recognized and understood. The course blueprints are intended to provide guidance regarding what is essential and encourage integrity and cohesiveness within the curriculum.

Step F: Developing Learning Activities
Theme teams are created to develop learning activities (Bevis, 2000; Hills & Watson, 2011). Using this approach ensures consistency between the program goals and the students' learning. Using the following established guidelines that have been tested over many years, faculty members are coached on how to develop these learning activities so that they can create an electronic repository of learning activities for every course (see Chapter 11).

The following guidelines for creating learning activities were developed specifically by Hills and Bevis (1992) to be used particularly in the development of the Collaborative Nursing Program of BC (see Chapter 11).

GUIDELINES AND STRUCTURE FOR DEVELOPING LEARNING ACTIVITIES

OVERVIEW

- Use a "hook" to grab the learner's interest.
- Describe why this learning activity should be chosen.
- Answer the question: So what?
- Describe how this learning activity is connected to other learning activities.

ENDS IN VIEW

- Outline the purpose of the learning activity.
- Describe the opportunities for learning it will provide.

IN PREPARATION

- Provide structure—this may be in the form of questions or readings.
- Ask student to reflect on previous experience.

IN CLINICAL OR REAL WORLD

- Provide experiential-based activity.
- Give clear instructions.
- Relate activity to ends-in-view.

IN SEMINAR

- Provide structure to analyze information.
- Consider how analysis will address:
  - Social justice and equity
  - Link to Caring Science
  - Nursing praxis
  - Ways of knowing
- Pose questions to help learner develop personal meaning.
- Remember that the purpose of analysis/synthesis is to:
  - Increase learner's ability to recognize patterns
  - Increase learner's ability to increase transferability
- Remember to include an elastic clause for student input:
  - How would you (the learner) like to change the learning activity?
  - What would you like to do instead that is comparable?

WRITE

Have students keep a journal throughout the course. Having opportunities to write encourages critical thinking and reflection.

DIALOGUE

- Encouraging students to have at least a learning partner or a study group is even more preferable. Discussing their ideas, writings, and experiences assists students to become knowledgeable about issues, confident in their own thinking, and reflective about their practice.
- With your learning partners or study group, discuss your experiences of having completed the learning activities for this course. Consider if there are other ways that you might structure a teaching/learning experience.

REFLECT

- Adding a reflection component to the learning activity assists students to become reflective practitioners and to develop insight into their learning and practice.

● This structure of learning activities has proven to be particularly helpful in the development of our collaborative curriculum; it provided faculty members with a way of maintaining some consistency in pedagogical practices across numerous sites and in the development of our courses for off-campus delivery.

CRITERIA FOR CRITIQUING LEARNING ACTIVITIES

The following criteria were developed by Hills and Bevis (1992) to be used to critique learning activities that were developed for the Collaborative Nursing Program of BC (see Chapter 11).

● The theoretical base is explicit—learning activities are scholarly.
● There are clearly labeled headings.
● The learning activity is explanatory—learners are provided with clear directions.
● The learning activity contains only one learning activity.
● Learning activities that belong together are arranged in clusters.
● There is an elastic clause—to provide flexibility for the learner.
● The learning activity is reality-based.
● The learning activity addresses critical aspects of the curriculum, program, or course.
● There is a similar format for the learning activities so that learners can anticipate what follows.

Faculty members can continue to add to this repository in the upcoming years. This strategy is a shared resource for all faculty and is particularly helpful to new faculty members teaching new courses.

Step G: Establishing Student Classroom and Practice Clinical Evaluation as Authentication
This step is critical because even if all other phases are congruent, if student evaluation methods are used that are not consistent with the philosophy, program goals, and the curriculum framework, the program will fail. Students will learn what they are evaluated on, so if students are learning to be caring and to use their clinical judgement, they need to be evaluated on those capacities. This is especially true with practice evaluation.

The evaluation team of the Collaborative Nursing Program of BC has developed a way of evaluating practice performance based on Benner's (1984, 2001) work which is consistent with a Caring Science curriculum (Hills, 1993, 2001). The team massaged Benner's domains of practice to fit better with Collaborative Nursing Program of British Columbia (CNPBC) (see Table 10.1). Also see Chapter 18 for a fuller description of classroom and practice evaluation.

Faculty will be introduced to this strategy and will be guided to develop their own clinical appraisal that is consistent with their philosophy, goals, framework, and context.

PHASE 4: DEVELOPING A PROGRAM EVALUATION PLAN

A program evaluation plan is an important aspect of the Caring Science curriculum development process. Although it is often presented last, as is being done now, it is imperative that the

TABLE 10.1 Benner-CNPBC Domains of Practice With Rationales

BENNER'S DOMAINS OF PRACTICE	CNPBC DOMAINS OF PRACTICE	RATIONALE
Helping Domain	Health/Healing Domain	to include health
Teaching/Coaching Function	Teaching/Learning Domain	to include learning from client
Diagnostic and Patient-Monitoring Function	Clinical Judgment Domain	combined as each involved aspects of clinical judgement
Effective Management of Rapidly Changing Situations		
Administering and Monitoring Therapeutic Interventions		
Monitoring and Ensuring the Quality of Healthcare Practices	Professional Responsibility Domain	to capture essence of the domain in language more congruent with curriculum
Organizational and Work-Role Competencies	Collaborative Leadership Domain	to incorporate language that more accurately reflected a Caring Science philosophy

CNPBC, Collaborative Nursing Program of British Columbia.

Source: Reproduced from Hills, M. (2016). Collaborative and emancipatory: Leading from beside. In W. Rosa (Ed.), *Nurses as leaders: Evolutionary visions of leadership* (p. 304). Springer Publishing Company.

plan be considered from the outset. It is advantageous to create an Evaluation Subcommittee to concentrate on program evaluation within Phase 2, although the majority of their work will not occur until later phases.

The program evaluation plan must be kept in mind throughout the curriculum development process. When this occurs, evidence can be collected throughout all phases of curriculum development and implementation. There are five emerging approaches to evaluation (Fetterman & Wandersman, 2005; Guba & Lincoln, 1989; Hills & Carroll, 2017; Patton, 2011). The Evaluation Subcommittee can be introduced to these approaches and choose an appropriate one for their program. Both quantitative and qualitative data can be collected. From our experience the latter is the more difficult to do well.

REFERENCES

Benner, P. E. (1984). *From novice to expert: Excellence and power in clinical nursing practice*. Addison Wesley.

Benner, P. E. (2001). *From novice to expert: Excellence and power in clinical nursing practice*. Prentice Hall.

Bevis, E. (2000). Teaching and learning: A practical commentary. In E. Bevis & J. Watson (Eds.), *Toward a caring curriculum: A new pedagogy for nursing* (pp. 217–259). Jones & Bartlett.

Bevis, E., & Watson, J. (2000). *Toward a caring curriculum: A new pedagogy for nursing*. Jones & Bartlett. (Original work published 1989)

Fetterman, D., & Wandersman, A. (2005). *Empowerment evaluation principle in practice*. Guilford Press.

Guba, E., & Lincoln, Y. (1989). *Fourth generation evaluation*. Sage.

Hills, M. (1992). *Collaborative nursing program of BC: Development of a generic integrated nursing curriculum with four partner colleges*. Report to the Ministry of Advanced Education. Centre for Curriculum and Professional Development.

Hills, M. (1993). Clinical evaluation: Creating a practice appraisal form. In M. Hills (Ed.), *Collaborative nursing project: Development of a generic integrated nursing curriculum in collaboration with four partner colleges.* Report to the Ministry of Advanced Education, Centre for Curriculum and Professional Development.

Hills, M. (2001). Using Co-operative Inquiry to transform evaluation of nursing student's clinical practice. In P. Reason & H. Bradbury (Eds.), *Handbook of action research, participatory inquiry and practice* (pp. 340–347). Sage.

Hills, M. (2016). Emancipatory and collaborative: Leading from beside. In W. Rosa (Ed.), *Nurses as leaders: Evolutionary visions of leadership* (pp. 293–309). Springer Publishing Company.

Hills, M. (November 2017). *Creating a Caring Science curriculum: Transcending the bio-medical & behaviorist paradigms.* Unpublished Keynote address. Global Human Caring Congress, Santiago, Chile.

Hills, M., & Bevis, E. (1992). Developing learning activities for the collaborative nursing curriculum of British Columbia. In M. Hills (Ed.), *Collaborative nursing project: Development of a generic integrated nursing curriculum in collaboration with four partner colleges.* Report to the Ministry of Advanced Education, Centre for Curriculum and Professional Development.

Hills, M., & Carroll S. (2017). Collaborative action research & evaluation: Relational inquiry for promoting caring science literacy. In S. M. Lee, P. A. Palmieri, & J. Watson (Eds.), *Global advances in human caring literacy* (pp. 115–130). Springer Publishing Company.

Hills, M., & Watson, J. (2011). *Creating a Caring Science curriculum: An emancipatory pedagogy for nursing* (1st ed.). Springer Publishing Company.

Iwasiw, C. L., Andrusyszyn, M.-A., & Goldenberg, D. (2018). *Curriculum development in nursing education* (4th revised ed.). Jones & Bartlett.

Jillings, C., & O'Flynn-Magee, K. (2007). Knowledge and knowing made manifest: Curriculum process in student-centered learning. In L. Young & B. Paterson (Eds.), *Teaching nursing: Developing a student-centered learning environment* (pp. 383–402). Lippincott Williams & Wilkins.

National League for Nursing. (1988). *Curriculum revolution: Mandate for change.* Author.

National League for Nursing. (2003). *Position statement. Innovation in nursing education: A call to reform.* http://www.nln.org/docs/default-source/about/archived-position-statements/innovation-in-nursing-education-a-call-to-reform-pdf.pdf?sfvrsn=4

Patton, M. Q. (2011). *Developmental evaluation: Applying complexity concepts to enhance innovation and use.* Guilford Press.

van Manen, M. (2014). *Phenomenology of practice.* Routledge/Taylor & Francis Group.

Creating Canada's First Caring Science Curriculum: The Collaborative Nursing Program of British Columbia

Whereas the schools' previous programmes had a biomedical orientation, the new programme focuses nursing practice on people and their health and healing experiences. Additionally, it shifts the focus of nursing education from a behavioural educational paradigm to a caring, emancipatory paradigm.
—Hills, 2001, p. 341

INTRODUCTION

In this chapter, we explain, and give examples of each of the components described in Chapter 10, in order to provide concrete examples of the phases of the curriculum development process. We describe a curriculum that used the processes outlined in Chapter 10 and the theoretical/philosophical framework described in Chapter 4. This curriculum was based in a Caring Science paradigm that originally was developed collaboratively by five schools of nursing in British Columbia (BC), Canada. This program was developed between 1989 and 1994 by a 13-member curriculum development team (Hills, 1992, 1993, 1998; Hills & Bevis, 1992; Hills & Lindsey, 1994; Hills et al., 1994). Each school of nursing partner had two representatives who attended all of the Collaborative Nursing Program of British Columbia (CNPBC) meetings and then returned to their respective partners and brought all of their faculty members up to date by engaging in a similar process that they had just experienced with the CNPBC curriculum team. This was a significant decision-making structure because it placed the coordinator as the leader of the CNPBC, not as a representative of any particular school of nursing. By 1993, the CNPBC had grown to include 10 partners. Subsequently, the CNPBC has undergone many changes in partners; however, the "continuity within the Collaborative committees persists over several PSI [Post Secondary Institutions] membership reformations. Shifts in the postsecondary legislation and institutional policy over time influenced the PSI participation in the Collaborative" (Zawaduk et al., 2014, p. 581).

This program was the first collaborative program in Canada and it was also the first Caring Science curriculum in Canada. While this program has undergone many iterations and has changed significantly over the years, including adding and changing partners, making many curriculum changes, and having many faculty member changes, some schools of nursing continue to offer this curriculum based on its original philosophical/theoretical foundation (Zawaduk et al., 2014). Also, see Chapter 12 for reflections on 30 years of experience with this collaborative Caring Science curriculum. Our purpose in sharing these experiences of this curriculum development process is to provide concrete examples of engaging in the early stages of developing a Caring Science curriculum. This particular chapter is notably based on the lead author's experiences and works. We want to acknowledge the several schools of nursing in Canada and elsewhere that continue to embrace this Caring Science perspective to this day.[1]

DEVELOPMENT OF A PHILOSOPHY

The philosophical statement, referred to as a "metaparadigm" by our team, consists of a statement regarding the faculty members' beliefs about nursing, health, and people and their views on teaching and learning—their theoretical and philosophical positions at a minimum. If you are creating a Caring Science curriculum, it should go without saying that a Caring Science philosophy and theory must permeate this philosophical position. At this point, you may want to review Chapters 1, 2, 3, and 4 of this book.

In the CNPBC, several months were spent articulating our philosophy. It is not easy for 13 people with different perspectives to agree on philosophical statements. We engaged in many healthy debates and we developed our "team" capacity by using different team-building exercises. This type of engagement, developing our ability to work as a team, created a sense of coherence with the group, even though we initially held varying perspectives and opinions. For example, we all participated in the Myers-Briggs Type Indicator® personality inventory. The results and discussions about our personality preferences gave the team members a way to express their discomfort in a situation without feeling "blamed." We also had discussions about the aspects of curriculum that were most important to us. The example of the philosophical statement that follows was one of the iterations that was developed early in our planning process. Reaching this consensus allowed the team to put the philosophy aside for a while so that we could engage in other aspects of the curriculum process.

THE COLLABORATIVE NURSING PROGRAM PHILOSOPHY

The philosophy of the collaborative nursing program is informed by humanistic, existential, phenomenological, and socially critical orientations. These orientations are reflected in the way in which the program views persons, health and healing, healthcare, nursing, and curriculum.

---

[1] These programs include: Laurentian University, Ontario; Nevada State University, Nevada; Universidad de La Serena, Chile; Nursing Education in Southwestern Alberta, Lethbridge, Alberta; York University, Ontario; Siena University, New York State; University of Western Ontario/Fanshawe; Vancouver Island University, British Columbia; to name a few.

PERSONS

"Persons" refers to human beings, whether they are in an individual, family/group, community, or societal context. They are holistic beings who bring unique meaning to life experiences. People make choices based on the meaning they attribute to their experiences, and their choices are influenced by both internal and external factors. Implicit in the choices people make is the responsibility to be accountable for the consequences of their actions. Although ultimately alone and self-responsible, people live in relationships with others and are constantly evolving as they interact, and strive toward health.

HEALTH

"Health" (as described by the World Health Organization [WHO], 1986) is the extent to which people are able to realize aspirations, satisfy needs, and to change or cope with the environment. The environment comprises all cultural, lifestyle, political/economic, interpersonal, structural, and other ecological factors. Health is a resource, not an object of living: it is a positive concept emphasizing social and personal resources as well as physical capabilities. Promoting health involves enabling people to increase control over and to improve their health (WHO, 1986). People in ill health (whether physical, social, psychological, or spiritual) may still consider themselves to be healthy if they are able to lead, what they consider to be, satisfying lives. Health and healing coexist and healing is not simply viewed as the movement along a continuum from illness to health.

HEALTHCARE

The right to "healthcare" for all is highly valued by our society and supported by the Canadian nursing profession. Accompanying this right is our belief in equal quality of, and access to, healthcare through fairly distributed resources within and among our communities. People should be full participants in making decisions about their health.

The complex and changing nature of healthcare has direct consequences for the way in which nursing is practiced. Nurses have a vital role to play in shaping and responding to the challenges of healthcare in our society. Nurses must strengthen their mandate and their ability to promote health through continuous professional growth.

NURSING

"Nursing" is the professionalization of the human capacity to care. Nurses are in a unique position to help people understand their health-related experiences and to embrace their ability to make informed healthcare choices. Through caring relationships, nurses inform and involve their clients. This relationship empowers clients to make the best possible choices for their health and enhances the healing process.

Nursing involves a highly complex process of simultaneously using reasoning and intuitive thinking while providing care. Nurses must know, care, manage the context, and deal with the unpredictable; they must assume responsibility for their decisions and their professional growth and be accountable to their profession's standards and ethics.

Nurses work with many other disciplines, and in this multidisciplinary healthcare context, nurses provide a unique perspective to client care. The unique role of nursing is the nurse's ability to understand people's situations from their perspective and to participate with them through a caring, informed relationship to promote health responses to life experiences.

CURRICULUM

The "curriculum" of the Collaborative Nursing Program of British Columbia is defined as the interactions that take place between and among students, clients, practitioners, and teachers with the intent that learning takes place. Therefore, the quality of the curriculum depends upon the quality of these interactions, and students, practitioners, and faculty members are equally valued as partners in the learning process. Learning is a reformulation of the meaning of experience and leads to changes in attitudes, feelings, and responses. Learning is critically affected by the learner's concept of self, which is itself learned. The self-concept is enhanced when learners have a need to know, perceive learning as relevant and meaningful, and believe they have a chance of success. It is further enhanced when the learner's past and present experiences are acknowledged, respected, and reflected upon. When learners share the responsibility for identifying learning needs, planning learning experiences, and evaluating programs, their self-confidence increases and they become increasingly self-directed. Learners learn best when they feel cared for and challenged and when they experience success.

Nursing is a discipline that values different ways of knowing. Knowledge is derived from the understanding of self, practice, theory, and research, with each way of knowing informing and influencing the other. This form of praxis is a dialectical process through which knowledge is both derived from and guides nursing practice.

In this philosophy, nursing is seen as "the professionalization of the human capacity to care and nurses are believed to be in a unique position to assist people in understanding their health-related experiences and to encourage them to embrace their ability to make informed health choices" (Hills & Lindsey, 1994, p. 160).

TIME OUT FOR REFLECTION

Go back and review Chapters 1, 2, 3, and 4 of this text.

Consider the beliefs, assumptions, and positions reflected in the philosophy just presented.

- How well does it fit with our current presentation of Caring Science as the disciplinary foundation for nursing?
- If you were to write a philosophical statement today, would you find it necessary to refer to other theories such as Critical Social Theory or phenomenology?
- Could you write a philosophical statement purely based on Caring Science?

PROGRAM PURPOSE AND GOALS

Once you have reached a place with your philosophical statement on which the team feels they have sufficient consensus to move forward, it is time to enter the next phase, developing the program purpose and goals. An example of a program purpose and program goals is provided to illustrate these concepts. This example was developed collaboratively by the members of the Collaborative Nursing Program of BC (Hills et al., 1994).

PROGRAM PURPOSE

The purpose of this program is to educate nurses to work with individuals, families, groups, or communities from a health-promotion perspective and an ethic of caring. The program will provide students with opportunities to develop sensitivity to people's experiences with health and healing. By being cognizant of nurses' professional role, students will learn to work as partners with clients and other healthcare providers. Through their understanding and participation in the changing healthcare system, graduates will be active participants in creating health for all.

PROGRAM GOALS

The graduate of the program will be able to

- practice nursing with a health promotion–caring perspective within a variety of contexts and with diverse client populations;
- be an independent, self-directed, self-motivated, and lifelong learner with a questioning mind and familiarity with inquiry approaches to learning;
- be self-reflective, self-evaluative, accountable, and make clinical judgments based on different ways of knowing, including critical thinking and intuition;
- create and influence the future of nursing practice at a political, social, and professional level by responding to and anticipating the changing needs of society;
- be prepared to meet the professional practice requirements as established by the appropriate legislative body.

TIME OUT FOR REFLECTION

Consider the following questions and record your responses in your journal.

- What relationships exist between the philosophy and the program goals?
- Are there concepts included in the philosophy that are not reflected in the program goals? If yes, create a goal to reflect the discrepancy.
- Consider the goals for your nursing program. Are they congruent with your philosophy? If not, change one or the other so that they are congruent.

CURRICULUM FRAMEWORK

This phase involves the delineation of core concepts and conceptual maps to guide the learning experience. Over the past several years, nurse educators have been asking, "If nursing education doesn't use a behavioral approach to curriculum design, what should it use?" In many ways, giving up the Tyler (1949) behavioral approach to curriculum design has created a void in nursing curriculum development and left nursing education struggling to fill that void. A Tylerian approach to curriculum is specific, concrete, and relatively straightforward. You develop your program goals and objectives, decide on terminal objectives for every term, for every course, and then you level the content over the years and semesters being guided by the principle of going from the simple to the complex. This may be an oversimplification, but it illustrates the point that rejecting this structure for curriculum development has provided a space for nurse educators to use their creativity and imagination to create innovative and more nursing-oriented approaches to curriculum development. As Jillings and O'Flynn-Magee (2007) suggest, the nursing concepts that are used to build an organizational framework could come from a nursing model, conceptual framework, nursing theories, or from the mission and outcome statements. "Using these elements as sources of major concepts ensures that the main ideas about nursing roles and competencies and concerns for the recipients of nursing care are included" (p. 395).

The collaborative curriculum team in BC was based on an ethic of caring and used a health promotion framework to develop a Caring Science curriculum (Hills, 1992, 1993, 1998, 2001, 2016, 2017; Hills & Cara, 2019; Hills & Lindsey, 1994; Hills et al., 1994; Zawaduk et al., 2014).

The curriculum team in BC used focus groups consisting of nurse educators, nurse administrators, and frontline nurses from hospitals and community, government representatives from the Ministry of Health, the nurses' regulatory organization, and the nurses' union to determine what knowledge, attitudes, and skills (know, be, do) nurses would need to have to practice in the 21st century (Hills, 1992, 1993; Hills et al., 1994). The participants of the focus groups were asked three questions:

- What will nurses need to know to practice in the 21st century?
- What will nurses have to be able to do to practice in the 21st century?
- What attitudes will nurses require to practice in the 21st century?

Similar questions were asked in a study of nurses using a Delphi technique who were not involved in the development of the curriculum, but from the general nursing population (Beddome et al., 1995).

IDENTIFICATION OF CONTENT THEMES, PERMEATING VARIABLES, AND CONCEPTS

Data from both experiences were analyzed using a thematic analysis (van Manen, 1990) and that resulted in the creation of four themes that could be used to organize the *nursing content*:

- People's experience with health
- People's experience with healing
- People's experience with self and others
- People's experience with professional growth

Two *permeating variables* that would be integrated in every semester were identified:

- Caring and health promotion

Four critical concepts that would be woven into every course were identified:

- Ways of knowing
- Personal meaning
- Transitions/time
- Context

Although some aspects of the curriculum have been updated, these themes, permeating variables, and core concepts remain visible in the current curricula of many schools of nursing.

DEFINITION OF CONTENT THEMES

These content themes were defined and the definitions were agreed upon by consensus by all members of the curriculum team.

1. *People's experience with health*—defined as the process whereby people realize aspirations, satisfy needs, and change and cope with the environment (World Health Organization [WHO], 1986).
2. *People's experiences with healing*—defined as the process of becoming increasingly whole, regardless of the medical diagnosis . . . it is the total organismic synergistic response that emerges within the individual and leads to the resolution of the health issue or a peaceful death.
3. *People's experiences with self and others*—defined as the process of understanding the meaning of relationship. Understanding relationships includes self-knowledge and knowledge of others that is achieved through self-reflection, introspection, and interaction. This knowledge of self and others results in the discovery of personal meaning.
4. *People's experiences with professional growth*—defined as the process by which nurses make a difference at a personal, professional, and socio-political level.

This framework provided the overall *structure* to organize the courses within the entire program and is depicted in the diagram of Figure 11.1. We used a Celtic knot to represent the interrelatedness of these themes, concepts, and constructs. In all Celtic knots there is no beginning and no end; they are continuous and totally connected. These knots could be said to represent eternity, whether this means loyalty, faith, friendship, or love. Only one thread is used in each design which symbolizes how life and eternity are interconnected.

CURRICULUM DESIGN: STRUCTURING AND SEQUENCING COURSES

Once the framework is in place to provide an overview of the program, courses need to be developed and decisions need to be made about the sequencing of the courses. In addition, electives from other disciplines must be considered and identified. Obviously, you cannot teach everything first and all at once. Several decisions need to be made about what to teach when, and what depth of understanding is required at different points in the curriculum; so you need to consider

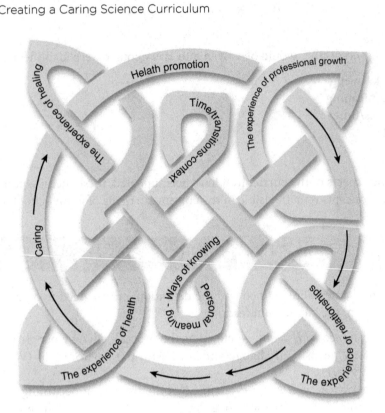

FIGURE 11.1 Framework for collaborative nursing program of BC.

how you will decide what to teach first and what will follow and in what order. This process can be very time consuming and challenging. Because this process, in some ways more than others, challenges our beliefs about learning, there is often much disagreement among nursing faculty members. This is also the time when decisions need to be made about how the nursing components will interface with the non-nursing aspects of the program, such as electives. For example, some nursing programs believe that students should take liberal arts courses in their first 2 years and do their nursing courses in the senior years of their program. Others believe that nursing courses should occur in every semester beginning with the first and be integrated throughout the curriculum. No matter what the decision, the program philosophy of caring must be visible in the decisions that are made. For the CNPBC, it was consciously decided to have nursing prominent at the very beginning of the program, a decision that would prove to be prudent.

In the development of Collaborative Nursing Program of BC, all nursing content was organized under the four themes just identified and these themes were sequenced and structured throughout the 4 years of the program. Initially, a matrix was created simply to place the different courses leveled/scaffolded throughout the curriculum into different semesters. For example, *Health 1* was placed in semester 1, *Health 2* in semester 2, *Health 3* in semester 3, and so forth. Each of the four themes was placed in the matrix in this way. These levels were always understood to have different levels of complexity, going from simple to complex.

Each course within a theme was then further developed by a predetermined focus. For example, the theme "people's experience with health and healing" occurred in each semester but had a different focus and level of complexity, semester to semester. In year 1, semester 1, the course on people's experiences of health and healing focused on health and what it means to be healthy. Students learn about health by examining their own health and that of others and by hearing people's perceptions of health. In year 1, semester 2, the course on people's experiences of health and healing focuses on people living with chronic diseases. The people and health focus is maintained but students learn particularly about people's experiences of living with a chronic disease such as diabetes, asthma, and so forth. In Year 2, semester 3, the course on people's experiences with health and healing focuses on people's experiences of living with episodic health challenges, such as pregnancy, and in semester 4, they learn about people's experiences of living with acute episodic health challenges. The point here was to reconceptualize medical descriptive language to describe nursing. It was like we were trying to stand on a balcony and look down on our nursing experiences. We were not trying to get a view from 3,000 feet; we were simply trying to get out of the weeds of medicine that were holding us down and just get another broader view; from above, from the balcony.

All themes of nursing content were distributed throughout the curriculum in a similar way (see Exhibit 11.1).

EXHIBIT 11.1 Course content by theme—Collaborative Nursing Program of British Columbia

	SEPTEMBER - DECEMBER		JANUARY - APRIL		MAY - AUGUST	
	SEMESTER 1		SEMESTER 2			
YR.I	HEALTH I (N)	(0-0-3-1)	HEALTH II (N)	(0-0-3-0)	PRACTICUM	
	PRO.GROWTH I (N)	(0-4-4-0)	S & O II	(3-0-0-0)	7 WEEKS	(0-20-4-0)
	HEALTH SCIENCE I	(3-0-0-3)	ELECTIVE	(3-0-0-0)		
	S & O I (PSYCHI)	(3-0-0-0)	HEALTH SCIENCE II	(3-0-0-3)		
	PACKAGE I••	(3-0-0-0)	NURSING PRACTICE I (N)	(0-8-2-3)		
	TOTAL HOURS	(24)	TOTAL HOURS	(28)	TOTAL HOURS	(24)
	SEMESTER 3		SEMESTER 4			
YR.II	HEALING W.S.I (N)	(0-0-0-6)	PROF.GROWTH II (N)	(0-0-3-0)	W.E. I (CO-OP)	
	NURSING PRACTICE II (N)	(0-12-4-0)	HEALING W.S.II (N)	(0-0-3-6)		
	HEALTH SCIENCE III	(3-0-0-0)	NURSING PRACTICE III (N)	(0-12-4-0)		
	PACKAGE II	(3-0-0-0)	HEALTH SCIENCE IV	(3-0-0-0)		
	TOTAL HOURS	(28)	TOTAL HOURS	(28)		
	SEMESTER 5		BRIDGE		SEMESTER 6	
YR.III	PROF.GROWTH III (N)	(0-0-3-0)	BRIDGE IN		HEALTH IV (N)	(0-0-3-0)
	PHILOSOPHY	(3-0-0-0)	HEALTH (N)	(0-0-3-0)	S & O III (N)	(0-0-3-0)
	HEALTH III (N)	(0-0-3-0)	PRO.GROWTH (N)	(0-0-3-0)	HEALTH SCIENCE V (N)	(3-0-0-0)
	NURSING PRACTICE IV (N)	(0-12-4-0)	HEALTH SCIENCE (N)	(3-0-0-0)	STATISTICS	(3-0-0-0)
	PROF.GROWTH IV	(3-0-0-0)	NURSING PRACTICE (N)	(0-6-3-0)	NURSING PRACTICE V (N)	(0-6-3-0)
			PACKAGE	(3-0-0-0)		
	TOTAL HOURS	(28)	TOTAL HOURS	(21)	TOTAL HOURS	(21)
			BRIDGE OUT			
			HEALING (3 WK.) (N)	(0-0-4-8)		
			PRECEPTORSHIP			
			(37.5 HRS. X 11 WK.) (N)			
			CONTINUING STUDENTS			
			W.E. II (CO-OP)			
			SEMESTER 7			
YR.IV	W.E.III		PROF GROWTH V (N)	(0-0-3-0)	W.E.IV	
			PROF. GROWTH VI (N)	(0-0-3-0)		
			PACKAGE III	(3-0-0-0)		
			S & O IV	(0-0-3-0)	Before the Bridge	
			NURSING PRACTICE VI (N)	(0-6-3-0)	Seminar	1: 32
			TOTAL HOURS	(21)	Clinical	1: 08
	SEMESTER 8				Lab	1: 10
YR.V	INDEPENDENT					
	CLINICAL STUDIES	21 HR. WK. x 13 WKS. (N)			After the Bridge	
	RATIO 1:20				Seminar	1: 32
					Clinical	1: 16
•• PACKAGE = CHOICE BETWEEN SOCIOLOGY, ANTHROPOLOGY, PSYCHOLOGY, PHILOSOPHY					Preceptorship	1: 20

(0-0-0-0) = 1 ST # REFLECTS CLASS ROOM: 2ND # REFLECTS CLINICAL: 3 RD # REFLECTS SEMINAR: 4TH # REFLECTS LAB

There are at least two important points about the structure and sequencing of these courses. The nursing faculty was committed to creating courses that truly reflected nursing, and that was accomplished by using language, concepts, and knowledge that are within nursing's domain of practice, not medicine's. This was a struggle because for at least 40 years we had been designing nursing curricula based on medicine's disease-treatment-cure model. Second, the nursing faculty wanted all courses to reflect its commitment to its philosophy and program goals. Again, that was accomplished by keeping an ethic of caring and a health promotion perspective at the forefront in all course development.

INSTRUCTIONAL DESIGN: COURSE DEVELOPMENT AND LEARNING OUTCOMES

In the Collaborative Nursing Program of BC, themes teams were constituted to develop each of the courses. Course content had already been articulated within each of the nursing content themes (Table 11.1) so the work now concentrated on sorting content over semesters and years of the curriculum.

Because this program was developed initially across five different nursing programs within five different institutions, the curriculum team worried about program integrity throughout the curriculum development process. One way that this was handled was for the team to focus on the nursing concepts to be taught and to develop learning activities (discussed in what follows) that would encourage the learning of those concepts. As a result, the team developed a "virtual extensive library" of learning activities for each course. A faculty member who was assigned to teach that course had multiple learning activities from which to choose, but they all were focused on learning the content, the competencies, and the skills for that course.

TABLE 11.1 Content Themes by Semester

EXEMPLARY CURRICULUM BASED ON HEALTH PROMOTION

	SEMESTER 1	SEMESTER 2	SEMESTER 3
Year 1	Health	Chronic Health Challenges	Practicum
Year 2	Episodic Health Challenges	Complex Episodic Health Challenges	Preceptorship/ Co-op Work
Year 3	Prevention	Preceptorship	Health Promotion
Year 4	Preceptorship/ Co-op Work	Societal Health	Preceptorship/ Co-op Work Experience
Year 5	Individual area of focus		

TEACHING METHODS

This phase has been covered quite extensively in Chapters 5, 6, 7, and 8, so there are only a couple of additional concepts that we need to add at this point. One of the most useful strategies for teachers who want to create a Caring Science curriculum and use relational emancipatory pedagogy is to learn how to develop learning activities. As Bevis used to always comment, "It is not what the teacher says or does that is important; it is what the teacher has the students do that is important in the overall scheme of education" (personal communication).

Bevis (2000) recommends that teachers become metastrategists; using teaching methods of engagement. We spend considerable time thinking about how to design teaching/learning experiences that will create the dance between theory and practice. We strategize about the types of questions to ask that will provoke critical reflection in ourselves and our students. Although it is important to have knowledge of the content area, we usually spend more time thinking about what we do not know about the topic or issue than about what we do know. We try to think about how we view an issue and why that is the case. We try to determine what questions we need to ask to better understand the relationship between the elements of the issue at hand. We become curious about why others think differently or the same as we do about an issue.

But, how do we give order to these questions so we know how to progress? You have already learned some strategies for doing this, such as Wallerstein et al. (2018) SHOWED method (see Chapter 7). Another way to structure teaching/learning experiences is by using learning activities (Bevis & Watson, 1989/2000). As you have experienced throughout this book, we use learning activities to structure teaching/learning encounters.

CREATING LEARNING ACTIVITIES

Engaging in critical dialogue requires considerable planning and thoughtfulness. We use learning activities to *structure* dialogue in a teaching/learning situation. Learning activities (Bevis & Watson, 1989/2000) as they are used here have particular meaning and structure and consist of several component parts as described in Chapter 10.

For examples of learning activities, see the Chapter 18 learning activities "Using the Connoisseurship Model to Access Learning" and "Developing Criteria for Evaluating Learning."

ESTABLISHING CLASSROOM AND PRACTICE (CLINICAL) EVALUATION AS AUTHENTICATION

Classroom and practice evaluation, originally created by Hills (1993, 2001) and other team members, is described and discussed fully in Chapter 18. The main point about evaluation, both from classwork and practice, is that it must be congruent with Caring Science.

EVALUATION PLAN

The final phase of the curriculum development process is the design of an evaluation plan. This plan should include strategies for evaluating individual courses and an overall strategy for evaluating the program. In addition, strategies for evaluating student classroom and clinical performance need to be developed as part of the plan. Although it is beyond the scope of this book to describe program evaluation, there are many excellent books, articles, and book chapters written on the subject (e.g., Fetterman and Wandersman [2005], Guba and Lincoln [1989], Patton [2011], Hills and Carroll [2017]). We have included concepts of evaluation related to assessing students' performance in Unit IV (see Chapter 18). However, it is important to note that the planning for evaluation occurs simultaneously with curriculum development.

In addition to the evaluation plan in which faculty members and schools of nursing are interested for their own purposes, nursing programs are regulated and are required to meet standards of practice guidelines designated by their governing bodies. An evaluation plan for this type of external evaluation must also be planned.

REFERENCES

Beddome, G., Budgen, C., Hills, M. D., Lindsey, A. E., Duval, P. M., & Szalay, L. (1995). Education and practice collaboration: A strategy for curriculum development. *The Journal of Nursing Education, 34*(1), 11–15. https://doi.org/10.3928/0148-4834-19950101-05

Bevis, E. (2000). Clusters of influence for practical decision making about curriculum. In E. Bevis, & J. Watson (Eds.), *Toward a caring curriculum: A new pedagogy for nursing.* (pp. 107–152). National League for Nursing.

Bevis, E., & Watson, J. (2000). *Toward a caring curriculum: A new pedagogy for nursing.* National League for Nursing. (Original work published 1989)

Fetterman, D., & Wandersman, A. (2005). *Empowerment evaluation principle in practice.* Guilford Press.

Guba, E., & Lincoln, Y. (1989). *Fourth generation evaluation.* Sage.

Hills, M. (1992). *Collaborative nursing program of BC: Development of a generic integrated nursing curriculum with four partner colleges.* Report to the Ministry of Advanced Education. Centre for Curriculum and Professional Development.

Hills, M. (1993). Clinical evaluation: Creating a practice appraisal form. In M. Hills (Ed.), *Collaborative nursing project: Development of a generic integrated nursing curriculum in collaboration with four partner colleges.* Report to the Ministry of Advanced Education, Centre for Curriculum and Professional Development.

Hills, M. (1998). Student experiences of nursing health promotion practice in hospital settings. *Nursing Inquiry, 5,* 164–173. https://doi.org/10.1046/j.1440-1800.1998.530164.x

Hills, M. (2001). Using co-operative inquiry to transform evaluation of nursing students' clinical practice. In P. Reason & H. Bradbury (Eds.), *Handbook of action research, participatory inquiry and practice* (pp. 340–347). Sage.

Hills, M. (2016). Emancipatory and collaborative: Leading from beside. In W. Rosa (Ed.), *Nurses as leaders: Evolutionary visions of leadership* (pp. 293–309). Springer Publishing Company.

Hills, M. (November 2017). *Creating a Caring Science curriculum: Transcending the bio-medical & behaviorist paradigms.* Unpublished Keynote address. Global Human Caring Congress, Santiago, Chile.

Hills, M., & Bevis, E. (1992). Developing learning activities for the collaborative nursing curriculum of British Columbia. In M. Hills (Ed.), *Collaborative nursing project: Development of a generic integrated nursing curriculum in collaboration with four partner colleges.* Report to the Ministry of Advanced Education, Centre for Curriculum and Professional Development.

Hills, M., & Cara, C. (2019). Curriculum development processes and pedagogical practices for advancing caring science literacy. In W. Rosa, S. Horton-Deutsch, & J. Watson (Eds.), *A handbook for caring science: Expanding the paradigm* (pp. 197–210). Springer Publishing Company.

Hills, M., & Carroll S. (2017). *Collaborative action research & evaluation: Relational inquiry for promoting caring science literacy.* In S. M. Lee, P. A. Palmieri, & J. Watson (Eds.), *Global advances in human caring literacy* (pp. 115–130). Springer Publishing Company.

Hills, M., & Lindsey, E. (1994). Health promotion: A viable curriculum framework for nursing education. *Nursing Outlook, 42*(4), 158–162. https://doi.org/10.1016/0029-6554(94)90003-5

Hills, M., Lindsey, E., Chisamore, M., Basset-Smith, J., Abbott, K., & Fournier-Chalmers, J. (1994). University-college collaboration: Rethinking curriculum development in nursing education. *The Journal of Nursing Education, 33*(5), 220–225. PMID: 8051573.

Jillings, C., & O'Flynn-Magee, K. (2007). Knowledge and knowing made manifest: Curriculum process in student-centered learning. In L. Young & B. Paterson (Eds.), *Teaching nursing: Developing a student-centered learning environment* (pp. 383–402). Lippincott Williams, & Wilkins.

Patton, M. (2011). Developmental evaluation: Applying complexity concepts to enhance innovation and use. Guilford Press.

The Myers & Briggs Foundation. (2014). *Myers-Briggs Type Indicator® Basics*. The Myers & Briggs Foundation. https://www.myersbriggs.org/my-mbti-personality-type/mbti-basics

Tyler, R. (1949). *Basic principles of curriculum and instruction*. University of Chicago Press.

van Manen, M. (1990). *Researching lived experience*. University of Western Ontario: Althouse Press.

Wallerstein, N., Duran, B., Oetzel, J., & Minkler, M. (2018). *Community-based participatory research for health: Advancing social and health equity* (3rd ed.). Jossey-Bass.

World Health Organization. (1986). *Ottawa Charter*. Author.

Zawaduk, C., Duncan, S., Mahara, M. S., Tate, B., Callaghan, D., McCullough, D., Chapman, M., & Van Neste-Kenny, J. (2014). Mission possible: Twenty-five years of university and college collaboration in baccalaureate nursing education. *Journal of Nursing Education, 53*(10), 580–588. https://doi.org/10.3928/01484834-20140922-04

Humanism in the Classroom: 30 Years of Experience With Caring Science

Lynn Rollison and Piera Jung

INTRODUCTION

In this chapter we provide an example of a fourth-year leadership course offered in a unique approach as part of a collaborative Caring Science program for nurses at Vancouver Island University (VIU) in British Columbia (BC), Canada. The evolution of this course restructure occurred over 7 years and was an exciting journey. In this chapter we share details of the course development. At the time, we had no idea that we would move the development of this course to re-embrace and revision a caring pedagogy in our own way. We discuss how we see ourselves living the Caring Science philosophy through various markers, as seen in Hills and Watson (2011), and how we altered and grew in our teaching approach by offering concrete examples from experience.

COLLABORATE PROGRAM: PHILOSOPHICAL UNDERPINNINGS

Our current collaborative-based philosophy and curriculum was developed by a 13-faculty-member curriculum committee with Hills as the director along with Em Bevis and Jean Watson as consultants during the period of 1989 to 1994 (personal communication with Dr. M. Hills). Since that time, we have seen many changes influencing our partnerships (see Zawaduk et al., 2014). Despite the changes and evolution of nursing in our current world, today we continue to embrace a curriculum that was developed utilizing pedagogy for a Caring Science curriculum. At times we have drifted from our philosophical moorings and have also found our way through some difficulties. Currently, we grant a nursing degree along with North Island College where we have a shared curriculum. Affiliation with previous partners of the Collaborative Nursing Program of British Columbia (CNPBC) and then later the Collaborative Academic Education in Nursing (CAEN) program has influenced and had a profound effect on us through a shared pedagogy and philosophy (Hills & Watson, 2011).

Philosophically our curriculum has been built and is underpinned by the Caring Science curriculum (Hills & Watson, 2011). Drawing strongly on many stellar writers embedded in all years of our four-year nursing education, including Watson, Chinn, Carper, Benner, and others, our students are well versed in epistemological thinking. Our program embraces a practice to prepare the learners for the ever-shifting needs of healthcare systems that include: anticipating changes in the role of the nurse; developing a critique of hegemonic practices in healthcare; strengthening leadership attributes; deepening knowledge to meet the challenges of the complexity of care in healthcare systems; and preparing students to engage with the evolving societal and environmental trends nurses face. Our program encourages students to become inquisitive practitioners, knowing that there are multiple ways of knowing and learning (Belenky et al., 1986). We believe that learners learn best when they feel respected and challenged and when they experience success (Vancouver Island University and North Island College, 2016). As faculty we value the students and what they bring with them; their unique experiences are the gifts they give to themselves, but also to the profession of nursing. As faculty, our leadership, over time, has supported looking to our philosophical roots when drifting from the curriculum was noted.

Our philosophy at VIU views teachers "as expert learners working with students in partnership, empowering them in equitable ways, drawing on student experience and on theory of various kinds to develop the content to be learned" (Vancouver Island University and North Island College, 2016). We try to be caring and gracious with our students and this is further supported by many in our faculty, previous graduates from the program, who bring the "lived experience" of the caring curriculum with them as they develop their teaching art (Vancouver Island University and North Island College, 2016). Over the years, we have developed access through various entrances into the program to licensed practical nurses, long-term care attendants, prior learning assessments, and other means. In 2005–2007, the CAEN curriculum was updated to reflect changes in healthcare and society. Components of inquiry, critical thinking, health promotion, case management, and leadership were infused more prominently into the curriculum. Caring became the central concept in our three relational practice courses (Vancouver Island University and North Island College, 2016).

COURSE DEVELOPMENT AND EVOLUTION

How did we, as two teachers, begin to find our way in identifying a path and our innovations in a leadership course? Early on we embraced an emancipatory pedagogy. According to Hills and Watson (2011), emancipatory pedagogy is what counts as knowledge and further is a "relational inquiry process that facilitates the transfer of consciousness through which learning and deep insight occurs" (p. 53). This consciousness occurs between students and teachers at the intersections of caring relationships that help to advance knowledge and support transformational learning environments. In the development of the leadership class, we have worked diligently to foster experiential learning, open discourse, shared leadership, and gave voice and deep understanding to the issues that students will face in their nursing careers.

One of the previous teachers for the leadership class took on the role of chair for our department and we put our names forth to teach this compulsory course as part of our workload. During the first year we offered the course as it was laid out by the interdisciplinary team that originally developed the course of study. It was rich with guest speakers and the content included depth into leadership theories. At first, we had separate classes of 36 students each but worked together to organize the weekly schedule and to bring the content alive while offering the same lessons and guest speakers. Perhaps, due to our naivety, we struggled to keep students interested and attending the classroom. Towards the end of the class, usually a 14-week class of 3 hours in length, we had only 12 and ten students respectively in each of our classes. We were dismayed as this is not a response we typically received with our decades-long history of teaching. With this sense of failure, we began to rethink our approach and to make the course our own, infused with our beliefs about learners and our personal philosophy.

IDENTIFYING ISSUES AND MAKING CHANGES: SHIFTING OUR VIEW

The classes lacked energy and students had limited engagement with the material presented. Classes were built on objectives, definitions, guidelines, and leadership theories for students to learn. The content of the classes was predetermined by the teachers, and at times, pre-arranged according to the textbook chapters that we were using. This way of structuring class information is teacher-centered rather than learner-centered. We used a textbook from the previous class that followed the course content to include examples of leadership styles, approaches, and case studies along with follow-up questions and answers. These activities fell like stones into a deep pond and became lifeless time wasters as well as uninteresting to read or comment on. Was it us, could we not bring this course alive? We knew something was missing but we did not know what. We started to inquire with students and with ourselves. At first, students were reluctant to share their thoughts with us. We worked on creating an open environment and culture where students felt safe and comfortable in sharing their ideas. We openly shared with the students that we were learners just like them. We articulated that learning was about change and change was uncomfortable because we had to admit to our own vulnerability. Each time we made a mistake we learned from it. We wanted to partner with the students so that they had a say on how and what they choose to learn. Working within the blueprints of the course, we began to look for opportunities to bring students' voices into the content and classroom. We also invited students to provide constructive feedback on our practice. This was humbling and liberating. We made a conscious effort in building connections with students both inside and outside of the classrooms. Students informed us that they needed to relate the learning to their experiences to make sense of the information provided in class.

As teachers, we were deliberate in reflecting on our teaching practices. Following each class, we met to unpack practices we deemed effective. We went around in circles until we asked ourselves the daunting question "What are we trying to achieve?" The answer slowly emerged from our muddled conversations. As faculty, we were conflicted with the demands of instituting academic rigor in nursing education while helping students with their learning. We struggled with the need to "measure" students' performance as the primary goal of determining success. Philosophically, both teachers shared the values and beliefs of success as nurturing students to maximize their abilities and strengths, focusing on the process of learning rather than the outcomes of learning.

With these insights, we started changing our way of being. We decided to combine our classes together (total of 72 students) to bring more opportunities for dialogue and discourse in the classroom. We began sharing our stories in class; it did not matter whether they were successes or failures, as failures held greater learning, posing questions for each other following the stories, and highlighting the strengths and resilience we noticed about each other from the stories. We repeated this format for a few classes and soon noticed a steady increase in attendance. In addition, we also recognized how we, as faculty, were enjoying the classes more and looked forward to the next class and more ongoing dialogue. We also observed that students were increasingly willing to share their stories and their questions. The learning environment that we were creating and experiencing was what we were striving for; being in relationship with students so that we can cocreate learning experiences that are meaningful.

Feelings of mutuality with the students and our success in our early efforts encouraged us to take more risks and we felt freer to try new assignments and teaching methods and to take more chances on our "out-there" ideas. We felt we could "play" a little more with innovations in our approaches and infuse the learning with the lens of emancipatory pedagogy.

INNOVATIVE CLASS FORMAT

At first, our classes were organized in a traditional format of one 3-hour session per week for a full semester. However, Piera proposed a move to a conference-style learning environment, similar to attending a workshop where participants come for 1 or several days to enhance or augment their knowledge and learning. We envisioned a reshuffling for students to attend seven full-day classes or one 6-hour-long class once per week for half of the fall semester. This reconfiguration took several years in order to make timetable changes fit into the organization and flow of student classes. We strongly believed that as these students would be our colleagues within the next semester, as registered nurses, we should show them respect and caring through a different approach in the classroom.

Once the altered teaching schedule of time was approved, we noticed how freeing it was to have a long period of time to work with various leadership concepts and activities. But it was also daunting to develop and create engaging activities to stimulate the students over 6 hours. We built the course with a wide variety of individual, small-group and larger group activities. We augmented the learning with invitations to guest speakers on résumé writing and how to conduct yourself during an interview, as well as professional colleagues, leaders in the community, professionals in practice, and previous graduates. Our hope was to provide the student nurses with as many supports and professional connections as possible. Guest speakers also included invitations to our licensing body, nursing union, and professional organizations to speak about their support for the graduate nurse in British Columbia.

Nourishing the Mind, Body, and Spirit

As with any conference, refreshments and snacks are usually available and we planned to have tea, coffee, and home-made foods for the class. This was also an uncomfortable point as we did not want to be seen to be influencing the students. Despite our small concerns we went ahead with sharing food. The homemade foods went over extremely well to the point of amazement. Our generosity resulted in weekly feelings of gratitude from the students that spread throughout the class thereby developing a mutual respect between students and faculty. Many students thanked us each class for this kindness, making us more committed to bringing food. This gesture also granted us respect for our efforts to welcome them into the learning environment we were trying to create. It seemed like such a little thing to do and yet it was successful, and our attendance in class continued to stay high.

Learning is about mind-body-spirit. The welcomed snacks nourished our students' bodies, while the active engagement of classroom learning fueled our students' minds and spirits. Partnering with students to create meaningful learning experiences was pure joy. Through the advocacy branch of the provincial Nursing Association (Nurse & Nurse Practitioners of British Columbia), we invited guests to share their personal experiences of what it is like to be stigmatized due to their living conditions. The guests became part of the teaching team by inviting students to walk beside them and see the world through multiple lenses. The intentional pedagogical experience enabled students to make sense of what they were feeling, thinking, and learning. The learning reflections from students were powerful and truly transformational.

Creative Activities and Developing Voice

Tapping into the students' creative side, we consciously remained open to alternate methods of students' work. In an assignment entitled "My Nursing Philosophy," students were invited to develop their voices by sharing their values and beliefs of what nursing means to them. Although the activity was worth only 10% of the entire course, our students put in much time and effort with deep reflections and thoughts. Students were proud of their work because it showed the human side of who they are as nurses. Some of the work was presented in written format; others were offered as poetry, artwork, and song lyrics accompanied by music! Taking the learning beyond the classroom, some of the students' nursing philosophy provided a symbolic backdrop for the pinning ceremony.

Nourishing students' spirits and hearts can be a fun and noisy affair. Nursing education is demanding and requires hard work. So often students do not get a chance to acknowledge and appreciate how their peers have helped them to be successful in their learning journey. In an appreciative activity students were invited to gift their peers with as many lollipops as they wished providing that each lollipop be accompanied by a statement of how the individual had made contributions to the student's learning journey. The experience started out slow and built to a synergistic caring experience in a matter of minutes. The results of this experience were unexpected, magical, contagious and it was hard to truly describe the feelings of positive energy, enthusiasm, kindness, and love that were palpable in the room. Recognizing that nursing is a demanding discipline we sincerely hoped that students would take these caring relationships with them as they transition into the work environment.

Class Community

One of the small but priceless choices we recently made was to create time in the classroom for announcements of various topics at the start of the class. As all graduating students are in one place, we had many requests from other years for 5 minutes of our class time from student groups in earlier years, faculty, and the various individuals within the department. At first this truly interfered with the timing of the class as presentations and simple messages ran longer than the short time they had requested. In addition to faculty and others wishing to connect with the group as a whole, students also needed time to share their planning and announcements. This included their Nursing Gala, graduation, fundraising events and activities, volunteer groups as well as updating activities from the student nurses' associations and other professional clubs. At present, we leave 30 minutes at the beginning of the class as well as additional time following breaks for class community time. Through validation, this much-needed arrangement to communicate allowed for students to have a voice into the schedule and demonstrated our respect for their needs.

Pecha Kuchas

During our early years we presented leadership theorists and approaches offering knowledge on how these ways of thinking were developed over time and how they are lived in organizations. Piera implemented a unique approach to learning leadership theory by asking groups of students to develop a "Pecha Kucha." The unique approach of Pecha Kucha was designed by Klein and Dytham (2020) in Tokyo and has been widely adopted by others as an alternative presentation style. Pecha Kucha asks the presenter or group to share 20 images for 20 seconds and the entire presentation lasted for exactly 6 minutes and 40 seconds. The authors of the presentation must know the information well and be succinct in the time allotted. In addition, at the end of each leadership presentation, our students were asked to develop a provocative question on the topic of the Pecha Kucha for the audience of students to engage with. At first, we did not allow enough time for this discussion to evolve but over time we learned to embrace the importance of creating a classroom based on dialogue where students feel safe to wrestle with ideas presented by peers and by teachers. It was amazing to watch the learning unfold as students began talking with each other in a professional manner where they openly asked for clarification of different comments, ideas, and perspectives. The depth of conversation enabled students to voice the personal meanings that were embedded in their assumptions, sharing their ideas out loud and in public, empowering them to own their values and beliefs. As teachers, it was heart-warming to hear students build on and/or demystify each other's comments to seek mutual understanding, developing trust and community—all on their own. We simply supplied time and space and watched the magic happen.

Leadership Challenge

Once we decided to change our teaching format and delivery of the leadership class (after our second year of teaching the course), we deliberated on sample textbook leadership case studies and wondered if we could use this idea and adapt it to a more dynamic approach including real-life case studies. Instead of prescribed cases that occurred as historical examples, we would invite leaders who were currently or recently implementing a significant change within their agency or healthcare center. Each of the seven community leaders invited would present their "Leadership Challenge" and set up the parameters of the issue, omitting outcomes, solutions, or resolutions to the problem. The situations from the invited community leaders were unique and complex; for example, one leader was implementing medical assistance in dying in her community; two leaders of multi-leveled long-term care residential facilities needed to organize how to move all the residents from old facilities to new buildings; and another leader was implementing electronic health records within an acute-care emergency department. Many of the leaders were either previous guest speakers, graduated students, or colleagues and there was a lot of energy and commitment to make this learning experience come to life.

Students were placed in groups of eight and given 2 weeks in which to "don" their leadership hats and develop a well-designed approach, complete research, and map out a plan to deal with the leadership challenge presented. The guest leaders would return to the class several weeks later for a second visit where students presented a summary on how they would handle the challenge, including rationale, any research pertaining to the approach, as well as identifying issues that were unresolved. The invited leaders would then give feedback to their plan and offer the approach to the challenge they implemented as well as the issues they faced or did not anticipate.

The assignment required a lot of organization and preplanning but overall, we were very pleased with the students' thoughtful plans and the depth of insight into the learning challenge. The community leaders were committed and engaged, and we repeated this activity the next year with many of the same leaders. Students, in their evaluations, stated that this activity was realistic and offered them insights into the world of leadership with examples of situations that face those who lead in healthcare settings. The students appreciated the unpredictability of the challenges and had to sort through numerous factors where they had only partial information. This level of experiential learning enabled students to be creative, to develop a high level of thinking skills, and test out their learning in real time.

During this time, we realized that we had exhausted this activity and began building other unique learning situations. The following year, we organized a Health Fair where eight healthcare agencies visited our students one afternoon presenting on what Health Authority can offer the new graduate as employment, educational incentives, and other topics. On-going change and development have become a part of the leadership course evolution.

Professional Learning Reflections

In the nursing program all practice courses, and some theory classes, ask students to submit professional learning reflections to show their thinking as they link their learning to nursing insights, practice, and beliefs systems. These submissions are due anywhere from two to four times per semester, depending on the needs and level of the learner. Reflective thinking and writing promote students to fully engage in the process of "meaning making" (Costa & Kallick, 2008; Mezirow, 1990). As faculty we understand that reflecting on learning is also intrinsically linked to metacognition and self-regulation that enhances the student's ability to integrate insights into their learning and life experiences as well as make better choices and improve learning. Self-reflection also has the added bonus of enhancing self-regulation, an imperative to the development of a professional nurse. Learning reflections are submitted to faculty members who then comment, question, name, and help students deepen their thinking. In the leadership class we have used reflections numerous times as a mechanism to evaluate student-learning modules, to provide self-identified evidence of the integration of theory into understanding, and as a way of valuing their thoughts and beliefs. When students engage in the practice of self-assessment, as part of the measurement of learning, they are taking full responsibility for their role as an active educational member.

Faculty Synergy

Through the years of working together, I (Piera) continued to be in awe of Lynn's capacity to show love and caring in the way she connected with students, not just a few but all of them. Lynn took time to know each student deeply, their strengths, or their challenges caused by internal and/or external factors. When students have a learning question, they would feel comfortable in speaking with Lynn, either in class or in office hours. It is through this connected knowing that students feel like they are being taught by someone who truly cares about them, opening themselves up for learning and change. In developing relationships with students, Lynn brought out each student's unique strengths, and respected their lived experiences as their truths. Lynn's genuineness in helping students to learn shines through in the way she nurtures the student's capacity. Instead of assuming the role of evaluator, Lynn takes on the role of a supportive coach to maximize each student's potential to do their best work.

Both of us have strengths, but Piera is a wise woman who shows a deep respect for others in a gentle and supportive manner. She listens in a way that is exceptional, hearing people in what they say, valuing them without criticism or judgment. She brings a wealth of knowledge and experience with her and has the uncanny ability to help link learning and concepts. She embraces Freire's (1985) ways of "being in" helping students name and identify their world. In this way they can speak about their concerns in an enlightened approach. The observation of strengths she provides in a calm and unhurried approach gives the students the feeling that she has all the time in the world for them. This is an unusual gift as many of us rush through our lives and forget that we are here to help students learn. She is a great example of embracing Socratic methods of questioning and probing and as a role-model, she lives the experience for others to see and feel. I believe it is within this mutual caring and respectful relationship that we share that enables us to provide a positive learning environment.

One common theme we share is our strong beliefs and values of students as learners; students as unique individuals who have lived great lives before stepping into our classrooms. The Caring Curriculum constantly reminds us to treat students as human beings and "one size does not fit all" when it comes to meaningful learning.

CONTENTIOUS INSTITUTIONAL DOGMA: GRAPPLING WITH THE ACADEMIC GRADING SCALE

The Caring Curriculum is rooted in consciousness that reciprocates between students and teachers. Learning is a conscious journey. Giving constructive feedback is an essential part of a nurse's work. Learning to give and receive feedback in ways that are supportive and meaningful has been a challenging lesson to learn. The academic grading scale has caused many points of tension for both of us as teachers involved in the leadership course. Questions that we posed included: How can I place a value on the learning process? As educators, our role and passion are to help students learn. Learning is a very personal experience and there are multiple paths. While it is easy to assign a grade based on a final destination, we question what other meaningful stops are missed by the evaluator. For example, driving through the mountains, there are so many vistas that one can easily miss if we focus only on a final destination. Through our struggles, we have learned to give respect and acknowledgement to the vista points that students have visited by having learning dialogues with them as part of the evaluation process. Seeking to understand the paths students have taken, either by choice or necessity, helps us to be cognizant of their journey. When we take time to dialogue and seek multiple truths, we are more open to appreciate the learning that students have gained along the way; their paths may be different than mine, but no less meaningful.

Over the past few years, we have been moving away from the notion of marking. It has caused the two of us to have many opportunities for discussion while grappling with institutional and departmental norms and what we believe is critical for learning and learners. Nursing is highly competitive and first-year nursing students state that they need to obtain straight As to gain entry into the program which sets them up for placing additional pressure on themselves throughout their course of study. We see this competition continue as they work through their 4 years of education. This belief system of "straight As" sets them up for unrealistic standards and increased stress when grades become the defining characteristic of success. However, marks are extrinsic motivators that create unnecessary competition when teamwork and caring are the goals we wish to foster in nursing students.

Over the past seven years we have consciously decided to focus more on providing meaningful, timely, in-person, and written feedback to nurture learning rather than measuring learning through rigid grade scales. We have developed a more relaxed notion of grades as we see them as not so important or even accurate estimates of learning. At the start of the semester we inform the learners that our goal is to help them grow and our focus is not on marks but on learning. We are thoughtful with grading and many students continue to achieve high marks. We will provide an example of one situation that exemplifies the absurdity of marking.

Most recently, we have worked through some alarming discomforts when marking students' work that has challenged our thinking. In one particular assignment we ask students to develop a paper, poem, or art form depicting their beliefs about nursing—their personal philosophy. Notably, in the assignments we grade personal reflections on what nursing means to the individual student nurse. During marking we found an overwhelming quantity (read most) of exceptional work that showed compassion, caring, and courage (two poems are included in this chapter). As teachers we have shared these profound stories with one another and cried at the insights and poignancy of many. We have been moved by individual's experiences as a child, or a family member with a heart attack, death of a grandmother or sister, that drew them to nursing. These are fascinating stories of rendered lives seen through the eyes of nursing and caring. Each student had their unique way of interpreting their beliefs and we were deeply moved. We feel that it is an honor to be reading these personal and intimate views on their life experiences that are shaping them as caring professionals. However, there was a powerful moral challenge that became more difficult as we read and grappled with questions of: "What grade do I give?" "Do I have a right to place a value on this paper?" "Who am I to say this is right or wrong, an A or a B paper?" As we struggled to think of what to do, we came to the realization that all students should be given full marks. This was the beginning of our shared philosophy shift from grading to ungrading (Stommel, 2018).

CARITAS: EVIDENCE FROM PRAXIS

Looking at our revisioning of the leadership class we wondered what markers we embodied that illustrate our commitment to a Caring Curriculum. Watson (2007) outlines 10 Caritas processes that are hallmarks to creating a caring environment. "Carita" is Latin for love and compassion. In reviewing each carita we explored our journey and mapped out the measure of how we each met these criteria. For instance, positive self-exploration can be a difficult task; as humans it is easier to find flaws, issues, and areas for improvement. Together we shared stories of kindness we saw in each other's work through teaching leadership that helped us create a classroom that is positive and formative for students' growth.

1. Practicing Loving-Kindness Within the Context of an Intentional Caring Consciousness

We believe that we live the reality of loving-kindness in our daily actions with students. In preparation for this piece of writing we shared with each other what we love and respect in the other.

We have embraced ways of being that support caring, loving ways. In particular, giving time outside the classroom to listen, individually, to students' concerns is something we have tried to build into the learning and in the assignments. Both of us have carved out time to review students' learning both individually and in working groups. For example, after the Pecha Kucha presentations, Piera meets with each group of students to review their work, providing positive feedback on content and delivery. She supports them in their learning and students are appreciative of her time and solid, supportive feedback. No group of students opts out of these meetings and I have heard lovely comments about Piera's meetings. As novel strategies work with groups, we then build in additional time to these approaches and look for new ways to value students either individually or in groups.

Another example is when Lynn meets with all the students who wish to review their résumé assignment and two letters: one of introduction and the other a thank you letter. In this way she helps students identify their assets and experiences that show their commitment to nursing, assessment, team building, leadership, or other strengths. These meetings are time consuming as they can take up to 45 minutes but offer real pleasure to Lynn. Through these meetings, Lynn has the opportunity to see the type of people we are educating and helping to shape the students' concepts of themselves through positive affirmations.

In writing letters to guest speakers, Lynn always envisions writing to the most valued person she knows and letting the deep feelings of fealty and respect show through. In this way letters are compelling and genuine heart-felt tributes to those who receive them.

In addition to giving time outside the classroom, we are both open to students' situations such as extending deadlines without penalty. Students have complex lives and at times find themselves in difficult situations. Last year, we had several young women who had experienced deaths in their families as well as experienced personal complex illnesses. We extended deadlines for assignments, provided the in-class exam as a take-home exam, and offered one-on-one opportunities to hear their stories and appreciate their situations. It is during these times that students offer their profound thanks to both of us for the way we offer the class and the deep learning they encountered.

2. Being Fully Present in the Moment and Acknowledging the Deep Belief System and Subjective Life World of Self and Other

In our classroom discussions we often take the lead on certain parts in which we have developed expertise. We each listen to each other speak, nodding and showing strong listening skills as a model for the students. It also shows respect and thoughtfulness. We enjoy listening to each other and to hear the stories the other offers.

During one class we had a cohort of licensed practical nursing (LPN) students within the group. My father had died 2 weeks prior and as Piera was speaking in class, I stopped listening, thinking of my father and my loss. I thought that I had quickly recovered, shook my head, and regained my composure and commenced listening. After class one of the LPN students came to my office and asked me how I was as she noted that I had looked far away and she knew something was wrong. I recalled looking at her, knowing she had seen me during this time when I was so distracted. I wondered if I should share, but then told her my father had recently died and I was thinking of him. I was so touched by her kindness in seeing me and recognizing something was wrong. Despite not knowing what that was she showed courage to ask me about myself. Later I wondered how many other students had seen my lapse and recognized something was wrong for me. I realized that this student and others see right through us. They also see our genuine respect for each other, that we like each other and are admiring of each other's gifts and knowledge. We are seen as authentic and students notice the mutual respect we share and lack of tension between us.

Piera has many strengths that she brings to the classroom; she is calm, provides thoughtful answers, never hurries to give an answer, speaks when necessary, supports others, never gossips, and is well respected by all. Piera's real strength is her ability to link the learning with what the student offers in classroom dialogue. In addition, she asks provocative questions which extend the student's thinking and pondering. Recently, she has been asked to be chair of the Evaluation and Curriculum committees, and most recently also asked to be cochair of our nursing department.

3. Cultivating One's Own Spiritual Practices With Comprehension of Interconnectedness That Goes Beyond the Individual

We strive to connect with students and to fully understand them as persons. For us it is not about the assignment, it is about who they are. We attempt to use a place of unknowing to connect with students, not treating them as if they are all the same. You must get to know them, and in getting to know them, you respect who they are and what they come with.

4. Developing and Sustaining Helping–Trusting, Authentic Caring Relationships

Over time, and collaboratively, we have developed our belief system to incorporate a trusting–helping way of being with students and each other. We have attempted to walk the same path and share the uncomfortable times when activities did not work out well, and envision ways to make change. The process continues, giving each other the courage to support to make those changes. We then deliberately try to notice things about each other and tell others. We often stay after work to work with students. We look at ways to meet the students' needs when they are overwhelmed with assignments or other issues as a way of caring. We role-model safe space for disagreement and by bringing forward different perspectives.

5. Being Present to and Supportive of the Expression of Positive and Negative Feelings Arising in Self and Others With the Understanding That All of These Feelings Represent Wholeness

We strive to be OK with what worked and what did not work in the classroom and to be able to laugh about it and give ourselves permission to move on. Our ultimate desire is to do the best we can for the learner. We see ourselves as nurses, with different and complementary strengths and understandings, and these attributes provide a wholeness in the classroom.

6. Creatively Using All Ways of Being, Knowing, and Caring as Integral Parts of the Nursing Process

Everyone loves a story and so do students or learners. It allows them to delve into the emotion of the moment and stories help to give examples to the content that we are trying to convey. As teachers, we both engage in storytelling to highlight the essence of what we are trying to teach and then they can grasp the concepts.

7. Engaging in Genuine Teaching/Learning Experiences That Arise From an Understanding of Interconnectedness

We have developed a mutual respect for each other that is recognizable. Teaching together has been the best teaching experience for both of us. Our shared working space is a safe environment; we trust each other wholeheartedly; it is authentic without requiring us to assume a different persona. We can be ourselves with each other.

8. Creating and Sustaining a Healing Environment at Physical/ Readily Observable Levels and Also at Non-Physical, Subtle Energy, and Consciousness Levels, Whereby Wholeness, Beauty, Comfort, Dignity, and Peace Are Enabled

A 6-hour class is a long time for anyone, so to add some distraction Piera came up with the idea of offering an energizer activity. We asked students if they would be willing, at certain points in the class, to offer an activity that would re-engage learners when they were tired after an intense guest speaker. This activity provided an opportunity for students to play a role in reawakening consciousness levels, appreciate one another and their gifts, plus provide some needed humor and connectedness. And it was fun. Activities included a sing along, physical movement, and guided meditation.

The nursing philosophy assignment offered a wondrous activity that embodies beauty, awakenings of inner potential, and peace (highlighted earlier). The assignment asked students to share their thoughts about what it means for them to be a nurse. This activity could take any form: art, music, poetry, writing, anything that spoke to the student. Students shared many aspects of their lives as part of the philosophy as the guidelines were not overly prescriptive. They shared why they became nurses, from experiences that perhaps were not positive to highly positive times during their lives, such as when a father was having a heart attack, personal hospitalization as a child, death of a mother or grandmother, giving birth, and such. Each student identified that coming into nursing gave them the opportunity to make something meaningful out of their experiences or life to date. One young woman sang a song, another prepared a collage, but all were moving and very personal.

As part of the learning, we invited guests to speak about antistigma and this provided students with an opportunity to hear about two individuals' experiences and what it is like to live in poverty and with addiction. The speakers challenged our students to undo and to re-create their previous assumptions. Later, some students made connections with these individuals to meet later in order to deepen their knowledge. This experience helped to develop consciousness to treat marginalized people in a different way. It also provided deeper conversations inside the classroom as well as in other classes and venues.

9. Administering Human Care Essentials With an Intentional Caring Consciousness Meant to Enable Mind-Body-Spirit Wholeness in All Aspects of Care; Tending to Spiritual Evolution of Both Other and Self

We were fortunate enough to attend the Caring Conference in Victoria in October 2019. The intentional caring consciousness happened for the two writers at the caring conference. It was a nurturing, inspiring time that energized us and we returned to our home institution speaking glowingly of our experiences. The conference helped to clarify our view of our program in a larger view and highlighted our current focus on health and our need to deepen teaching on healing aspects.

As we have said in Caritas #1, we see the students as people and provide caring to them in terms of reorganizing exams and assignments in the event of family deaths, illnesses, and other situations that delay or interfere with their classroom or assignment deadlines, without penalty.

10. Opening and Attending to Spiritual-Mysterious and Existential Dimensions of Existence Pertaining to Self and Others

As women, we are comfortable with where we are in life. We are open to different ways of seeing the world. We embrace taking a stance and working outside of the boundaries that are created for us within the institution. Within the last year, we moved into a new, state-of-the-art building and one of the rules was that we were not permitted to put anything on the walls. This was made clear only after I had hung a painting outside my office, made by a student in an art contest. The painting is small, colorful, animated, and emotional. Despite finding out about these rules, I have not taken this picture down. In addition, we hung a photograph of the four faculty who attended the Caring Conference along with Marcia Hills and Jean Watson, signifying our attendance and announcing our pleasure and dedication to the foundation of our curriculum.

How do you measure the learning and meaning that students give to the classroom environment? Of course, we use midterm and end-of-semester feedback to help guide our planning for the next year to improve and refine what worked and what did not. However, a real marker for our success is seen in our invitation for previous graduates to come and speak with the leadership students. Each year we have a surprising number who swap shifts, take a day off, or take their lunch hour in order to come and speak about their experiences as new graduates. It is such a rich experience for the students, and us, to hear sage words from people who were sitting in their seats only 1 year ago. Students are riveted by the dialogue and sharing of words of wisdom such as "NCLEX® prep," adapting to the workplace, being charge nurse, and other topics. Each year we allow more time for the question and answer period to satiate the students' questions.

NEXT STEPS: KEEPING US ON OUR TOES

As we move through our discomfort with assignments and exams, we enlisted assistance from colleagues within the institution who support innovative approaches to learning and teaching, called Centre for Excellence in Learning (CIEL). We individually attended an "Unmarking" session to help faculty unravel from the vicious cycle of marking to instead providing feedback. Then we met again with CIEL to help us further alter our thinking and ways of being in the Leadership classroom. This was highly productive in helping us see alternatives to reduce the marking and to add more ways of giving feedback.

In the coming year, we plan to continue our understanding of unmarking and engage with students' work through feedback rather than grading. We plan to develop what Freire calls the "problem-posing" educational approach whereby more questions are asked than answered. When students are requested to share their ideas, we all engage in a space rich in relationships and dialogue. Students are asked to complete reflections throughout the course to see how their learning is unfolding throughout the half-semester and to assign a grade to their efforts.

Interestingly, when an individual is asked to assess their own work or performance on an assignment or project, most give a fair or lower estimate of what we might assign. Our sense is that most students will provide a fair and honest assessment of their learning throughout the term. We also reserve the right to elevate or reduce a mark a student has self-assigned. In some of the literature, what is most commonly seen is that students tend to give themselves lower marks than a faculty member might assign. We look forward to sharing this approach with our students this fall and anticipate some discomfort in their responses. Being aware of student concerns and answering their queries will be important to how this works. We believe that learning in communities should be a "nonhierarchical vision of human connectedness" (Gilligan, 1982, p. 62).

SUPPORTING A CARING CURRICULUM

As faculty who have taught in the Caring Curriculum nursing program for many years, we have seen a drift from the intended philosophical underpinnings that guide the curriculum. Many questions arise as to why the drift has occurred, such as: Are the faculty well-versed in the tenets of the curriculum? What does it look like to live these beliefs and to support the students' learning? What is it that new faculty need to be conversant and confident about and to work with the philosophy and feel ready? In the early years of the Caring Curriculum, conferences were held annually to connect faculty across different schools to share dialogue, practices, and to learn from each other.

We feel new and seasoned faculty need to be well versed in the curriculum and its under-pinnings in order to help students pull through concepts in their learning and ready them for changing practice situations. Nursing education has become more complex, continuously evolving such that academic institutions need to recognize that nursing is a discipline that requires scholarship, research, and creativity. The need to have dedicated time for curriculum dialogue and discourse has become ever more important to create common understandings of how to shape and take ownership of the Caring Curriculum. It is imperative that we take on the opportunity to clearly identify what we (as nurse educators) value as nursing and how we choose to advance the discipline when there is immense pressure to conform to an industrious way of providing care. Content saturation in the nursing curriculum is counterproductive to the caring culture of students' learning environment because students learn in relationships with their teachers. A bonsai tree is admired for its enduring strength and beauty with just a few thoughtfully chosen branches. A concept-based curriculum is well-positioned for our students to pivot and thrive in a complex environment. Together, we need to ask, "How are we living the curriculum?" "What does caring look like, sound like, and feel like in nursing educa-tion and in nursing practice?" "What if we make learning less stressful and more impactful?" "What if we spend more time measuring learning in terms of caring practices than measuring for grades?" "What if we reclaim nursing as Caring Science?"

FINAL THOUGHTS

Aligning ourselves with the students' learning needs and developing relationships rather than focusing on the content has become our focus. We are also looking at ways to avoid the "throw-away" assignment and to develop activities that continually build on students' knowledge and leadership development. We see our responsibility is to organize challenges and opportunities for students to "try on roles" of leadership, decision-making, delegation, and confrontation. We continue to search for novel ideas and learning situations that are uniquely nursing and to provide students realistic examples to work through. We continue to scrutinize ourselves, "go out on a limb" with ideas, cogitate and share thoughts that encourage innovation and daring in activities to enhance and stimulate learners. The work to continue to develop our teaching philosophy and put it into action is stimulating and ever changing; while exciting and rewarding, it is well worth the effort.

PHILOSOPHY OF NURSING: EXAMPLES OF EXCELLENCE

We have included two poems from previous students, now graduates, who have agreed to share their names and their work on their nursing philosophy.

My Nursing Philosophy by Rachel Hollett
Shaking hands, knees knocking
Deep breath, "Good morning. . .
I'll be your nurse."
No answer, forewarning
Shake off my tiredness
Forget my hunger
It doesn't seem like you have much longer

Wash your face,
Comb your hair
Your son comes in
I find him a chair
I come back in the room
And he is crying
Tucked into bed, you lay drowning
Gurgling, muffled,
Agonizing breaths
"Is she in pain?"
The chase of death

I hold your hand
As you lay dying
Look at your family
Realize we're all crying
And then it comes
Sweet relief
Gone the flicker of life
Our time together so brief
I close your eyes
Releasing your stare
Care for you gently,
Like you're truly still there

Half the days gone,
I'm back sitting at home
You're gone now,
But I'm not truly alone

> My focus, my efforts, everything I could do
> A tiny piece of my heart
> You've taken with you

We had the privilege of speaking with Rachel most recently and she reflected on her first year as a registered nurse and her thoughts, today, on her poem. She was deeply moved as she recalled and began to speak about her poem and reflected on her practice and how these feelings coalesce in her daily work. She shared tidbits about working as a new nurse: the support from teammates, the enjoyment and pleasure she finds in nursing, the positive work environment, the need to debrief with colleagues, walking on night shift to gain a sense of proportion, and healing while on shift and to gain wellness. What was truly amazing was her appreciation for the patient, speaking of the profound responsibility and honor it is to care for people. Rachel also offered that the poem was written as a compilation of the experience of the death of her grandmother as well as a patient she had cared for during a practicum.

Below is another poem, shared by Autumn. In her words, Autumn summarizes her reasons for becoming a nurse: My decision to become a nurse was influenced following the time I spent at a pediatric hospital. My son fell very ill with bacterial meningitis when he was 6 months old. He went undiagnosed for 6 days in a local hospital but when he became septic, we were flown to a tertiary center. The care we received was phenomenal. The nurses integrated me, as the mother, in all my son's care. They empowered me by listening to my fears and concerns. The nurses inspired my desire to become a nurse so that I could provide the same compassionate care for other people. When I reflect on the care we received, I can now see how purposeful and therapeutic it really was. I will forever be grateful for the nurses who cared for us.

Nurses – Superheroes in Scrubs by Autumn McIvor

> My son fell very ill and weak
> I knew there was something wrong.
> I took him to the hospital,
> We were admitted before too long.
>
> He was very dehydrated,
> So they tried to start an IV.
> Seven tries before they got it in
> It was so impossibly hard to see.
>
> He cried in weak whimpers,
> I sobbed to see him so.
> I remember my distress like it was yesterday,
> although this was years ago.
>
> I wouldn't leave the room,
> I wouldn't leave his side.
> Too scared that I would lose him.
> For days and days, I did bide.

The nurses came and assessed him,
They hid their fear quite well.
My baby was so sick,
This time for me was hell.

Nurses asked how I was coping
In my darkest hour.
When they saw I wasn't taking care of myself?
They made me take a shower.

When the nurse saw I was scared to hold him
With all the tubes and lines.
She picked him up and put him in my arms
To remind me he was mine.

The nurses trusted my intuition,
Advocated to the doctors about my fears.
When I was feeling overwhelmed,
They stayed to dry my tears.

The nurses kept me informed
About what was going on.
They involved me in my baby's care
So, I wasn't just a pawn.

When it came time to be discharged
I was frightened to take him home with me.
They encouraged and showed their faith
To show how capable I would be.

I remember how the nurses made me feel,
How they cared for me and my son.
They inspired me to become a nurse,
So I could pass the same compassion on.

REFERENCES

Belenky, M. F., Clinchy, B. M., Goldberger, N. R., & Tarule, J. M. (1986). *Women's ways of knowing: The development of self, voice, and mind* (Vol. 15). Basic books.

Bevis, E. O., & Watson, J. (1989). *Toward a caring curriculum: A new pedagogy for nursing*. National League for Nursing.

Costa, A. L., & Kallick, B. (Eds.). (2008). *Learning and leading with habits of mind: 16 essential characteristics for success*. Association for Supervision and Curriculum Development.

Freire, P. (1985). *The politics of education*. Bergin & Garvey.

Gilligan, C. (1982). *In a different voice: Psychological theory and women's development*. Harvard University Press.

Hills, M., & Watson, J. (2011). *Creating a Caring Science curriculum: An emancipatory pedagogy for nursing* (1st ed.). Springer Publishing Company.

Klein, A., & Dytham, M. (2020). *Pecha Kucha*. https://www.pechakucha.com/about

Mezirow, J. (1990). How critical reflection triggers transformative learning In J. Mezirow & Associates (Eds.), *Fostering critical reflection in adulthood: A guide to transformative and emancipatory learning*. Jossey-Bass.

Stommel, J. (March 11, 2018). *How to ungrade* {Blog Post]. https://www.jessestommel.com/how-to-ungrade

Vancouver Island University and North Island College. (2016). *Bachelor of Science in nursing curriculum guide*. British Columbia, Canada.

Watson, J. (2007). Watson's theory of human caring and subjective living experiences: Carative factors/*caritas processes* as a disciplinary guide to the professional nursing practice. *Texto & Contexto - Enfemagem, 16*(1), 129–135. https://doi.org/10.1590/S0104-07072007000100016

Zawaduk, C., Duncan, S., Mahara, M. S., Tate, B., Callaghan, D., McCullough, D., Chapman, M., & Van Neste-Kenny, J. (2014). Mission possible: Twenty-five years of university and college collaboration in baccalaureate nursing education. *Journal of Nursing Education, 53*(10), 580–588. https://doi.org/10.3928/01484834-20140922-04

Evolution of a Caring-Based College of Nursing

Anne Boykin, Theris Touhy, and Marlaine Smith

HISTORY AND BACKGROUND OF THE PROGRAM

The story of the evolution of the nursing program in the Christine E. Lynn College of Nursing at Florida Atlantic University (FAU) was originally described in a book written by the faculty and edited by the dean: *Living a Caring-Based Program* (Boykin, 1994). Following is a description of the early years of the program as presented in Chapter 1 of that book. Our evolution is a story of commitment, passion, innovation, and caring for an idea of nursing and helping it grow. The program began in 1979 with the establishment of an upper-division nursing program for registered nurses, the first such program at a public university in our area. Although our numbers were small (four faculty members, a consultant director, and 10 registered nurse [RN] to bachelor's degree [BSN] students), we were blessed with an opportunity that allowed us the freedom to create our concept of nursing and to explore innovative teaching strategies. We were not yet aware of the many implications of our task, nor were we bound by what had come before.

Our talented RN to BSN students were leaders in the nursing community and masters of their skill. They had achieved a high level of success in the profession, and they challenged us with the question: "We are expert nurses; what more do we need to learn about nursing?" They forced us to continually think about nursing as a concept, apart from skills, techniques, and the medical model in which we had all been schooled. We shared our ideas about what was important in nursing practice and our hopes and dreams for how nursing practice could be improved. As we studied the concept of nursing and its essence, we began to filter nursing from non-nursing content in an effort to articulate the essence of our discipline. Among our early influences were the values and teaching work of Sid Simon and Jay Clark (1975) and Diane Ustal's (1977) work on values clarification in nursing. Our teaching/learning philosophy was one of openness and mutuality, which yielded a healthy respect for learning from and with each other. The theories of Martha Rogers (1970), Madeline Leininger (1981), Jean Watson (1979), and Paterson and Zderad (1976) assisted us to more fully reflect on the discipline of nursing. Caring for self and other emerged as an essential framework for nursing in those early years.

With plans to begin a generic program in 1982, additional faculty members were hired and a full-time director was appointed. The dialogue on caring as a concept of great depth in the discipline took on new dimensions. Our original curriculum, like many others at that time, was organized using a general systems theory framework. Yet, our philosophy at that time hinted at our real values, as illustrated in this statement from the 1981 philosophy: "The foundation of professional caring is the blending of humanistic, scientific, and nursing theories. Humanistic caring is the creative, intuitive, and cognitive aspects of the helping process." Through the process of preparing for accreditation, faculty members began to identify those aspects of the philosophy, and particularly the framework for the curriculum, which did not fully express where we were in our thinking about nursing.

This was an exciting time for faculty members to focus on the essence of the discipline, our beliefs about nursing, and how we could create a program of study that reflected these beliefs and values. Faculty members began to ask difficult questions, such as: do we want to continue teaching nursing as we have been, or shall we take the risk and ask the question: what is the content of the discipline that should be taught? All faculty members realized that the classroom content being taught was predominantly medical science. We struggled to know what, in fact, was the content of the discipline. The process of discovery began by evaluating the syllabi for existing courses. The first step was easy. All the content that was not specific to nursing was sorted out. A decision was made to place all of the pathophysiology, pharmacology, and assessment content into separate courses. The question became, what content would fill the remaining gaps? If we were no longer approaching the study of nursing through diseases, then what was the content of the discipline to be studied?

We began to meet regularly, and by sharing our individual stories of nursing practice, we began to believe that if they were shared with students, the content of nursing would be known. This process was long, confusing, exciting, scary, and continuous. Omission of its de- tails should not lead the reader to believe the process was simple and without painful struggles. Throughout our dialogue, the importance of caring as a unique concept in nursing continued to unfold. Many factors nurtured and influenced the growth of this concept. Mayeroff's book, *On Caring* (1971), was and continues to be a required text in our program because it offers a generic way of knowing self and other as caring person. Paterson and Zderad's book, *Humanistic Nursing* (1976), also had a significant influence on the evolution of the curriculum. Their ideas about the phenomenon of nursing, nursing situations, and call and response seemed to fit with our concept of nursing. Carper's (1978) ways of knowing helped broaden our understanding of the range of knowledge needed to study and practice nursing. We questioned: what it means to be caring; how caring is lived in nursing; can caring be taught; and how best to teach caring? Roach's exquisite works describing the manifestations of caring and the attributes or qualities demonstrated in the professionalization of caring helped us answer these questions and move forward to establish a program of study grounded in caring. The works of many other scholars were brought forward for ongoing dialogue. The theory of Nursing as Caring (Boykin & Schoenhofer, 2001) has had a significant influence on our philosophy and programs of study. However, our faculty did not ascribe to any particular framework; instead, we created our own statements of belief on caring.

Many things have changed in the 40 years since we began caring for an idea of nursing and helping it grow. What has not changed is our passion for nursing, the love of nursing as a unifying body, and the belief that nursing offers a unique and invaluable service to human persons—caring. Through the scholarly work of our faculty members and our students, we continue to reflect upon, develop, celebrate, and share the values that called each of us to the human service of nursing. We continue to evolve in our understanding of teaching nursing grounded in caring and extending and developing the study of the concept of caring. It is our belief that without a focus on caring as an essential domain of nursing knowledge, the nature of nursing cannot be fully understood. Our commitment to creating a College founded on caring includes not only the study of nursing but the cocreation of an environment to foster knowing each other as caring persons and the gifts we bring to this process.

CREATING A CULTURE OF CARING

Beliefs and values of the faculty not only guide the design, implementation, and evaluation of a caring-based program, but they also frame a way of being in relationship with self and other. The Dance of Caring Persons (Boykin & Schoenhofer, 2001) is the model used to express caring relationships. This model (Figure 13.1), etched in the terrazzo floor of the lobby of the College of Nursing building, serves as a constant reminder of right ways of relating grounded in respect for and valuing of each person. The flat aspect of a circle conveys that each dancer brings unique gifts to the work of the College. No one person's gifts are more important than another's—just different due to role. In this way, the College's structure is not represented in a traditional organization chart, but a circular, flat structure depicting interrelationships rather than hierarchy. Each person is viewed as special and caring. Each role is essential to accomplishing the mission and goals of the College. The circle is open as there is always room for others to join the dance. The intent of all dancers is to know other as caring person and support each other in living caring uniquely. The ongoing challenge is to be open to knowing caring in the moment. One aspect of the dance is that each person is engaged in the lifelong process of growing in knowing self and other as caring person. An explicit understanding of what it means to be a person provides direction for being in all relationships—personal and professional.

The declaration that all persons are caring and engaged in caring relationships calls for an understanding of what it means to live caring both in the ordinariness of life and uniquely in the practice of nursing. Mayeroff's (1971) caring ingredients offer a helpful framework for knowing self and other as caring. These ingredients include: knowing, honesty, courage, hope, trust, humility, and alternating rhythm. Faculty members and students reflect on how each of these ingredients is lived uniquely in their lives. This reflection fosters an understanding of self living caring moment to moment. Our commitment to the belief that all persons are caring called for us to intentionally come to know self as caring person in order that we may know others as caring. This personal knowing changed ways of relating. It brought forth the realization that expressions of caring are lived uniquely by each person and the challenge is to grow in an understanding of what it means to live caring.

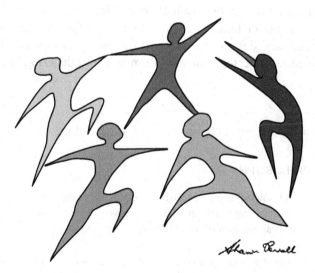

FIGURE 13.1 The Dance of Caring Persons.

Examples of strategies as a faculty to facilitate knowing of self as caring include:

- Retreats that focus time on centering self in order that one may have heightened awareness of unique ways of living caring;
- Structured time for informal dialogue with colleagues on what it means to be a faculty member in a caring-based program;
- Designated time for meditation;
- Opportunities to experience various ways of caring for self, that is, through yoga classes or participating in therapeutic touch sessions offered at the College;
- The study of nursing with students focused on knowing self and other as caring person.

Opportunities for students to know self as caring are integrated throughout their program of study. Students are first introduced to the concept of caring as they tour the College. The building itself was designed to be a "teacher" of caring. When we received the remarkable $10 million gift from Christine E. Lynn (matched by the state of Florida), we decided that our new home would be an expression of caring. It is a healthy, healing place built on principles of sustainability and a commitment to transform nursing education through creation of healing spaces. It is a structure that celebrates and honors the traditions of nursing. Many spaces were intentionally designed to support reflection and knowing of self as caring person. These spaces include a sacred space for meditation, several "outdoor" rooms embraced by a garden with a labyrinth, and a holistic practice area. Students systematically focus on knowing self as caring. The course Caring for Self was created to engage students in exploring knowing self as caring person and in examining the literature on caring for self. Each student is their own "laboratory," experiencing and learning how to make choices supportive of personal well-being. With a curriculum revision the concept of Caring for Self is initiated from the very beginning of the curriculum and culminating course, Creating Healing Environments, invites the student to broaden the knowledge of caring for self in cocreating caring/healing environments for self and other.

THE SHARED STUDY OF NURSING

The shared study of nursing (commonly called the "curriculum") is derived from our philosophy and is based on the understanding of nursing as a professional discipline grounded in caring. The unique focus and defining characteristic of nursing as a social and human service is nurturing the wholeness of persons and environment through caring (Exhibit 13.1). Caring

EXHIBIT 13.1 Florida Atlantic University Christine E. Lynn College of Nursing

STATEMENT OF PHILOSOPHY

Nursing is a discipline of knowledge and professional practice grounded in caring. Nursing makes a unique contribution to society by nurturing the wholeness of persons and environment in caring. See https://nursing.fau.edu/about/college-at-a-glance/philosophy.php

Source: From Philosophy of the Christine E. Lynn College of Nursing (2020). https://nursing.fau.edu/about/college-at-a-glance/philosophy.php

is the essential value held dear to those who choose to be members of a helping profession. To study nursing is to study caring, to grow in understanding of self and other as caring person, and to be committed to the development of caring knowledge and the value of caring to the health and wholeness of persons nursed (Boykin & Schoenhofer, 2001; Touhy & Boykin, 2008).

NURSING SITUATIONS: THE CONTEXT FOR KNOWING NURSING

The concept of the nursing situation guides the study of nursing for faculty members and students in all nursing courses. Faculty members believe that the experience of nursing takes place in nursing situations: lived experiences in which the caring between the nurse and client fosters well-being within a cocreative experience (Christine E. Lynn College of Nursing, 2020). The nurse enters the world of the person nursed with the intention of knowing the other as caring person and coming to know how the other is living caring in the situation and expressing hopes for growing in caring. Within the nursing situation, the nurse attends to calls for caring and creates caring responses that nurture personhood (Boykin & Schoenhofer, 2001).

In each nursing situation there are calls for nursing and a response from the nurse. Identification of the calls for nursing arises from the nurse's intentional full engagement with the one nursed and from the ability of the nurse to draw on a broad knowledge base in order to understand the particular situation. Through authentic presence, as caring person, the nurse is able to enter the world of the other, come to know the other, hear calls for nursing, and respond appropriately to nurture wholeness. Inquiry into nursing situations facilitates student understanding of nursing as a discipline and a professional practice grounded in caring.

In the study of nursing situations, there are no "standard" calls or responses—no predetermined goals or plan of care based on a medical diagnosis. The person nursed is always the focus of the nursing situation. Boykin and Schoenhofer (2001) reflected:

> The challenge for nursing is not to discover what is missing, weakened, or needed in another but to come to know the other as caring person and to nurture the person in situation-specific, creative ways. We no longer understand nursing as a "process" in the sense of a complex sequence of predictable acts, resulting in some predetermined desirable end product. Nursing is, we believe, processual, in the sense that it is always unfolding and that it is guided by intention. To characterize nursing situations with a nursing diagnosis and to portray the situation as a linear process driven by diagnosis or problem to be addressed with a pre-envisioned outcome would be to rob the situation of all the beauty of nursing. (p. 30)

The nurse responds to each call for nursing in a way that represents the uniqueness of the nurse and their own expressions of caring. Each response to a particular nursing situation would be slightly different and would portray the beauty of the nurse as caring person. It is in this way that the art of nursing is created by each nurse in each situation. Sharing this art deepens our understanding of the richness of our practice and provides an opportunity to reflect on the range of knowledge essential to expert nursing care. The following nursing situation, *Where Are They Now*, was created by one of our RN to BSN students. This is an example of a situation which could be used in class to study the nursing of persons who are dying.

Where Are They Now?
Jaime Castaneda, BSN

Hello my friend, my dying friend.
There you lie, an old man, weak and all alone
resting in a bed of thoughts, staring back in time,
gasping for every bit of life you have left,
with no one here to ease your moment but me, your nurse.
I wonder who hides behind such a hopeless look and blank stare.
Were you a crying baby once introduced into this world
by a proud mother,
who showered you with hugs and kisses, hopes and dreams?
Or perhaps a playful child full of energy and imagination
who would grow up to become a teenager in love?
Were you someone's brother, husband, or maybe even a father?
Did you have any friends?
Where is everybody now? Does anybody care?
As we've come to meet, I watch death take you away
and the light within you subsides.
Each breath becomes weaker, and each pulse an eternity.
The moment freezes in time as darkness engulfs your light.
Thus, I watch you being absorbed.
Yet, there is nobody else here but me, your nurse,
to ease your path, share your moment,
hear your silent cry, and bring hope to those hopeless eyes.
The hope that you are not alone, and
that behind the darkness there is a light.
Somehow we've come to meet, as the
writings of your life come to an end,
the terminal lines of your final chapter
become the introductory ones of mine.
Your past, unknown to me,
for the mystery of life is yours to keep.
I witness the pages of your past vanish deep
into your memory and become part of your soul.
Your present, I've come to meet.
An old man dying quietly in a hospital bed,
illuminated by the dim light of a sealed window,
and in the absence of fresh air for your soul to fly away.
Surrounded by an empty room filled with loneliness, and
crowded with memories, with nobody else here but me, your nurse.
Allow me to share this moment with you
and bridge your passage into that new place of endless dreams,
where love, energy and playfulness reign.
Where those arms, that once proudly introduced you into this world,
are anxiously waiting for you,
to shower you again with hugs and kisses, hopes and dreams.
My friend, my old, dying friend.
I wish you could see that you are not alone
and hear my thoughts of you, the patient, the child, the man.
As I contemplate your life for what it might have been
and offer my friendship,

hoping to illuminate the way
to your death with my presence, my true presence.
Good bye my friend.

Students studying this nursing situation might reflect on the following questions:

- Who is the nurse as caring person?
- Who is the person nursed as caring person?
- How is the nurse expressing caring in this moment?
- How might the student's personal knowing or study of the dying experience influence knowledge necessary to understand the nursing situation?
- What empirical knowledge is essential to hear the calls and create responses that nurture wholeness through caring in this situation (e.g., approaches to being-with and communication guided by nursing theories, imminent signs of death, pain assessment and treatment, evidence-based practice protocols and nursing research about care of dying persons, and research questions that might be generated related to spiritual caring, presence, and touch)?
- What ethical knowing is inherent in this situation if nursing is practiced from the perspective of caring? What ethical dilemmas present in care of persons at the end of life and what ethical frameworks would be useful in guiding responses?
- What kind of healing environment ought to be created for dying persons?
- What are the possibilities for growth and nurturance of personhood in this situation?
- What are the hoped-for outcomes of nursing care?

As the nursing situation is retold and relived, nursing knowledge emerges and is developed and shared; knowledge from nursing research and evidence-based practice guidelines are discussed; questions for research are generated; students and faculty members grow in their understanding of caring and caring relationships; and the richness of nursing as a discipline and practice emerges. Studying nursing in this way assists students in developing and celebrating nursing knowledge. They grow in their substantive understanding of caring and their appreciation of caring as nursing's unique contribution to the health and wholeness of persons.

Knowledge from prerequisite and supporting courses in the program of study such as pathophysiology, pharmacology, assessment, technical skills, literature, or psychology is brought to the study of the nursing situation as part of the range of knowledge necessary to hear calls and design nursing responses. This approach appropriately uses content from other disciplines to understand and practice nursing. However, as Touhy states, "while nurses respond to sequelae of illness, these responses should not take precedence over care of persons" (2004, p. 45). Emphasis in nursing courses is on critical reflection and integration of knowledge in specific nursing situations, and creation of nursing responses. The study of caring is integral to knowing nursing and is a focus in each nursing course at all levels of the program. The study of caring requires critical reading of meaningful substantive literature, reflection, dialogue, and incorporation into thoughtful practice (Schoenhofer, 2001).

Nursing situations are clustered within courses based on traditional and social expectations. In the undergraduate program, particular nursing situations from a common setting are grouped by course.

In the master's program, students study nursing situations experienced by nurses at the advanced practice level in a variety of settings depending on the designated major focus or track chosen by the student. Nursing education majors study nursing education in a caring- based curriculum; nursing administration majors focus on the creation of healthcare environments grounded in caring; and nurse practitioner students study caring in nursing situations in primary care and with clients of all ages, depending on the nurse practitioner focus.

The College has two doctoral programs: the Doctor of Philosophy (PhD) and the Doctor of Nursing Practice (DNP). Students in the PhD program focus on the development of Caring Science through research and theory development. Each PhD dissertation contributes to the growth of Caring Science. DNP students focus on transforming systems of care that reflect caring values in their roles as nurse practitioners or nurse administrators. Curriculum plans for all programs of study are accessible on the College's website. The elaboration of the curriculum has been published by Smith (2019).

Evaluation of Caring in Practice

A question often asked is how does one evaluate the professionalization of caring? When the undergraduate program was developed, a Collaborative Nursing Practice Evaluation Tool organized around Roach's "6 Cs" (1987) of compassion, competence, confidence, conscience, commitment, and comportment was developed for student self-evaluation and faculty and preceptor evaluation of the student. Each of the "Cs" was operationalized into expected competencies that students were required to demonstrate at an acceptable level. Table 13.1 provides an example of outcome indicators of "conscience." Students rate themselves on a numerical scale on each of the competencies, and the faculty and preceptor also rate the student both at midterm and at the end of the semester. From the "6Cs," 12 critical behaviors were selected that students were required to demonstrate at a satisfactory level.

The evaluations of graduate students in practicum courses also reflect caring competencies for advanced-practice nursing, administration, education, or advanced-holistic nursing, and are conducted collaboratively with the students, preceptors, and faculty members. Graduate students are expected to journal weekly on their experiences, reflecting on how they came to know the person nursed and how they integrated ways of knowing in hearing and responding to calls for nursing. They also prepare a written or oral presentation of a nursing situation.

TABLE 13.1 Caring Competencies and Outcome Indicators		
CARING COMPETENCIES AND OUTCOME INDICATORS	**MIDTERM RATING**	**FINAL RATING**
Conscience: the morally sensitive self, attuned to values and integral to personhood	self:	self:
	faculty:	faculty:

- Plans care in partnership with patient, honors human dignity, and respects patient's rights and choices
- Demonstrates accountability for own actions
- Analyzes ethical and legal issues in each nursing situation
- Supports fairness, equity, and nondiscrimination in healthcare
- Demonstrates professional caring by considering how to influence systems and policies impacting healthcare
- Demonstrates role of the nurse as advocate in the nursing situation
- Always plans for continuity of care, effectively teaches patients and families

Pedagogical Practices

Pedagogical practices are developed to be consistent with the College of Nursing philosophy on the nature of learning and the Dance of Caring Persons described earlier. Nursing situations studied in class represent the actual lived experience of students and nurses in nursing practice settings. They may come from the experience of the faculty member or the student and may be presented in various art forms (Barry et al., 2015). Students are encouraged to reflect on the uniqueness and beauty of their nursing situations and represent them through some aesthetic form. These aesthetic projects, integrated through all programs of study, illustrate through deep reflection the caring expressed in a nursing situation. Following is a representation of a nursing situation by graduate student Patricia LaMedica.

Human Tide

Together as birth waters broke
Together as your tide recedes
Solid earth moving under waves
Here, riding out this last bit of your storm
Between the living and the dying we touch
Mother-Daughter
Nursed-Nurse
You are slipping away
Like so many grains of sand in my hand
I need you to stay
I whisper for you to go
Oh, your ragged breath
The heaving of your body
In and out
Hypnotic swells that rise and fall
Rogue wave rises up and crashed upon the shore
Angry foam rushes in, swiftly recedes
Your life water whisked away
Leaves me bereft upon the shore.

Other examples of aesthetic representations can be found in Barry et al. (2015). Through the study of nursing situations, students continually focus on who they are as caring persons in a particular nursing situation and how the caring between the participants enhances personhood and nurtures wholeness for both the nurse and person nursed. Through the study of nursing situations, students learn to conceptualize, reflect, think critically, come to know self and others as caring, value and respect person, and ground nursing responses in caring.

Nursing practice course expectations include care maps, weekly reflective journals, facilitated dialogue, and simulated learning. Care maps are completed in undergraduate nursing practice courses. They invite the student to tell the story of the one nursed, identify knowledge needed to practice in this situation using multiple ways of knowing, reflect on self and other as caring person, identify calls for nursing, nursing responses, and evaluative data. These care maps are used instead of a traditional care plan based on the nursing process. The intent is to foster knowing of the one nursed as caring person.

Reflective journaling provides students the opportunity to appreciate the beauty of the nursing experiences they have encountered. Here is one example of a set of questions used in reflection:

- What are the calls for nursing?
- What possible nursing responses might be considered?
- Who is this person as caring person?
- How does this person live caring day to day?
- What is it like for me as student to be in this situation?
- How has reflection on the nursing situation enhanced my knowledge of nurturing the wholeness of person through caring?

Excerpt from a student's reflective journal:

> As I walked into C.J.'s room, I was struck by the contrasting images of a seemingly healthy boy hooked up to so many different machines. Pictures of him, his family and his girlfriend scattered around the room like glimpses of a distant memory, C.J. lay in his bed, almost as if waiting to be woken up by his mom before school. As I approached his bed, he began to convulse in the way that my nurse preceptor had warned me he might. As I watched him, I was moved by the necessity of the caring philosophy in such a time as this. Medically, there was little we could offer C.J. as he was on the proper medications and receiving the appropriate treatment. A student nurse trained in the holistic care of persons, I suddenly realized there was something I could offer him: my authentic presence. Although C.J. was unable to communicate effectively with us, he was still a person complete in that moment and as his student nurse, I was committed to nursing his whole person. Thus, I turned on his cooling blankets, sat by his side and spoke with him. I told him how important he was to the nurses here and how I could tell how important he was to his family and friends without even meeting them. Our conversation may have been one-sided verbally, but somehow I feel that he knew what I was saying to him and it made a therapeutic difference in the large picture enveloping our young man. (Marissa Bradford, undergraduate student)

The Canvas course platform is used successfully for engaging students in discussions of living caring in nursing practice and articulation of how patterns of knowing were integrated into their study of nursing situations. This format allows all students in the course to share their learning, growth, and insights and learn from each other. Presentation of a nursing situation that has been experienced during the course and postconference discussions about nursing situations experienced are also utilized to enhance learning. In postconference discussions, students share: the response to the direct invitation to care (inviting the nursed to help them come to know what matters most; Boykin & Schoenhofer, 2001, p. 59), the range of knowledge necessary to come to know the person nursed, and respond to calls and design responses, the hoped-for outcomes, and their understanding of the mutuality of the caring between.

Simulation is an integral part of practice learning. In each of the courses in the undergraduate program, and several in the master's program, faculty members have created scenarios that are staged in the simulation lab or virtual Lynn hospital with the human patient simulators. These scenarios are developed to engage students in hearing and responding to calls for nursing that include competent performance of technical skills, assessment, and decision-making regarding changes in a patient's vital signs, or providing authentic presence and touch during a time of anguish or fear. Faculty members or graduate teaching assistants assume the roles of family members and other health professionals as the scenario is enacted so that students respond to the totality of a dynamic situation. In the debriefing following enactment of the scenario, students are asked to reflect on the calls for nursing presented in the situation and how their responses reflected Roach's 6 Cs (1987), Mayeroff's (1971) caring ingredients, or concepts from Nursing as Caring (Boykin & Schoenhofer, 2001), or other theories. In this way, students are engaged in reflecting on the salience of caring knowledge to their practice.

Advancing Caring Through Research, Practice, and Service

With the mission, vision, and values of the College grounded in caring, the centrality of caring goes beyond the teaching mission and the educational programs of the College to infuse the research, practice, and service missions as well.

CARING AND THE RESEARCH MISSION

The research mission of the College of Nursing is advancing the body of knowledge of caring in the discipline of nursing. This mission is realized through the organizational structure, faculty recruitment, and a mentoring program for new faculty members. The College of Nursing has an Office of Nursing Research and Scholarship whose purpose is to support faculty members in advancing their programs of research. This Office has an associate dean for Research and Scholarship and two research administrators who support faculty members in preparing grants and in postaward grant management. A well-funded intramural grants program exists to support pilot work with the expectation that this work will lead to proposals for external funding. The criteria for awarding this intramural funding include the development of an explicit connection to advancing caring knowledge. The guidelines for applicants ask, "how does the proposed work emerge from a caring philosophy and fit into your ongoing research program?" Caring knowledge can be conceptualized as particular caring theories or explicit philosophical values that are common to a variety of theoretical perspectives. It is the responsibility of the researcher to establish the connection between their work and the advancement of Caring Science; in this way, the College encourages faculty members to shape their research trajectories within a caring framework.

Faculty recruitment is influenced by the caring values of the College. When prospective faculty members apply for positions, interview questions include queries about their understanding and appreciation of the philosophy and how they view their work within the context of advancing caring knowledge. These questions offer prospective faculty members the opportunity to be reflective and intentional in their choice to join our community. The goal of pursuing research and making scholarly contributions to the body of knowledge related to caring in nursing is understood. For example, faculty members have pursued research programs related to: supportive spousal communication patterns when one of them has dementia; the use of HeartMath® Techniques to reduce stress in parents of preschool children, engaging in integrative nurse coaching to decrease sarcopenia in older women, exploring what matters most to caregivers of people with mild to moderate dementia; and enhancing cancer screening in underserved minority populations. In each of these diverse research projects, the faculty members have made some explicit relationship to caring theories, values, and advancing Caring Science.

Each new faculty member enters a structured mentoring program designed individually to transition the faculty member into this College culture of caring. The program involves engagement of the faculty member with a mentorship team. The team consists of senior faculty members who focus on the new faculty member's growth in all three missions and who can guide the faculty member toward success. Research mentors help new faculty members identify an initial trajectory including sources of funding. Faculty members' growth is nurtured by the associate dean for Research and the research mentors; they support the development of manuscripts, identify opportunities for faculty development in key areas through attendance at educational programs, and guide the faculty members in grant writing. Faculty members are oriented to the College of Nursing philosophy including the salient literature related to caring. Monthly dialogues on integrating caring into teaching are held, and new faculty members are encouraged to attend. New faculty members are connected with more senior faculty members who may be working in related areas. Currently there are four major research focus areas in the College: healthy aging across the lifespan, holistic health, health equity, and transforming healthcare environments. All four of these focus areas have a strong explicit relationship to advancing Caring Science.

Caring and the Practice Mission

Although not identified as a mission distinctive from service, it is useful to focus on practice separately because of its importance to nursing as a professional discipline. The College has focused on its interrelationships with practice through the development of several centers and through partnerships with healthcare organizations. Two centers in the College deliver care to the community. One is the Louis and Anne Green Memory and Wellness Center, whose unique mission is grounded in the College's philosophy of caring. "The mission of the Center is to meet the complex needs of persons with memory disorders and their families through a comprehensive array of services, compassionate and innovative programs of care, research and education" (nursing.fau.edu/outreach/memory-and-wellness-center/index.php). Noteworthy programs, such as caregiver support and art therapy, acknowledge the wholeness and inherent healing capacity of persons and families. The explicit intention of the Center is to "treat the whole person with dignity and respect, enabling each client to function at his or her personal best and to maximize his or her quality of life" (nursing.fau.edu/outreach/memory-and-wellness-center/index.php). The Center's building was specifically designed to house a diagnostic clinic, a dementia-specific adult day center, and counseling and educational and research activities. Baccalaureate, master's, and doctoral students in the College have practice experiences at the Center. In this way, students can witness and engage in nursing practice that reflects the College philosophy. The Center becomes a laboratory where caring is studied and lived.

The FAU College of Nursing Community Health Center is a nurse-led interprofessional practice that provides integrated primary and mental healthcare, and specialty diabetes care to an underserved diverse population with complex healthcare needs. The Center provides social services and telehealth to promote access to care in remote areas. A caring-based model guides the practice.

The Initiative for Intentional Well-Being is located in the College of Nursing and offers programs related to holistic health. For example, yoga classes, healing touch, Reiki classes, and other practices have been offered through the Initiative. The purpose of the Initiative is to integrate holistic caring practices into nursing education and practice.

The Anne Boykin Institute for the Advancement of Caring in Nursing was established in 2011 to serve as a global catalyst for promoting the universal visibility and significance of caring in nursing. Its mission is to provide global leadership for nursing education, practice, and research grounded in caring; to promote the value of caring across disciplines; and to support the mission of the College. The Institute has developed Caring Science resources available for public use and hosts an annual Summer Academy that engages those interested in Caring Science in topics such as Caring Science–based research, teaching from a caring perspective, inteprofessional practice grounded in caring, and social justice and caring (nursing.fau.edu/outreach/anne-boykin-institute/index.php).

Faculty members provide service to the local, state, national, and global communities that reflects the philosophy of the College. For example, several faculty members provide primary care to underserved communities in the geographic service area. Students participate in service learning by partnering with communities to complete projects that are priorities for these communities. Our student organizations are engaged in multiple service projects throughout our communities. One faculty member, Dr. Rhonda Goodman, has developed a thriving study-abroad program in Guatemala and Ecuador focused on service learning. The caring-based model that she developed is being adopted by six other nursing programs.

LOOKING TO THE FUTURE

Several trends affirm the directions taken by our College in building a school dedicated to caring: advancing the science, practicing the art, studying its meaning, and living it day to day. One indicator is that hospitals on the journey toward Magnet® status designation or those with Magnet status (http://www.nursecredentialing.org/Magnet.aspx) must articulate a practice model. Caring frameworks, including Nursing as Caring (Boykin & Schoenhofer, 2001) have been adopted by several hospitals in Florida. Many hospitals across the country are implementing professional practice models based on Watson's theory. Educational-practice partnerships are the logical way to bridge the practice/education gap through transforming practice environments and educating students in real practice laboratories directed by caring theories.

Another example of this growth in interest in bringing Caring Science into the nursing workplace is the Watson Caring Science Institute (www.watsoncaringscience.org) and the consortium of hospitals guided by Watson's theory of human caring. These organizations provide evidence of a movement to change the current healthcare environment to reflect values of compassion, relationship, and creating healing environments.

Next, the Carnegie Report (Benner et al., 2010) on the future of nursing education calls for reforms that have been foundational to the caring-based approach to education within the Christine E. Lynn College of Nursing. This report calls for a situated, contextual approach to learning through the use of narratives, patient interviews, and case studies that engages students in clinical reasoning and clinical imagination. They recommend greater attention to the integration of theory and practice in both classroom and clinical settings. This is consistent with the use of nursing situations in both classroom and clinical learning in clinical conferences. The nursing curricula of the College build upon a strong foundation in arts, humanities, and the sciences and integrate this knowledge, including aesthetics, into learning. Increasing the use of simulation is another recommendation; we have been developing simulations that reflect caring values and provide opportunities for students to integrate caring knowledge within practice. This unique approach to simulation transforms it from an exercise in technical know-how and critical thinking to a rehearsal of ethical comportment and growing ontological competencies (Watson, 1999) so important to living caring in practice situations.

Finally, the College has established the Archives of Caring in Nursing with the mission of preserving the history of Caring in Nursing, inviting the study of Caring, advancing Caring as an essential domain of nursing knowledge, and creating meaning for the practice of nursing. Descriptions and indexes to the collections are accessible on the College's website at nursing.fau.edu/outreach/archives-of-caring. We are committed to securing the papers of Caring scholars and developing and maintaining the Archives to provide access to primary sources. This preserves the caring knowledge of the past as a springboard for knowledge development for the future.

It is evident that the Christine E. Lynn College of Nursing has laid the foundation for the future. The focus on Caring is a part of the organizational structure and culture. It is reflected in the mission, vision, values, and philosophy and is explicitly present in curricular themes, program, and course objectives. The culture of living caring is strong, and as in any culture, it will endure with mentoring and orientation programs.

Our doctoral program focuses on Caring Science. With this emphasis we are establishing a future for the advancement of Caring Science within the discipline and beyond. Those prepared at the doctoral level will bring their research program and the values and approaches to knowledge development underpinning it to other schools of nursing, seeding and growing these ideas in other locations.

With an increasing number of national and international nursing scholars studying Caring, we are considering alternative educational models that can be offered to those who want to study Caring. This could be in the form of a certificate program or an Institute for Caring studies. Sustaining a Caring-based program across time will take a committed group of scholars, continuous reflection on the mission of the College, and consistent community building and outreach. For those of us who believe that the work is essential for the future of the discipline of nursing and the lives of those we nurse, it is a labor of love.

REFERENCES

Barry, C. D., Gordon, S. C. & King, B. M. (2015). *Nursing case studies in caring: Across the practice spectrum.* Springer Publishing Company.

Benner, P., Sutphen, M., Leonard, V., & Day, L. (2010). *Educating nurses: A call for radical transformation* (Carnegie Foundation for the Advancement of Teaching. Preparation for the Professions Program). Jossey-Bass.

Boykin, A. (Ed.). (1994). *Living a caring-based program.* National League for Nursing Press.

Boykin, A., & Schoenhofer, S. (2001). *Nursing as caring.* Jones & Bartlett.

Carper, B. (1978). Fundamental patterns of knowing in nursing. *Advances in Nursing Science, 1,* 13–24. https://doi.org/10.1097/00012272-197810000-00004

Christine E. Lynn College of Nursing. (2020). *Philosophy.* https://nursing.fau.edu/about/college-at-a-glance/philosophy.php

Leininger, M. (1981). *Caring: An essential human need.* Slack.

Mayeroff, M. (1971). *On caring.* Harper & Row.

Paterson, J., & Zderad, L. (1976). *Humanistic nursing.* John Wiley Biomedical Publication.

Roach, S. (1987). *The human act of caring.* Canadian Hospital Association.

Rogers, M. (1970). *An introduction to the theoretical basis of nursing.* F. A. Davis.

Schoenhofer, S. (2001). Infusing the nursing curriculum with literature on caring: An idea whose time has come. *International Journal for Human Caring, 5*(2), 7–14. https://doi.org/10.20467/1091-5710.5.2.7

Simon, S. B., & Clark, J. (1975). *More values clarification: Strategies for the class-room.* Pennant Press.

Smith, M. C. (2019). Advancing caring science through the missions of teaching, research/scholarship, practice and service. In W. Rosa, S. Horton-Deutsch, & J. Watson (Eds.), *A handbook for caring science: Expanding the paradigm.* (pp. 285–301). Springer Publishing Company.

Touhy, T. (2004). Dementia, personhood and nursing: Learning from a nursing situation. *Nursing Science Quarterly, 17*(1), 43–49. https://doi.org/10.1177/0894318403260639

Touhy, T., & Boykin, A. (2008). Caring as the central domain in nursing education. *International Journal for Human Caring, 12*(2), 8–15. https://doi.org/10.20467/1091-5710.12.2.8

Ustal, D. (1977). Searching for values. *Image, 9*(1), 15–17. https://doi.org/10.1111/j.1547-5069.1977.tb01593.x

Watson, J. (1979). *Nursing: The philosophy and science of care.* Little, Brown.

Watson, J. (1999). *Postmodern nursing and beyond.* Churchill Livingstone.

Creating a Caring Science Curriculum: The Siena Experience

Donnean Thrall, Lisa Lally, and Jennifer Thate

INTRODUCTION

The Journey Begins: The Who and the Why

It is critical to note that a program that espouses a Caring Science curriculum cannot exist within program outcomes or course learning objectives without it first living within the faculty who facilitate the program. It is about who we are, as much as, if not more than, what we do. For our students to learn Caring Science, such that they can practice Caring Science, they must first experience it. And that in many ways is dependent on the faculty's way of being, both in and outside the classroom. To that end, we begin with our stories of how we each came to Caring Science and to Siena College to begin a program that is built upon a Caring Science philosophy.

I (JT) came to nursing purposefully after obtaining a degree in biology and chemistry. I had traveled to Haiti on a medical mission trip as an undergraduate and was struck by the need for something more than medical treatment and cure. I knew very little about nursing at that time, but after taking a position as a patient care technician in a local Catholic hospital, I began to understand that nursing, as a profession, was unique in what it brought to the care of patients and to healing through a holistic lens. I met powerful nurses during my time as a technician, who demonstrated how the power of their presence helped to place patients in a position to heal. It was after that experience that I decided to pursue a degree in nursing. While I was not able to fully articulate it, I developed a sense of nursing as a discipline that had caring at its core. As I moved through practice positions, graduate school, and eventually to a faculty role, I began to try to answer the questions: What is caring? How can it be taught? Can the ability to care and its impact on healing be measured? Attempting to find answers to these questions has led me to like-minded colleagues and eventually led to my taking a position at Siena College where I have had the opportunity to participate in the creation of a nursing program rooted in Caring Science. In the second semester of my first year at Siena, I began the Caritas Coaching Education Program (CCEP). This program expanded my understanding of Caring Science and Caritas and has impacted my way of being in my faculty role. It has also caused me to evaluate how the contextual aspects embedded in the function and structure of the academic department impact the implementation of a program rooted in Caring Science.

As a faculty we have continued to explore this and have sought to ensure that, not only our classes and pedagogies reflect Caring Science, but that also our departmental structures reflect and facilitate caring practices.

I (LL) was led to nursing from a very early age after a hospitalization where the nurses truly impacted my life. The deep calling for the need to help and care for others was evident in my desire to work at a local hospital from my teens as a candy striper through my work as a nurses' aid, LPN, RN, advanced practice nurse and nurse educator/administrator. I started my academic teaching career as an extension of my love for nursing and desire to share with new students. What I know now, that I did not know then, was that my inherent way of being as a nurse wanted to teach new generations of "the how" of being a nurse: not only the skills needed to be a clinically savvy nurse, but the importance of being fully present with another while that is done. My theoretical framework of nursing and educating nurses was illuminated during my doctoral program when I wrote a paper exploring my personal nursing educational philosophy. It was then that I had words to describe my way of being as a nurse and educator, which as I learned, was immersed in the foundational components of Caring Science theory. While living this reality within my nursing courses and students, I had a unique and wonderful opportunity to start a brand new nursing program at Siena College. With a large leap of faith, I jumped at the opportunity to begin a nursing program not only with all I had learned through my years as a nurse and educator, but most importantly, to start a program that lived and breathed Caring Science. The journey of the development of a postlicensure nursing program immersed in the theory of human caring began as a solitary one, with Dr. Hills and Dr. Watson's first edition of this book, *Creating a Caring Science Curriculum: An Emancipatory Pedagogy for Nursing,* by my side. I then went to Wisconsin to meet these two amazing women for a one-day conference on building a Caring Science curriculum. From there, my love deepened for the work they have done and I wanted to further my understanding of unitary Caring Science and pedagogy development. That year, I began a 2-year postdoctoral fellowship in Caring Science with Dr. Jean Watson which truly was life changing as I not only learned more about the theory, but developed life-long friendships and colleagues in Caring Science. This leads me to today, with a flourishing nursing program at Siena College, wonderful colleagues and Caritas friends, and the desire to continue to shed light on the importance of theory-grounded nursing practice.

Twenty years ago I (DT) started my journey with Caring Science in the doctor of nursing (ND) program at the University of Colorado. After completing an undergraduate degree in health sciences and working in the natural products and herbal supplements industry, I was searching for a graduate program in holistic healthcare. I considered many different fields of study, including naturopathic medicine, physician assistant programs, nutrition and nursing. When I found the ND program at the University of Colorado and its unique, holistic approach to nursing education, I knew I had found my path into a career in healthcare. It was through the curriculum of this program that I was introduced to Dr. Jean Watson and the Theory of Human Caring. As one of only a few holistic programs at the time endorsed by the American Holistic Nurses Association, our course work was deeply rooted in caring theory, reflective practice, complementary therapies, and narrative inquiry. As time went on, I found that I was eager to engage more deeply in the work and sought out opportunities to engage with it even more. A classmate and I did an independent study in nursing theory with Dr. Watson in 2002; we would meet at Dr. Watson's condo, the old nurse's quarters for the Boulder Colorado Sanitarium on Mapleton Avenue, and talk about nursing theory and nursing practice in her living room every couple of weeks. This experience of connecting with

Dr. Watson on such a personal level helped me to start my nursing career deeply rooted in a theoretical basis for my practice. I was not even licensed as a nurse yet and Dr. Watson made me feel like I had so much to offer the profession and that I had the ability to take my vision for nursing practice grounded in theory out into the world and be a change agent. It was a remarkable experience and one that I am very grateful for. From there I went on to take the certificate in caring and healing courses that Dr. Watson and her Caring Science colleagues from the University of Colorado offered at Naropa University in Boulder, CO before returning to New York to raise our children near their grandparents. After many years of working in hospital and educational settings where I did not always feel fully supported or celebrated for who I was as a caring/healing theory–guided nurse, I found my way to a teaching position in the Baldwin Nursing Program at Siena College. Siena was seeking a nursing faculty member with experience in a Caring Science curriculum. I knew this was the perfect position for me to advance my work in Caring Science, both personally and professionally. As part of my continued growth in building my Caritas literacy, over the past few years I completed a 2-year postdoctoral fellowship in Caring Science with Dr. Watson, graduated from the Watson Caring Science Institute's Caritas Coach Program and achieved board certification as an advanced practice holistic nurse (AHN-BC).

BUILDING A PHILOSOPHICAL AND THEORETICAL FOUNDATION

The nursing program at Siena College began in 2016 with the development and approval of a postlicensure bachelor of science degree in nursing. Siena College, with its strong Franciscan heritage, saw nursing as a perfect fit for the small, private, Catholic liberal arts college. The decision to start a nursing program at Siena came to fruition through the work of visionary leaders of the college and a local hospital system that offered an associate's degree in nursing. In response to the Institute of Medicine (2011) report on the Future of Nursing, these leaders recognized the need to prepare more nurses at the baccalaureate level and thus set out to bring the two institutions together to provide a means to offer a 4-year degree in nursing utilizing the resources from each organization. It is through these partnerships that students in our region have greater access to baccalaureate education while maintaining the high-quality associate's degree institution's program as a strong and viable option for entry into practice.

The addition of nursing majors at Siena College aligns seamlessly with the mission and history of St. Francis. Franciscan values related to healthcare can be traced back to the 13th century and the teachings of St. Francis and St. Clare of Assisi. The importance of caring for the health and well-being of vulnerable populations is manifested in the compassionate work of St. Francis in the care of lepers. The care for those who are sick and suffering is an integral part of Franciscan tradition (Monti, 2013). Dominic Monti (2013) states, "For all Franciscans, our attitude and behavior towards those who are sick forms an essential part of our call to Gospel conversion" (p. xi.). In the earliest writings of St. Francis and St. Clare of Assisi, one learns that caring for the sick, especially those vulnerable populations of the poor and marginalized, are thought of as one of the basic characteristics of the Franciscan movement (Monti, 2013). The integration of nursing at Siena College contributes to that movement in the current day.

Theoretical Grounding

The development of the Siena College postlicensure nursing tracks leading to a bachelor of science degree in nursing have intentionally been created based upon a theoretical foundation in Jean Watson's Theory of Human Caring. As such, we seek to embrace and fully integrate a human-Caring Science model within a nursing disciplinary framework, which mirrors our mission as a Franciscan college. This purposeful inclusion of nursing theory and the language of nursing within our curriculum makes explicit the disciplinary knowledge of nursing. Theories and philosophies of nursing science are what frame our disciplinary knowledge, so without being explicit, we risk losing the distinctiveness of our discipline (Watson, 2018a). Smith (2019) agrees with this position and notes that we are currently in a time where nursing is losing its identity as a discipline. Many schools of nursing are not fully integrating the foundational tenets of our discipline that define nursing's distinct theory-informed knowledge. If nursing is not grounded in theory-guided practice and nursing research, Smith (2019) posits that we are using the knowledge of other disciplines (e.g., natural and social sciences) to direct the care of our clients, instead of our own nursing theory which has been informed by nursing practice. It is therefore critical to integrate our theoretical foundation into our curriculum in order for nursing to continue as a distinct discipline. The nursing department at Siena College fully embraces this and has purposefully integrated the language of nursing theory into our program.

In addition to nursing theory we see the integration of the liberal arts, natural, and social sciences as an integral part of a well-rounded baccalaureate education, contributing to the development of critical thinking and broadening how our students view and engage with the world around them. Thus, this multifaceted education provides students with the tools to engage with the theoretical disciplinary perspective in nursing. To that end, we sought to integrate a strong nursing theoretical and disciplinary foundation with a diverse liberal arts education when developing the curriculum and instructional pedagogy for our postlicensure nursing program. One of the first steps in this process was the creation of a praxis model to visually and relationally depict the importance of the synergy between nursing immersed in Caring Science and the Franciscan values of our college. Lally Flack and Thrall (2016) developed this model using the works of Watson (2008a, 2012), Hills and Watson (2011), and the Siena College Franciscan values. See Figure 14.1.

Our Praxis Model

Chinn and Kramer (2018) define "praxis" as a synthesis of thoughtful reflection, caring, and action within a theory and research-driven practice. Watson's (2018a) notion of praxis reaches beyond reflection and knowledge-guided action to embodying a moral and ethical commitment to human caring, healing, health, and the universe. Watson goes on to describe praxis as a philosophical search for truth, beauty, aesthetics, with a movement toward a moral community of caring/healing and peace that nursing has always represented (Watson, 2008a). This expanded vision of praxis has guided us in the development and implementation of our unique praxis model; a model which remains fluid and will evolve over time through faculty and students engaging in intentional reflection-in-action and reflection-on-action (Hills & Watson, 2011; Horton-Deutsch & Sherwood, 2017; Schön, 1987; Tanner, 2006). See Figure 14.1.

The model begins with the inner circle of the *engagement of the heart* through transpersonal human caring. This is the core of the discipline of nursing and the Franciscan tradition. Franciscan education at Siena is incarnational, personal, communal, transformative, engages the heart, develops servant leaders, and pursues wisdom (Siena College, 2020a). These Franciscan values include the development of understanding hearts of compassion. Franciscan education has as much to do with opening the heart to love as it does with opening the mind

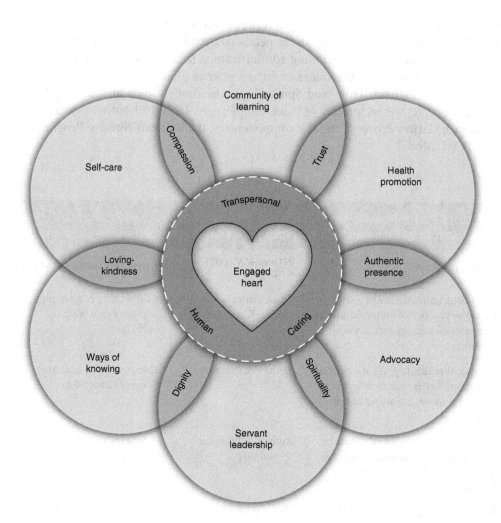

FIGURE 14.1 Baldwin Nursing Program Caring Science praxis model.

Source: Praxis model courtesy of the Nursing Dept., Siena College. Lally Flack, L., & Thrall, D. (2016). *Baldwin Nursing Program praxis model.* Siena College Department of Nursing Handbook.

to truth, and we must do so with humility and intellectual honesty, with courage and perseverance (Siena College, 2020a). The synergy of the Franciscan values and the theory of human caring is evident. Watson describes *transpersonal human caring* as the central component of the caring relationship between the nurse and patient that extends beyond time and place (Watson, 2008a). Leading us "to realize that maybe this one moment, with this one person, is the very reason we're here on earth at this time" (Watson, 2008b). This caring relationship is nurtured through the application of the Caritas Processes®, bringing our full authentic self to each encounter, showing loving-kindness and equanimity to ourselves and the other person, thereby changing the life experience of both the nurse and patient, student and educator, and beyond (Watson, 2008a).

Emerging from the engaged heart and transpersonal human caring at the center of this model, the outer circles of the praxis model relate to foundational components included in our curriculum (Community of Learning, Ways of Knowing, Servant Leadership, Advocacy,

Health Promotion and Self-Care) and reflect the *outward manifestations* that shape our program at Siena College. The smaller inner petals reflect the *intrinsic values* that live within each of us in our department, including administrators, faculty, staff and students and demonstrate the embodiment of the values of Caring Science (Authentic Presence, Compassion, Dignity, Loving-kindness, Trust, and Spirituality). The dashed lines surrounding the center of the model depict the reciprocity of these components. Table 14.1 outlines the relationship between each Caritas Process® and the components of the Baldwin Nursing Program Caring Science Praxis Model.

TABLE 14.1 The Relationship Between the Caritas Processes® and the Components of the Baldwin Nursing Program Caring Science Praxis Model

CARITAS PROCESS®	INTRINSIC VALUES (PETALS)	OUTWARD MANIFESTATION
1. Sustaining humanistic/altruistic values by practice of loving-kindness, compassion, and equanimity with self/others	Compassion Loving-Kindness	Community of Learning Servant Leadership Self-Care
2. Being authentically present, enabling faith/hope/belief system; honoring subjective inner, life-world of self/others	Authentic Presence	Community of Learning Servant Leadership
3. Being sensitive to self and others by cultivating own spiritual practices; beyond ego-self to transpersonal presence	Authentic Presence Spirituality	Advocacy Community of Learning Servant Leadership Ways of Knowing
4. Developing and sustaining loving, trusting/caring relationships	Compassion Trust	Community of Learning
5. Allowing for expression of positive and negative feelings—authentically listening to another person's story	Authentic Presence Compassion Dignity Loving-Kindness Trust	Community of Learning Servant Leadership
6. Creatively problem-solving-'solution-seeking' through caring process; full use of self and artistry of caring/healing practices via use of all ways of knowing/being/doing/becoming	Authentic Presence Compassion Trust	Advocacy Community of Learning Servant Leadership Ways of Knowing
7. Engaging in transpersonal teaching and learning within context of caring relationship; staying within other's frame of reference; shift toward coaching model for expanded health/wellness	Transpersonal Human Caring/Engaged Heart *	Advocacy Community of Learning Health Promotion

(continued)

TABLE 14.1 The Relationship Between the Caritas Processes® and the Components of the Baldwin Nursing Program Caring Science Praxis Model (*continued*)

CARITAS PROCESS®	INTRINSIC VALUES (PETALS)	OUTWARD MANIFESTATION
8. Creating a healing environment at all levels; subtle environment for energetic authentic caring presence	Transpersonal Human Caring/Engaged Heart *	Community of Learning Self-Care
9. Reverentially assisting with basic needs as sacred acts, touching mindbodyspirit of other; sustaining human dignity	Transpersonal Human Caring/Engaged Heart *	Community of Learning Servant Leadership
10. Opening to spiritual, mystery, unknowns;allowing for miracles	Transpersonal Human Caring/Engaged Heart *	Community of Learning Self-Care Ways of Knowing

Transpersonal Human Caring/Engaged Heart incorporates all intrinsic values.

Intrinsic Values

Loving-Kindness for self and others is a foundational component of Watson's Theory of Human Caring. "Loving-kindness gives birth to a natural compassion. The compassionate heart holds the pain and sorrow of our own life and of all beings with mercy and tenderness. . . that has the power to transform the world" (Kornfield, 2002, p. 102). Watson speaks to loving kindness throughout her work and has referenced the work of Kornfield to further define *Caritas Process® #1*. All caring must be grounded in love and kindness, first for oneself, so it can extend out to others (Watson, 2008a). This is a key component of our Caring Science philosophy at Siena College. For our nursing students to become caring nurses, it is imperative that they first learn to care for themselves with loving kindness.

Compassion is related to the ability to embody loving-kindness and is a core component of the praxis model and Watson's theory. The transpersonal nature of the relationship between the nurse and patient, the educator and student, or between colleagues is dependent upon compassion which supports the development of a trusting relationship.

> When we come to rest in the great heart of compassion, we discover a capacity to bear witness to, suffer with, and hold dear our own vulnerable heart the sorrow and beauties of the world. (Kornfield, 2002, p. 102)

Not only is compassion a precursor to caring for others, it also is necessary to care for oneself. Our program emphasizes the development of self-care practices with the hope that the students and faculty will continue this as a life-long practice. As a Franciscan college, compassion for self and others is a key core value. As compassionate leaders, both as faculty and students, we strive to "lead by putting others first, through our commitment to social justice, service with others, and concern for the poor and vulnerable" (Siena College, 2020b).

Authentic Presence is one of the foundational premises of Watson's theory. It can be described as an awareness of one's own consciousness of being in a caring moment. Watson speaks of authentic presence as the experience of fully "being in" the moment with another, which does not preclude the nurse from performing necessary tasks and procedures. This being present in the now, or *Caritas Consciousness*, is biogenic, both life giving and life receiving. From this experience of authentically "being with" another, each person's life history and the energetic field changes through that transpersonal caring moment (Watson, 2008a). As Watson (2012) states, "In the sense of a caring moment, caring is a moral ideal rather than an interpersonal technique, and it entails a commitment to a particular end. The end is the protection, enhancement, and preservation of the person's humanity and human dignity, which helps to restore inner harmony, wholeness, and potential healing" (p. 71).

Spirituality: Nurses are entrusted to care for patients as whole persons—body, mind, and spirit. To be fully present and "see" who that spirit-filled person is beyond the outer physical elements, it is important for the nurse to give attention to their own personal spiritual development. The development of one's spirituality is integral to becoming a compassionate, caring, and authentically present nurse (Watson, 2008a, p. 68). According to Watson, we have thoughts, feelings, and a body, but we are more than our thoughts, feelings, and physical body; we are embodied spirit (Watson, 2008a). Once spiritually self-aware, one can become more present to others with a fully engaged heart and approach their patients with loving-kindness (Watson, 2012). Therefore, the education of a nurse must be all-encompassing and reflective to include both the cultural and spiritual needs of all, including self. Siena College's Franciscan mission and the Baldwin Nursing program recognize that and embrace the full education of each student, including spiritual growth.

Dignity of the Human Experience and Trust: Respect for human dignity is a provision within the Code of Ethics for Nurses. "A fundamental principle that underlies all nursing practice is respect for the inherent dignity, worth, unique attributes, and human rights of all individuals. The need for and right to health care is universal, transcending all individual differences" (American Nurses Association, 2015, p. 1). To include the term "dignity" in the praxis model was intentional, as preserving human dignity is a universal right and is central in the worldview of nursing, Franciscan values, and Watson's theory. This is the premise of the trusting/caring relationship between the nurse and patient (Watson, 2012).

As noted, the outer circles of the praxis model relate to foundational components reflected in our curriculum (Community of learning, Ways of knowing, Servant leadership, Advocacy, Health promotion and Self-care). These outward manifestations are further described in "The How of Creating a Caring Science Curriculum" section and demonstrate how the intrinsic values are lived out in our Caring Science curriculum.

Our Mission

This praxis model also informs the philosophy and mission of the nursing program at Siena College. The mission statement was birthed out of deep thought and reflection that included not only meeting the identified requirements of a bachelor's program in nursing, but also the inclusion of our deep-seated Caring Science philosophy. Recognizing that the future of nursing is dependent on educating nurses who embrace a Caritas consciousness, we developed our departmental mission to reflect what we envision for our students and faculty. This includes what we experience in our community of learning and the being and becoming of a Caritas nurse.

Department of Nursing Mission (Siena College, 2017)

It is the mission of the Department of Nursing to co-create a community of learning that fosters an engaged heart in the process of transpersonal human caring. This is realized through our commitment to living a Caring Science curriculum.

We embrace Siena College's core Franciscan values to create lifelong learners, compassionate leaders, and innovative professionals.

We honor the unique lived experience of all people, including the student and faculty. Caring for self is integral to this process and we believe this supports the development of effective, compassionate, and authentic practitioners.

We are dedicated to graduating students who embrace servant leadership by partnering with our community to promote health through advocacy and service.

The experience of a Caring Science curriculum results in graduates who are full partners on the healthcare team and who uphold the ethical, moral, and professional responsibilities within the discipline of nursing to be guardians of human caring.

THE LIVED EXPERIENCE OF BEING AND BECOMING: THE "HOW" OF CREATING A CARING SCIENCE CURRICULUM

Caring Science theory serves as an undergirding to all that we do at Siena College in our nursing program. As we just described, it has influenced the development of our program's philosophy, praxis model, and mission. It can be seen in our course descriptions and learning outcomes. It has also shaped our pedagogies and classroom environments. Finally, it has impacted our departmental structure and function as well as the development of our tenure and promotion guidelines. In this section we share some specific examples and strategies that we have used as we have sought to develop a program that fully embraces Caring Science theory.

Living Out the Praxis Model

First and foremost, the intrinsic values in our praxis model that reflect the Caritas Processes® inform the outward manifestations that shape our program. At the center of how we teach nursing is bringing our true *authentic presence* into the classroom and to each individual student encounter. It can not be understated that by modeling caring with our students, it changes their outlook on nursing education and the nursing profession. The practice of *loving-kindness* is a central component to all we do with our students and each other by encouraging reflection and self-care throughout the program. This leads to a greater awareness of self and the ability to engage in transpersonal human caring with a fully engaged heart. This is done both through core course experiences and through the integration of deep reflective practices in the nursing coursework.

In the nursing department, it is our belief that the relationship between the student and the faculty is also built upon *trust*. We respect each student's lived experiences, and create a safe, nonjudgmental learning environment where each voice (student and faculty) is heard. We feel that a trusting environment, similar to the nurse/patient environment, inspires growth and creative problem solving. The cocreation of a *community of learning* is key to a Caring Science pedagogy. We believe that learning should be cocreated with our students and based upon mutual respect. Within this learning environment, we embrace all *ways of knowing*. As both a student and a practitioner, it is critical for nurses to utilize multiple ways of knowing to help guide their practice. Based upon the sentinel work of Carper (1978), empirical, personal, ethical, esthetic patterns of knowing are fundamental and conceived as necessary for achieving mastery in the discipline, but none of them alone should be considered sufficient.

As educators, we model a Caring Science philosophy through *servant leadership*. "Leadership" has been defined as a multifaceted process of identifying a goal or target, motivating other people to act, and providing support and motivation to achieve mutually negotiated goals (Porter O'Grady, 2003). While this is an important definition of leadership, we are challenged to take this further to the notion of servant leadership. In the Franciscan tradition, leadership has been described as an encounter with those other than those within our own "familiar circle" in a manner that awakens our empathy and compassion and enlarges our sense of belonging, power, and hope; then "us versus them" is transformed into "we." In nursing, both in practice and education, we are in a unique position to be servant leaders who guide our students with compassion and equalize the power in the relationship (Lally Flack & Thrall, 2019).

Self-care practices are the actions you take to care for your body, mind, and spirit and are a key component of our program's philosophy and our lived experience. Watson's theory speaks of the need to care for oneself so one can care for others. Self-care practices increase the nurse's ability to find more fulfillment in their work and life (Watson, 2008a). Furthermore, nurses are very knowledgeable on how to "do" the job; however, more effort needs to be directed towards how to "be" while doing the real work of the job (Watson, 2008a). This includes taking the time to care for oneself and centering prior to giving care to others. We do this in our program through inclusion of self-care practices in the coursework, as well as through the use of centering/meditation practices in the classroom (Lally Flack & Thrall, 2019). The first step of *health promotion* is to care for oneself, so care can be given to another. In our nursing program, health promotion is an outward manifestation in our praxis model and serves as an important component of our curriculum. By modeling healthy self-care practices in and out of the classroom, students in turn begin to model those same practices in their personal and professional lives. Health promotion can then naturally move beyond a focus on individual behavior towards a wider range of social and environmental interventions guided by the Sustainable Development Goals which aim to "to ensure that all human beings can fulfill their potential in dignity and equality in a healthy environment" (World Health Organization, 2018, p. 7). Similarly, *advocacy* for self, one's patient, and the profession is another outward manifestation of our praxis model. In our program we seek to create an environment that increases the individual and collective voice of nurses to influence policy and practice. Nurses are exposed to this concept through all of the coursework, but in particular, in the public health and health policy courses.

Our Curriculum

There are two tracks of the postlicensure nursing program, one for working nurses (RN to BS) and a Dual Degree Nursing Program (DDNP) for traditional college students through partnerships with local associate's degree programs. The nursing program began with a small cohort of 10 students in the RN to BS track in Fall 2016. This track of the program is offered in a hybrid format in which nurses come to campus one day per week to take both nursing and liberal arts coursework. In this reduced seat-time track, nurses are able to take one consistent day-off from work to come to campus and then complete the remaining coursework online.

The curriculum in our DDNP track is unique in that it is a collaboration with partner schools that offer prelicensure courses for an associate degree in nursing, while concurrently at Siena, we offer all of the liberal arts, core, prerequisites, and upper-level postlicensure nursing courses for a bachelor's degree in nursing. We have developed and received approval for two of these partnerships with associate degree nursing programs in the Capital Region of

New York state. These partnerships create a seamless pathway for students to earn both their associate and bachelor of science degrees in nursing while living and learning on the Siena College campus all 4 years. In this track, students begin their education in year one at Siena College taking nursing prerequisite courses in the natural sciences and social sciences as well as core courses in philosophy, history, creative arts, religious studies, quantitative analysis, and English. At Siena, students also take core courses in Franciscan heritage, diversity, social justice, and nature. These core courses at Siena reflect the Franciscan mission of the college and serve to prepare students to be in right-relation with self, humanity, and our physical and spiritual world. In year two, students begin taking nursing classes at one of our partner schools. While at the partner school, our students continue to take classes at Siena College to complete the core and nursing prerequisite courses and begin some upper-division nursing courses including our nursing theory course. Once students complete the prelicensure sequence at the partner school at the end of year three, they graduate with an associate's degree in nursing and take the National Council Licensure Examination (NCLEX-RN® exam) over the summer. Upon returning for their senior year on the Siena campus, students finish the upper-division nursing coursework and any remaining core classes and graduate with a baccalaureate degree in nursing.

We work closely with our partner schools to ensure a seamless academic curricular flow that is inclusive of Caring Science pedagogy. Both partner schools embrace Watson as a primary theorist to ground their curriculum. The director and/or faculty at Siena College have gone to both partner schools to deliver workshops to share our philosophy and pedagogical methods. These workshops provide an opportunity for our partner schools to identify how Caring Science is already informing their current curriculum. During this time, we share methods to enhance their practices and also encourage the importance of intentionally using the language of Caring Science throughout the curriculum. In order for our program to fully embrace Caring Science, it is important to continue to come alongside partner programs to ensure that Caring Science is infused in these first nursing classes.

PROCESS OF CURRICULUM REVIEW

In order to ensure that we maintain fluency with Caring Science throughout the curriculum, we have incorporated reflection on our Caring Science practices within our annual course-reporting process. In these course reports we include standard elements such as enrollments, attrition, materials used, proposed changes to the course, and an evaluation of these changes. In addition, we also include a section in which we reflect on how Caring Science has influenced a teaching activity, an assignment, or a pedagogical approach. In doing this, we maintain an intentional connection to our theoretical foundation. We believe that this will be increasingly important as our department grows quickly in the coming years. Table 14.2 provides samples from our course reports demonstrating the links to Caring Science.

THREADING OF CARITAS LITERACIES THROUGH THE CURRICULUM: EXEMPLARS

The Siena nursing curriculum begins in the spring of year two with *NURS 300 Advanced Concepts of Professional Nursing*. See Appendix A for Course Description and Student Learning Outcomes. This course lays a foundation for our Caring Science curriculum and is the starting point for the student's personal journey into the disciplinary foundation of nursing. Students explore concepts in caring, healing, and health from a holistic perspective for both themselves and the populations they care for. The content is nursing theory–based, rather than based in

TABLE 14.2 Excerpts From Course Reports on Links to Caring Science

YEAR IN PROGRAM	SIENA COLLEGE NURSING COURSE	EXAMPLE OF LINK TO CARING SCIENCE (FROM COURSE REPORTS)
2	**Advanced Concepts of Professional Nursing**	*Vision Board and Self-Care Summary Presentation* Culminating project integrating multiple ways of knowing into an aesthetic project representing the student's vision of where they have been and what they are striving for in the future. Application of Caritas Process® #1, 2, 3, 4, 6 Holistic Nursing Core Value #1 Holistic Philosophies, Theories and Values, #2 Holistic Nurse Self-Reflection, Self-Development, and Self-Care, and #3 Holistic Caring Process.
3	**Health Assessment and Health Promotion Across the Life Span**	*Video Recording of Head to Toe Assessment* Students use critical reflection techniques to review their own video and complete a self and peer evaluation using the scoring tool. This method of allowing the student to record their assessment for submission as many times as they want to, reduces the anxiety and vulnerability that students often feel when they have to complete their assessment in front of an instructor. This transforms the assignment from a high-stakes, fear-based exercise to one that gives the power back to the student. They use reflective practice techniques when they complete their self-assessment and also when they view their partner's video and discuss their scoring of each other. This method supports the Caring Science curriculum because it allows for equalization of power in the course and has the student engage in reflective practice by doing a self and peer evaluation. Students also write about their experience using Tanner's (2006) Clinical Judgment model as a guide, specifically writing about their reflection-in-action and reflection-on-action. The student engages in *Caritas Process®* #5 when they are present to, and supportive of, the expression of positive and negative feelings of their own and their partner during the CPE experience and Caritas Process® #1 offering loving-kindness and equanimity to themselves and others during this difficult culminating course project/assessment. Application of Caritas Process® #1 & 5. Supports Holistic Nursing Core Value #2 Holistic Nurse Self-Reflection, Self-Development, and Self-Care.

(continued)

TABLE 14.2 Excerpts From Course Reports on Links to Caring Science (*continued*)

YEAR IN PROGRAM	SIENA COLLEGE NURSING COURSE	EXAMPLE OF LINK TO CARING SCIENCE (FROM COURSE REPORTS)
3	**Research to Promote Evidence-Based Nursing Practice**	Class discussion on *Paradigms (positivist vs. constructivist) and reading "What counts as evidence?"*
		This discussion sets the stage for the course by exploring how research is defined and what counts as evidence. Facilitates reflection on feelings regarding research and the value of both quantitative and qualitative research as evidence for informing practice. Encourages individual reflection on one's own worldview/paradigm.
		Supports Holistic Nursing Core Value #2 Self-reflection and Core Value #5 Holistic education and research; Caritas Process® #6 Use of all ways of knowing in "creatively problem solving" informing evidence use in practice.
4	**Pathophysiology and Pharmacology for Nursing Practice**	*Service Opportunity With Homeless Veterans*
		In alignment with our Franciscan mission, students visit a homeless shelter for veterans twice at the end of the semester to provide education on medications, nutrition, and well-being. During the first visit they interview a veteran and identify healthcare educational needs of the client. During the second visit, they return with an educational plan inclusive of medications (with a medication reconciliation sheet), nutritional issues and/or other educational items. The students intentionally identify and exhibit Caritas Processes during the time spent with the veteran. These Caritas Processes serve as a foundation of their paper which describes the patient's perception of health and understanding of their medications/nutrition.
		Application of Caritas Processes® #1, 2, 3, 4, 5, 7, & 9.
		*This course is being redesigned as Holistic Pharmacology to include 50% herbal medicine and dietary supplements content supporting Holistic Core Value #5 Holistic Education and Research.

(*continued*)

TABLE 14.2 Excerpts From Course Reports on Links to Caring Science (*continued*)

YEAR IN PROGRAM	SIENA COLLEGE NURSING COURSE	EXAMPLE OF LINK TO CARING SCIENCE (FROM COURSE REPORTS)
4	**Caring and Advocating for the Older Adult**	*Elder Interview* Using the *Life Interview Questions Toolkit* from the Legacy Project, students conduct an Elder Interview with an older member of their family. This assignment is intended to expand the student's view of the role of elders in our society through narrative inquiry. It provides them with the opportunity to have a deeply connected personal experience with someone in their family whom they might not otherwise ask to share such specifics about their life without a class assignment. Application of Caritas Process® #2, 3, 4, 5, 10 and Holistic Core Value #3 Holistic Caring Process and #4 Holistic Communication, Therapeutic Relationship, Healing Environment and Cultural Care.
4	**Population and Public Health Nursing Perspectives**	Semester-long clinical *Community Assessment Project* This project guides students through the process of seeking to understand the various dimensions of an identified community and how these variables contribute to the health of the community. Students spend time exploring the physical environment as well as epidemiological trends and related community data. Students align these findings with feedback garnered from listening to community members, including both formal and informal leaders in the community. In conjunction with community members, students identify a priority health need and a related intervention to address this need. This project encourages the student to provide patient-centered Human Caring as evidenced by engaging with communities in a way that promotes "equanimity with other"; "creatively problem solving" by partnering with community members as stakeholders; and "engaging in transpersonal teaching" by "staying with other's frame of reference." Application of Caritas Process® #1, 6, 7 and Holistic Core Value #3 Holistic Communication, Therapeutic Relationship, Healing Environments, and Cultural Care.

(continued)

TABLE 14.2 Excerpts From Course Reports on Links to Caring Science (*continued*)

YEAR IN PROGRAM	SIENA COLLEGE NURSING COURSE	EXAMPLE OF LINK TO CARING SCIENCE (FROM COURSE REPORTS)
4	**Health Policy in Nursing Practice**	*Discussion Board: Ethical Dilemmas, Ethnic and Racial Disparities: Using Your Voice* This discussion brings to light the power of the student's voice. They have learned about ethical principles that are used in practice and policy as well as the related ethnic and racial disparities. Students select one of these two questions to further explore these concepts: Describe a clinical ethical dilemma you have witnessed or read about related to healthcare. Utilize the ethical terms discussed in the assigned reading. What actions could healthcare professionals take to address ethnic and racial disparities from an ethical perspective? Utilize the terms discussed in the assigned reading. Application of Caritas Processes®: #2, 3, 5 and Holistic Core Value #1 Holistic Philosophies, Theories, and Ethics.
4	**Transformational Nursing Leadership**	*Discussion Board: Communication, Teamwork, and Civility: Lessons From Geese* Students analyze "Lessons from Geese" (which is a powerful way to demonstrate transformational leadership through the example of geese flying in formation and loyalty) and broadly discuss how this could be used to create and support a caring organizational culture that values and uses effective team concepts to improve clinical practice. Share an example of this lesson from your leadership clinical and/or your clinical experience. In addition, reflect upon your work environment. Is it a welcoming civil workplace? How can what you have learned in this part of the course on leading change and managing conflict apply to the culture of your workplace to enhance a caring environment? Give examples of what could change and how you as a leader can manifest that change. Application of Caritas Processes®: #1, 2, 3, 4 & 6 Holistic Nursing Core Values #1 Holistic Philosophies, Theories and Values, #2 Holistic Nurse Self-Reflection, Self-Development and Self-Care, #3 Holistic Caring Process, and #4 Holistic Communication, Therapeutic Relationship, Healing Environment, and Cultural Care.

knowledge reflecting other disciplines (Manhart Barrett, 2017). Each class starts with a breathing exercise, relaxation technique, mindfulness meditation, or a reading to ground us in our work and shift our focus so that we can be authentically present in the moment together. Educators who embody and share mindful practices encourage learners to develop a level of presence and attention which helps to facilitate the engaged, spirited inquiry of active learning that serves to shape their nursing practice (Horton-Deutsch & Sherwood, 2017). The students are also introduced to Dossey's (2015) Integrative Health and Wellness Assessment tool to establish a baseline measurement of where they are with their self-care at the start of the semester and they compare that with where they are at the end when they reflect on their experience in the course in the self-care summary and philosophy paper at the end of the semester. With a focus on self-care, self-awareness, and contemplative practices threaded throughout the course and in our relationships together, students engage with the concepts on a deeply personal level. According to Watson (2020), it is possible to read, study, learn about, and even teach caring theory, but to truly "get it," one has to experience it personally. A module on values based on the work of Brene Brown (2018) provides a starting point for each student's unique perspective on their development as a holistic nurse grounded in Caring Science. Students write an affirmation statement in the introductory module of the course. This then informs the process of developing their culminating personal nursing philosophy paper which is grounded in nursing theory. A simple classroom exercise to write their own definition of nursing gets them thinking about the importance of language and how we describe our work. According to Watson (2018a), words matter and language defines reality. "Any profession that does not have its own language in this day and age does not exist" (p. 137). We need to use nursing language to name and document the phenomena of Caritas to make visible that which is otherwise invisible (Watson, 2018a). The students also begin to understand the role of the nurse *as* the healing environment and develop a greater sense of self in the process (Quinn, 1992; Watson, 2008a).

The faculty facilitates classroom and online discussions about readings on Watson's Theory of Human Caring including the 10 Caritas Processes® and Transpersonal Caring Moments. Practice exemplars and integration of the theory in both personal and professional life are covered. Caritas Literacy micropractices are introduced such as pausing before entering the patient's room, reading the field, being authentically present, suspending role and status, and seeking to *see* and *hear* the person behind the diagnosis, treatment, or disease (Watson, 2018b).

To support the application of Caritas Process® #1 *Cultivating the Practice of Loving-Kindness, Compassion and Equanimity with Self and Other*, students spend time discussing, experiencing, and reflecting on their own and their classmate's self-care practices. Understanding that self-care is more than pampering, students engage in life-changing experiences exploring autonomy, boundary setting, asking for help, and letting go (Richardson, 2019). A sample assignment related to self-care is in Table 14.3.

TABLE 14.3 NURS 300 Self-Care Discussion Board

Consider what you have been learning as you have read *The Art of Extreme Self-Care* by Cheryl Richardson (2019) and answer the following questions:

Describe two things that have resonated with you from the book and explain why they are significant to you.

How does your self-care and self-knowledge affect how you care for others?

Include an image or piece of artistic work (aesthetic knowing) in your post that represents how you care for yourself.

TABLE 14.4 NURS415 Fundamental Patterns of Knowing in Leadership Discussion Board
After reading the articles for this week,
Discuss ways you have seen leaders both in your clinical practicum and/or work experience, either support or hinder the application of evidence-informed practice at the bedside. What was the impact? You learned the basics about Carper's (1978) *Fundamental Patterns of Knowing* in NURS300. Now consider these Ways of Knowing in the context of nursing leadership and evidence-informed practice. . .
What are ways you as a leader would promote the application of theory-guided, evidence-informed practice (empirical and beyond) in a caring work environment? Lastly, broaden your scope beyond "the bedside" and consider our role in nursing as visionary leaders advocating for the health of individuals, families, and communities. Leadership roles in nursing can go beyond that of hospital management. Consider your potential as a *nurse activist*. . .
Where would you like your voice to be heard? What are you passionate about? How could you bring the voice of nursing to that cause and use evidence and theory to inform that work?

An additional key concept introduced in this first course is Carper's (1978) Fundamental Patterns of Knowing and the expanded work on the ways of knowing in the nursing literature. In an online discussion forum, students are asked to apply Caritas Process® #6 *Creative problem-solving/solution-seeking through Caritas—Use of all ways of knowing* to compare and contrast the sole use of empirical knowledge with the use of multiple ways of knowing in nursing practice. They are asked to describe how multiple ways of knowing impacted their lives and share an example where they have integrated at least three ways of knowing in some aspect of their personal lives. Again, this brings them to first think about how they experience this on a personal level before they integrate it into their practice.

During the senior year, in *NURS 415 Transformational Nursing Leadership,* the curriculum comes full circle and ties in the concepts threaded through the previous courses. See Appendix B for Course Description and Student Learning Outcomes. In a module on evidence-informed practice in leadership, students revisit an article on the ways of knowing from *NURS 300 Advanced Concepts of Professional Nursing* and reflect on how they now see this work in the context of their role as a nursing leader. See Table 14.4 for a sample assignment.

Students also take an even deeper dive into their personal knowing by completing many self-evaluation/assessment tools on emotional intelligence, personal style, and leadership capacity assessments. This encourages the student to dig into more reflection on who they are as a person and how that impacts how they show up as a nurse and leader.

In an overall culminating assignment in the program, students write a final reflection paper. In this paper the students, who are now licensed registered nurses, review their philosophy paper from their sophomore year and reflect on the evolutionary process of being and becoming a Caritas nurse. See Table 14.5 for the final reflection paper assignment.

NEXT STEPS: CONTINUED CURRICULUM EVOLUTION

As we live and experience this curriculum as faculty and reflect on the learning we see occurring in our students, we continue to explore how our curriculum might evolve to more deeply

TABLE 14.5 NURS 415 Transformational Nursing Leadership Reflection Paper

Begin by reviewing your *Philosophy of Nursing* paper submitted during your first semester in the Baldwin Nursing Program.

Reflect on how your philosophy has evolved over time (before this program, after the first semester/year, and now).

Reflect on the role of a transformative Caring Science nurse leader. Describe what style of leadership you embrace (or hope to) in the role of a caring leader.

Include your current definition of caring (informed by theory) and how this is integrated into your role as a nurse leader today and/or in the future (even if that role is at the bedside).

Describe ways in which the Caring Science curriculum and the Baldwin Nursing program mission impact your vision of the art of caring in professional nursing and nursing leadership.

In addition, consider your *Vision Board* and *Self-Care Summary* you created in your first semester and review the *Self-Care Assessment Tool* you completed at the beginning and end of this semester.

Reflect on where you were when you began nursing school, where you are now, and hope to be in the future. Have your self-care practices evolved in some way or have your practices been reaffirmed?

This culminating paper is designed to help you synthesize all that you have learned while working on a baccalaureate degree in nursing grounded in Caring Science.

---

reflect Caritas Literacies. We also remain open to other like-hearted theoretical and conceptual frameworks to help us further live out the intrinsic values represented in our Praxis model and the embodiment of Transpersonal Human Caring. One such endeavor is to seek holistic program endorsement through the American Holistic Nurses Credentialing Corporation (AHNCC). We started work toward this process by meeting the AHNCC criteria for certification, by supporting one faculty member (DT) in achieving board certification as an advanced practice holistic nurse (AHN-BC). Currently, a second faculty member (JT) is eligible to sit for the examination to achieve certification and hopes to complete this in the coming year. Next steps include review of course descriptions, outcomes, and assignments, in order to further integrate the core values described in the *Holistic Nursing: A Handbook for Practice*.

Another area for future development is to more formally evaluate the growth in our students as Caritas nurses as a result of their experiences in our program. Currently we collect feedback through a question that has been added to our end-of-semester course evaluations. While our students describe experiencing Caring Science throughout the curriculum, we believe that work needs to be done to ensure that all the course descriptions and outcomes more explicitly reflect Caring Science concepts and the Caritas Processes®. We have also posited that the students' feedback on their experiences of Caring Science is likely most impacted by faculty's way of being and the pedagogical approaches applied in the classroom as opposed to material that is taught. These approaches are described in the following.

The Classroom Environment

It is critical to the development of a Caring Science pedagogy to set up the environment in a way that is conducive to a safe and welcoming community of learning (outward manifestation of the praxis model). To do this, faculty need to be immersed in the pedagogy of Caring

Science to create an online and classroom environment that encourages the student voice, reflection, and active learning. This includes the hybrid nature of our courses, physical set up of the classroom, hierarchical structure, civility, and self-care (Lally Flack & Thrall, 2019).

The upper-division nursing courses are delivered in a hybrid format, ranging from 30% to 50% online. We meet with students in person each week to engage with course material and the hybrid portion serves as preparation for that week's lessons. By having students write and reflect on their experiences with the material, we are able to hear much more of their individual voices than if the class were only in person. We have discovered that students who tend to be more reserved and quiet in the classroom are able to express the full breadth of their knowledge and experience in the online environment. We use the Digital World Caring Communication Exemplars of offering full presence, acknowledge the awareness of shared humanity, attend to the individual, ask for and provide frequent clarification, demonstrate flexibility, and point out favorable opportunities yet acknowledge challenges to guide our online classroom environment (Sitzman & Watson, 2016).

We are also intentional in how we set up our in-person teaching and learning spaces, and try, whenever the physical space allows, to sit in a circle with our students. This demonstrates our intention to limit the power differential between students and faculty alike and emphasizes the value that each person brings to the learning environment. This arrangement allows us to see one another's faces as we share our stories and our unique knowledge born of our own experiences. In addition, this environment allows our students to gain a sense of having a voice (Lally Flack & Thrall, 2019). The works of Freire (2010), De Lissovoy (2010), Chinn (1989), Hills and Watson (2011) support this pedagogy where the relationship is participatory and liberating with power being shared.

Actualizing the physical setup of the environment has proven difficult at times within the constraints of our facilities. In our upper-level courses, we aim to keep class sizes small. This results in being assigned to small classroom spaces that do not always allow for this sort of seating arrangement; however, we continue to advocate for more classroom space to support this style of teaching as we believe (aesthetic knowing) that the physical environment can significantly impact the experience of learning.

In our communities of learning, it is imperative to create a culture that is civil and free from lateral or vertical violence. Lateral and/or vertical violence is a significant professional issue in the workplace and refers to overt or covert discord between nurses, usually within a power differential (Sanner-Stiehr & Ward-Smith, 2017). When related to nursing education, the concept of lateral or vertical violence takes on a new meaning to include student to student, student to faculty, faculty to faculty, and faculty to student interactions. In our caring community, it is critical for all faculty to model the expectation that there will be civility between all parties in the classroom and beyond. We introduce this critical concept and model civility in the classroom to establish a framework grounded in caring theory to encourage growth of critical thinking, clinical judgement, and student voice. In doing so, we are hopeful that it will find translation into the workplace (Lally Flack & Thrall, 2019).

Another tool employed in our classrooms is the use of quiet meditation or centering exercises at the start of the class or during a transition in class. This looks different as applied by different unique faculty. Some use a commercial app to do guided meditation. One faculty began using a "Check-in" as described in Chinn's (2008) *Peace and Power* when facing a particularly challenging semester in which the classroom community was tense. This process contributed to the facilitation of relationship building and provided a structured way to bring the students and faculty together in order to work towards being fully present during class. This is something we have continued to use in both the classroom and in our department meetings to begin our time together.

The cocreation of classroom norms has also been used to establish a learning environment that reflects the unique composition of each class. A process to cocreate the ground rules for class meetings and discussions with students has been used by some of our faculty (Eberly Center for Teaching Excellence, n.d). By doing this during the first class session a mutual community of learning is established which provides a safe place to engage with one another as we engage with the material. Some examples from these norms include: "Assume good will; address any concerns with the individual directly"; "Ask for clarification if you are confused. It's okay to say you don't know" and "Speak from your own experience, without generalizing."

Methods of Evaluation

One of the significant challenges we have been faced with has been how to apply the equalization of power aspects of our Caring Science philosophy in regard to grading and evaluation. Our program is part of a traditional liberal arts college with conventional grading and evaluation methods in use across the campus. As noted by Chinn (2007), we are becoming increasingly dissatisfied with the inherently patriarchal nature of traditional grading and grading practices, a process that sets up a difficult power-over relationship between teachers and students. We are investigating different evaluation methods and learning about concepts such as "ungrading" (Blum, 2017) and "authentication" (Hills & Watson, 2011). This is an evolutionary process that we are beginning to explore further. In support of this evolution, during the second year of our program one faculty member piloted a different method for online discussion boards that shifted the focus from a faculty-graded activity to a self-reflection exercise at the conclusion of the course. This new grading plan included a revised discussion board rubric and portfolio submission. This evaluation method has been adopted across the curriculum to lessen the top-down approach to grading and encourage self-evaluation and reflection. Through this feminist pedagogical approach, we seek to call forth the best in every student rather than police or oversee what might be wrong (Chinn, 2007). See Tables 14.6 and 14.7 for Discussion Board Portfolio instructions and grading rubric.

For many assignments in our courses, students complete a self-reflection using the grading rubric when they submit their assignments. In our experience thus far, we have seen students grade themselves equal to where the faculty member scores them or they underestimate their performance, submitting a more highly critical appraisal of their level of achievement. An additional benefit of this approach is that faculty members are more available to participate in or read and bring online discussions into the classroom rather than focusing on grading each online post, resulting in deeper, more meaningful learning experiences.

Within the Faculty and the Department

The structure and function of the nursing department itself contributes to the working, teaching, and learning environment. As such, it can either provide fertile ground for the faculty's way of being or come in conflict with caring practices. Careful attention has been given to the elements that make up the structure and function of our department, in order to support caring practices within and among the faculty and staff. These elements include: hiring practices; a model for Faculty to Faculty Coaching; personal development through participation in the Caritas Coach Education Program® (CCEP); clear, nonfear-based tenure and promotion

TABLE 14.6 Discussion Board Portfolio Assignment Instructions

Directions for Discussion Board Assignments and Discussion Board Portfolio

The discussion boards that are assigned in this course will serve as your online course work/class time. Therefore, it should account for approximately 1.5 to 2 hours of work per week depending on the course and depth of the assignment. The rest of your online class time will consist of other various online assignments, learning modules, and online quizzes.

Please create all posts and follow-up posts in a Word document. You will need these to compile a portfolio for grading at the end of the term. You will also want to copy out the post from the classmate you are responding to so that you can include it in your portfolio.

1. For each discussion board post, follow the instructions listed in Canvas for that particular topic.
2. Your initial post (250-word minimum) is due in the forum by Saturday at 1159pm before the assigned week so your classmates have time to read and respond.
3. Responses to two other student postings (100-word minimum) should be completed by the due date at 1159pm.
4. Initial post and responses must reference course readings or other materials.
5. Remember to use APA-formatted citations for any references used.
6. Compile a portfolio of selected posts. Select three (3) examples of your high-quality posts and responses (include a copy of the post you are responding to) and paste these into a single document.
7. Use the provided rubric to complete a self-evaluation of your posts. You will select a grade for each category and provide supporting comments.
8. Give yourself an overall grade for your discussion contributions as reflected in your portfolio.
9. Submit your portfolio and self-evaluation to the dropbox in Canvas by the due date.

guidelines; department bylaws that reflect equanimity among members of the department; and meeting and gathering practices. It is our belief that our way of being in the department in turn impacts our way of being and caring practices with and among our students.

TABLE 14.7 Rubric for Discussion Board Portfolio

POST #S SELECTED _____	SUPERB (A)	EXCELLENT (B)	VERY GOOD (C)	NEEDS IMPROVEMENT
Timely 10 x _____	Initial posting for every assignment is on time and follow-up posts are completed when the thread is still active and flowing prior to assignment due date. (90–100)	Most contributions are made when the thread is still active and flowing so the majority of students can profit from the information. (80–89)	Typically one of the last to respond to an active thread. (70–79)	Messages posted after the thread due dates. (69 or below)

(continued)

TABLE 14.7 Rubric for Discussion Board Portfolio (*continued*)

POST #S SELECTED	SUPERB (A)	EXCELLENT (B)	VERY GOOD (C)	NEEDS IMPROVEMENT
Thoughtful & Significant 30% x _____	Posts reflect analysis and synthesis of course content and related sources. Clearly stated opinion supported with rationale. Stimulates discussion through insightful comments. (90–100)	Posts are informative and/or original. Opinion stated but may lack supporting rationale. (80–89)	Posts summarize topics without much original content or insight. Opinion included but may be less clear or lack supporting rationale. (70–79)	Posts are missing or simply restates topic without insight or opinion. (69 or below)
Follow-Up Posts 30% X _____	Presents strong follow-up posts with depth of knowledge and reasoning. Opinion stated in a highly collegial manner. (90–100)	Provides adequate follow-up posts with rationale. Opinion stated in a collegial manner. (80–89)	Follow-up posts are simplistic and lack depth of knowledge. (70–79)	Weak follow-up posts. Lacks supporting rationale. Opinion not stated in a collegial manner. (69 or below)
Clarity, Grammar & Spelling 20% X _____	No errors. (90–100)	A few errors that do not impede understanding. (80–89)	Some errors that may impede understanding. (70–79)	More than four (4) errors that impede understanding. (69 or below)
Citations Included 10% X _____	Included in full. Link included to any articles not found in course materials. (90–100)	Some citations and links are missing. (80–89)	Many citations and links are missing. (70–79)	Citations and/ or links are not included. (69 or below)
Overall grade: _____				

HIRING PRACTICES

Our advertisements for faculty positions explicitly describe the philosophical foundation for our program and invite applicants to submit a Caring Science teaching philosophy. Our preference for a research doctorate acknowledges our commitment to disciplinary-specific nursing knowledge (Smith & McCarthy, 2010). It is our intent to hire faculty who have the capacity to introduce our students in the baccalaureate program to nursing philosophies, theories, and research to enable our graduates to engage in reflective praxis.

Sample from our job posting:
About the Baldwin Nursing Program at Siena College:
The Baldwin Nursing Program at Siena College provides an education that is congruent with the Siena College mission and learning goals and offers nurses a broader humanistic caring perspective of the discipline of nursing. The Nursing Program integrates a Caring Science curriculum with Franciscan values and a strong education in the liberal arts and sciences. With a focus on mindful learning, reflective practice, and the importance of self-care, our Caring Science teaching/learning philosophy creates an authentic environment to enhance the student's understanding of social, cultural, economic, and political issues that impact healthcare.

Requirements:
The ideal candidate will have a research doctorate (PhD, DNS, or other) and a MS in nursing. Applicants must demonstrate a commitment to excellence in teaching (both classroom and hybrid platforms) using a Caring Science philosophy and an active scholarship program. A minimum of three (3) years teaching in baccalaureate nursing is preferred. In addition, the ideal candidate will have experience with Dr. Jean Watson's Theory of Human Caring and Caring Science.

As part of the interview process, we ask candidates to give a 20- to 30-minute presentation of their teaching that reflects the integration of Caring Science pedagogy *or* a presentation of their research, including how it reflects inclusion of the disciplinary knowledge of nursing. This approach is critical to learning more about the potential each candidate has to be successful in integrating into our Caritas community.

MENTORING THROUGH COACHING

Once hired, how we support faculty as they transition to their new role is another key element of our departmental functions. To address this, we have developed a faculty to faculty coaching model to mentor new faculty. Our two initial full-time tenure track faculty (DT & JT) participated concurrently in a CCEP cohort at the end of JT's first year. Through this process these faculty reflected on the relationship they developed when JT was hired. Being the only two faculty, these two fell naturally into a supportive relationship. Both had several years of teaching experience in higher education and were not novices in their faculty role or in their commitment to caring philosophies and theories. In spite of these similarities, each brought unique strengths and desires for growth. DT was hired a year prior to JT and therefore had institutional knowledge regarding Siena; also, as noted previously, she had extensive immersion in Caring Science. JT came with a strong background in curricular design and assessment and had recently finished her doctoral education, thus bringing skills in theory-guided research. As a result, there was relational mutuality in care, benefit, trust, and support.

Through the CCEP program, the pair documented their reflections on the lived experience of the Faculty Coaching relationship that had formed during JT's first year at Siena. This resulted in an initial scaffolding for the Faculty to Faculty coaching model that would be used with all newly hired faculty. Elements of this model include: self-care assessments and discussions on how to maintain self-care while fulfilling all three traditional aspects of faculty role (teaching, scholarship, and service); a self-inventory of strengths and areas for growth; values clarification; and employing the practice of "calling out" Caritas in action as seen in one another. The self-inventory of strengths and areas for growth supports mutuality in the coaching relationship as noted previously. To accomplish this, faculty reflect on their own stories to identify how they each can contribute to the development of the other. Mixer et al. (2013) described this as comentoring. Through these coaching relationships we continue to explore ways to help deepen our own understanding of Caring Science and related nursing theories. We continue to explore how to integrate readings and discussions via these coaching relationships such that they become a part of regular departmental work. At the writing of this text, the two initial faculty (DT & JT) are now in coaching relationships with two new faculty in the department. It is our intent that this approach, of pairing existing faculty with new faculty, will contribute to sustaining a Caring Science curriculum as our program grows and new faculty are added.

TENURE AND PROMOTION

The process to obtain tenure and promotion can be wrought with fear and power differentials promoting a structure that degrades the person behind the process. It is our belief that one can delineate clear standards and guidelines for tenure and promotion while supporting the individual's care of self and others. In our experience, lack of clear standards and guidelines or the criteria by which the faculty member would be evaluated, fostered an environment where "striving to please many masters" motivated rather than focused efforts to grow and develop as a teacher and scholar. To counter this, the two initial hires in the program (LL & DT) created unambiguous criteria for promotion and tenure in the realms of teaching, service, and scholarship. We have made explicit what constitutes scholarly activity in nursing and utilized a point-based scholarship equivalency table. In our guidelines, the number of scholarly equivalencies to advance from assistant to associate professor with tenure and associate to full professor are clearly delineated, thus removing fear from the process. This has allowed faculty to be confident in their progress toward tenure. The Scholarship Equivalencies Table was created to give a clear description of and assign points to each type of scholarship (Table 14.8). For example, depending upon the level of promotion, faculty need to produce at least six (6) units (tenure and promotion to associate professor) or at least twelve (12) units (for promotion to full professor) from a peer-reviewed publication or equivalent as defined in Table 14.8 under either Categories I and II. Faculty also need to have an additional three (3) units from Categories III–VI, for a minimum *total* of nine (9) units for tenure and promotion to associate professor or at least fifteen (15) total units for promotion to full professor. These units of scholarship are fully explained in the Scholarship Equivalencies Table from our tenure and promotion criteria found in Table 14.8.

TABLE 14.8 Table of Scholarship Equivalencies

CATEGORY I: SIX UNITS OF SCHOLARSHIP

Author of first edition of peer-reviewed **book** that is published or in press (Additional units may be awarded at the discretion of the department for a maximum of 12 units.)
Editing or coediting a peer-reviewed book that is published or in press (Additional units may be awarded at the discretion of the department for a maximum of 12 units.)

(continued)

TABLE 14.8 Table of Scholarship Equivalencies (*continued*)

CATEGORY II: THREE UNITS OF SCHOLARSHIP

Peer-reviewed journal articles and book chapters that are published or in press
Development of peer-reviewed multimedia products and/or curricula which are sold by an academic publisher on a national level
Editing a peer-reviewed journal (three units per year of appointment)

CATEGORY III: TWO UNITS OF SCHOLARSHIP

Papers, poster sessions, and symposia selected competitively through peer review for national or international conferences
Securing grants: Applies to external grant awarded on a competitive basis of an amount above $3,000 (Additional units may be awarded based on prestige and amount of grant for a maximum of four units.)
Revised editions of peer-reviewed books (two units for each new or revised edition)
Serving on editorial advisory board (two units per year of appointment per board)

CATEGORY IV: ONE UNIT OF SCHOLARSHIP

Papers, poster sessions, and symposia selected competitively through peer review for regional or local conferences
Securing grants: Applies to external grant awarded on a competitive basis of an amount of $500–$3,000
Securing a Siena grant or fellowship: awarded on a competitive basis of an amount above $1,000 (max of one unit in this category per evaluation period)
Evidence of significant work on a submitted external grant that was not awarded or that has not yet been reviewed by the granting agency
Postdoctoral Fellowship: (one unit per year)
Postdoctoral Coursework and Certifications (i.e., CNE, CCEP, AHN-BC): (one unit per course/certification)

CATEGORY V: HALF UNIT OF SCHOLARSHIP

Unpublished articles and manuscripts with evidence that the faculty member is actively working toward publication (e.g., a "revise and resubmit" letter from an editor)
Unpaid consulting: Half unit per project only if the faculty member obtains acceptance from the Department of the value of the project to the faculty member's academic advancement (Maximum of one unit of scholarship is allowed for this category.)
Reviewing manuscripts as ad hoc reviewer for journals, publishers, and/or conference proceedings (up to half unit per year).

CATEGORY VI: ONE UNIT "ADD-ONS" FOR SCHOLARSHIP

First authorship
Publication in a Tier 1 Journal (defined as having a minimum 80% rejection rate)
Editor of a Tier 1 Journal
Student collaboration: Peer-reviewed publication or conference proceeding with a Siena student listed as a coauthor or copresenter
Recognized as a national expert **in one's field:** Defined as research cited or product of interview appears in a major magazine or news outlet, invited to deliver a presentation or webinar to practitioners or scholars at a local/national/international event (Maximum of one unit of scholarship is allowed for this category.)

For each scholarship category in this table, other scholarly activity may be recognized at the discretion of the Nursing Department.

DEPARTMENTAL BYLAWS

In a similar method to the creation of our tenure and promotion guidelines using a Caring Science framework, we are currently developing our nursing departmental bylaws. Through this work we have reflected on how caring philosophies influence the daily workings of the department. In particular, to decrease the potential for a power differential between faculty, staff, and leadership, we use consensus building for decision-making thereby creating equanimity between all. In our bylaws, we are explicit in the departmental membership, voting membership, curriculum and program development responsibilities, teaching assignments and scheduling, tenure/promotion and sabbaticals, faculty searches and appointments, and so forth.

An example of this in action is during our nursing department meetings and curriculum meetings. We use the tenets of Chinn's *Peace and Power* by starting meetings with a centering activity, check in, and then discuss each faculty's priority for the meeting. This way, each individual faculty has an opportunity to be heard and have their needs met along with the overarching needs of the department.

REFLECTING ON THE JOURNEY: SUSTAINING A CARING SCIENCE CURRICULUM

The journey to create a living, breathing Caring Science philosophy within our nursing department and curriculum has been a labor of love and discovery. It must encompass all that we "do" and "are" as educators and administrators to have the effect we so desire on our graduates and ultimately the patients they serve. Breaking down the barriers of the patriarchal behaviorist pedagogy, that for so long has dominated nursing education and subsequently the profession of nursing, is critical in order to bring joy back into nursing. We are intentional in our process to assemble a department with faculty and staff who are fully committed to embracing this philosophy and developing their personal and pedagogical practices through further education in Caritas literacy either through the Caritas Coach Education Program® program or the Watson Caring Science Postdoctoral Scholar program. As previously noted, we currently have two members of the department who are Watson Caring Science Postdoctoral Scholars (LL and DT) and two who completed the Caritas Coach program (DT and JT). It cannot be understated that having faculty who are immersed in the philosophy of Caring Science is critical to the success of a praxis in nursing that synthesizes action and reflection (Hills & Watson, 2011, p. 118) and whereby theory informs and is informed by the lived experiences of our faculty and students. We are committed to having all faculty in our department take part in education that further develops their Caritas literacy. "In this awakening of the unitary field, the personal *is* the professional. We practice who we are, we teach who we are, we live who we are as a person—thus, this work requires a personal transformation for our own journey to a higher level of consciousness" (Watson, 2018a, p. 46).

We have structured our program so that both students and faculty can find tangible ways to bring this theory to life in all that we do, both personally and professionally, and to reflect on how their practices contribute to the theoretical basis for nursing. It is one thing to read the work on your own, it is an entirely different experience to engage in structured coursework and commit to the very personal journey that is the work of Caring Science. Students often start the rigorous nursing program with expectations informed by past experiences from other educational settings. Often, we have encounters with students who are distraught and frightened about the intensity of the nursing program. Listening to another person's story without judgment, demonstrating empathy, shows the person that you care. Sometimes all a person needs is for someone to listen, rather than fix the situation. When students have apologized for being distraught or overwhelmed or angry, reminding them of Caritas Process® #5—allowing for the expression of positive and negative feelings—authentically listening to another person's story, demonstrates how one lives out Caritas. Doing this has validated their experience and allows the student to hear faculty give credence to their feelings through the Caritas Processes®. It also de-escalates most difficult situations. This experience for the student affirms their value and voice as a nurse and preserves dignity for the student. According to Watson, a caring attitude is not transmitted from generation to generation by genes but rather it is transmitted by the culture of society (Watson, 2008a, p. 18). We are committed to transmitting a culture of caring through our community of learning at Siena College.

REFERENCES

American Nurses Association. (2015). *Code of ethics for nurses with interpretive statements.* Author.

Blum, S. (2017). Ungrading. *Inside Higher Ed.* https://www.insidehighered.com/advice/2017/11/14/significant-learning-benefits-getting-rid-grades-essay

Brown, B. (2018) *Dare to lead.* Random House.

Carper, B. (1978). Fundamental patterns of knowing. *Advances in Nursing Science, 1*(1), 13–24. https://doi.org/10.1097/00012272-197810000-00004

Chinn, P. (1989). Feminist pedagogy and nursing education. In National League for Nursing (Ed.), *Curriculum revolution: Reconceptualizing nursing education.* (pp. 9–24). Editor.

Chinn, P. (2007). Reflections on feminist pedagogy in nursing education. In P. M. Ironside (Ed.), *On revolutions and revolutionaries: 25 years of reform and innovation in nursing education* (pp. 155–161). National League for Nursing.

Chinn, P. (2008). *Peace and power: Creative leadership for building community* (7th ed.). Jones & Bartlett Publishers.

Chinn, P. L. & Kramer, M. K. (2018). *Knowledge development in nursing: Theory and process* (10th ed.). Elsevier.

De Lissovoy, N. (2010). Rethinking education and emancipation: Being, teaching, and power. *Harvard Educational Review, 80*(2), 203–221. https://doi.org/10.17763/haer.80.2.h6r65285tu252448

Dossey, B. M. (2015). Integrative health and wellness assessment. In B. M. Dossey, S. Luck, & B. G. Schaub (Eds.), *Nurse coaching: Integrative approaches for health and wellbeing* (pp. 109–122). International Nurse Coach Association.

Eberly Center for Teaching Excellence. (n.d.). *Ground rules.* https://www.cmu.edu/teaching/solveproblem/strat-dontparticipate/groundrules.pdf

Freire, P. (2010). *Pedagogy of the oppressed.* The Continuum International Publishing Group.

Hills, M., & Watson, J. (2011). *Creating a Caring Science curriculum: An emancipatory pedagogy for nursing* (1st ed.). Springer Publishing Company.

Horton-Deutsch, S., & Sherwood, G. W. (2017). *Reflective practice: Transforming education and improving outcomes* (2nd ed.). Sigma Theta Tau International.

Institute of Medicine. (2011). *The future of nursing: Leading change, advancing health.* The National Academies Press. https://doi.org/10.17226/12956

Kornfield, J. (2002). *The art of forgiveness, loving-kindness and peace.* Bantam.

Lally Flack, L., & Thrall, D. (2016). *Baldwin nursing program praxis model.* Siena College Department of Nursing Handbook.

Lally Flack, L., & Thrall, D. (2019). Values and philosophies of being. In W. Rosa, S. Horton-Deutsch, & J. Watson (Eds.), *A handbook for caring science: Expanding the paradigm.* Springer Publishing Company.

Manhart Barrett, E. A. (2017). Again, what is nursing science? *Nursing Science Quarterly, 30*(2), 129–133. https://doi.org/10.1177/0894318417693313

Mixer, S. J., McFarland, M. R., Andrews, M. M., & Strang, C. W. (2013). Exploring faculty health and well-being: Creating a caring scholarly community. *Nurse Education Today, 33,* 1471–1476. https://doi.org/10.1016/j.nedt.2013.05.019

Monti, D. V. (2013). Franciscans and our healthcare: Our heritage. In E. Saggau (Ed.), *Franciscans and healthcare: Facing the future* (pp. xi–31). Franciscan Institute Publications.

Porter-O'Grady, T. (2003). A different age for leadership. *Journal of Nursing Administration, 33*(10), 105–110. https://doi.org/10.1097/00005110-200302000-00007

Quinn, J. (1992). Holding sacred space: The nurse as healing environment. *Holistic Nursing Practice, 6*(4), 26–36. https://doi.org/10.1097/00004650-199207000-00007

Richardson, C. (2019). *The art of extreme self care: Transform your life one month at a time.* Hay House.

Sanner-Stiehr, E. & Ward-Smith, P. (2017).Lateral violence in nursing: Implications and strategies for nurse educators. *Journal of Professional Nursing, 33*(2), 113–118. https://doi.org/10.1016/j.profnurs.2016.08.007

Schön, D. A. (1987). *Educating the reflective practitioner.* Jossey-Bass.

Siena College. (2017). *Baldwin nursing program: Mission statement.* https://www.siena.edu/programs/nursing/mission

Siena College. (2020a). *The Franciscan tradition.* https://www.siena.edu/visit/about/catholic-franciscan-tradition

Siena College. (2020b). *The mission of Siena College.* https://www.siena.edu/visit/about/mission

Sitzman, K., & Watson, J. (2016). *Watson's caring in the digital world: A guide for caring when interacting, teaching and learning in cyberspace.* Springer Publishing Company.

Smith, M. C. (2019). Regenerating nursing's disciplinary perspective. *Advances in Nursing Science, 42*(1), 3–16. https://doi.org/10.1097/ANS.0000000000000241

Smith, M., & McCarthy, M. P. (2010). Disciplinary knowledge in nursing education: Going beyond the blueprints. *Nursing Outlook, 58*(1), 44–51. https://doi.org/10.1016/j.outlook.2009.09.002

Tanner, C. (2006). Thinking like a nurse: A research-based model of clinical judgment in nursing. *Journal of Nursing Education, 45*(6), 204–211. https://doi.org/10.3928/01484834-20060601-04

Watson, J. (2008a). *Nursing: The philosophy and science of caring.* University Press of Colorado.

Watson, J. (2008b). The Caring Moment. *Caritas Meditation CD.* Watson Caring Science Institute.

Watson, J. (2012). *Human caring science: A theory of nursing.* Jones & Bartlett Learning.

Watson, J. (2018a). *Unitary caring science: The philosophy and praxis of nursing.* University Press of Colorado.

Watson, J. (2018b). Unitary caring science: Universals of human caring and global micro practices of caritas. *NSC Nursing, 4*(1), 1–7. https://doi.org/10.32549/OPI-NSC-22

Watson, J. (2020). Jean Watson's theory of unitary caring science and theory of human caring. In M. C. Smith (Ed.), *Nursing theories and nursing practice* (5th ed., pp. 311–331). F. A. Davis.

World Health Organization. (2018). *Promoting health: Guide to national implementation of the Shanghai declaration.* https://www.who.int/publications-detail/promoting-health-guide-to-national-implementation-of-the-shanghai-declaration

Appendix A

NURS 300

ADVANCED CONCEPTS OF PROFESSIONAL NURSING COURSE DESCRIPTION AND STUDENT-LEARNING OUTCOMES

This course serves as the foundation for the nursing program to introduce the student to the philosophical and theoretical framework of the Baldwin Nursing Program at Siena College. Caring Science is explored as a foundation for being, doing, and becoming a holistic nurse. Historical and contemporary social forces that are key to the current roles of the professional nurse are introduced. Principles of holistic nursing theories are examined, including the creation of caring/healing relationships through the use of authentic presence and integrative health practices. Students experience the significance of self-care and reflection in order to apply these concepts to their practice as a holistic nurse.

1. Understand various theoretical frameworks in nursing for integration into nursing practice.
2. Identify the core values of the Caring Science curriculum of the Siena College Baldwin Nursing program as an integral component of professional nursing care.
3. Examine the historical and social foundations of professional nursing.
4. Explore concepts of patient-centered care, professionalism, communication, health promotion as they relate to the role of the holistic nurse.
5. Appraise how the holistic nurse shapes the profession through the application of Caring Science in leadership, systems, and quality improvement.
6. Synthesize major concepts of professional nursing into an individual nursing philosophy to be used as a foundation for making professional nursing judgments.
7. Demonstrate understanding of professional codes of conduct and professional standards.
8. Develop reflective practice and scholarship through writing assignments.

NURS 415

TRANSFORMATIONAL NURSING LEADERSHIP COURSE DESCRIPTION AND STUDENT-LEARNING OUTCOMES

This capstone course is designed to give the student the opportunity to assimilate the theoretical disciplinary knowledge of nursing with the core values of a Franciscan education within the context of the role of the professional baccalaureate-prepared nurse leader. This course prepares the nurse to be a Caritas-conscious leader through the application, synthesis, and evaluation of concepts and nursing issues. Experiences promote the development of knowledge and skills needed for leadership and management roles within a culturally diverse healthcare system. The Caritas nurse leader evaluates strategies to manage resources and apply transformational leadership principles to create compassionate, caring work environments. The continuation of self-care strategies learned throughout the program are further explored to support lifelong integration both personally and professionally. Students are encouraged to reflect on how "being, doing, and becoming" a Caritas nurse transforms their role as a nurse leader.

1. Synthesize the theoretical disciplinary knowledge of nursing with the core values of a Franciscan education to become a leader with Caritas Consciousness.
2. Compare and contrast the role of leadership and management theories, including transformational leadership principles, in creating a caring, compassionate work environment.
3. Develop techniques to authentically communicate with nurse leaders, nurses, and staff to effectively lead a culturally diverse work setting.
4. Value the need for the nurse leader to provide a culture of mutual trust, teamwork, and open communication for effective delegation and creation of a caring workplace.
5. Examine how a nurse leader can use Caritas consciousness to contribute to the interprofessional team in order to better advocate for quality, safety, and improved patient outcomes.
6. Appraise current leadership trends and their impact on nurses, the practice of nursing, and healthcare.
7. Evaluate the role of the nurse leader as a driving force in the promotion of a dialectical relationship between theory and practice.
8. Demonstrate civic responsibility and leadership skills using a Caritas lens when engaging in professional and community service activities for a vulnerable or underserved population.
9. Compose a personal philosophy of transformative nursing leadership that reflects a synthesis of concepts learned in the baccalaureate program.

Developing Caring Consciousness in Nurse Leaders

Lisa Lally

INTRODUCTION

This chapter describes the background leading to the development and implementation of the Transformational Nursing Leadership capstone nursing course at Siena College. Chapter 14, Creating a Caring Science Curriculum: The Siena Experience, showcased the development of our Caring Science philosophy within the curriculum and departmental processes. This chapter further addresses how the curriculum is structured, and more specifically the capstone course, to develop nurse leaders with caring consciousness. The theoretical foundation and processes of this course will now be shared along with student voices that beautifully articulate the results of our curriculum at Siena College.

LEADERSHIP IN NURSING

There is a longing for leadership that creates a path back to that sense of meaning and impact—that connection with our deepest human purpose that brings out the best in us and unites us all in a common mission. There is a longing for caring leaders who bring clarity of voice and moments of peace and joy to environments of turbulence, constant change, firefighting and adrenaline addictions. (Johns, 2016, p. xviii)

What more do we need in today's world than to have a leader who demonstrates caring, compassion, and guides with an egoless heart? This is truly needed not only in the world at large, but in our nursing profession. The way we educate our nurses can have a large impact on the future generations of nurse leaders to come. Watson's Theory of Unitary Caring Science frames the discipline of nursing within a heart-centered relational approach. Can this experience be transcended to the faculty/student, student/student relationship? I posit that it actually can. . .and this is changing the way new nurses are approaching and becoming leaders in the profession. Not only is the relationship between the nurse and the patient a critical component of nursing, but the relationship between the educator and student should be equally important to develop nurses to be strong leaders with caring consciousness. Leaders with caring consciousness are authentic, genuine, and have an understanding of the importance of the human connection and relationship (Sitzman & Watson, 2018). This chapter explores that very relationship in the context of nursing education and nurturing the growth of our nurses to become caring leaders.

Leading With Caring Consciousness

How does one define a good or great leader? Everyone is capable of being a leader and nurses are well known as trusted leaders at all levels of our profession. Each person has the capacity to be a leader as long as one has the passion to make things better, be a kind and compassionate colleague, show vulnerability, and face the challenges of the workplace. As President Roosevelt said in my life mantra quote, *The Man in the Arena*:

> *The credit belongs to the man who is actually in the arena*, whose face is marred by dust and sweat and blood; who strives valiantly. . . there is no effort without error and shortcoming. . . who spends himself in a worthy cause. (Roosevelt & Thomsen, 2003, p. 1)

They go on to express that the "man in the arena" knows at last

> . . . the triumph of high achievement, and who at the worst, if he fails, at least fails while daring greatly, so that his place shall never be with those cold and timid souls who neither know victory nor defeat. (Roosevelt & Thomsen, 2003, p. 1)

We are in that position in nursing. We need to find our collective voice. We need to teach our students to have that voice and be that woman or man in the arena. Facing the fight, giving our best, showing our heart, and most importantly supporting each other. It takes courage to be a leader, as Brown (2018) points out in her book *Dare to Lead*. (This book has become an important part of our curriculum at Siena College.) Brown (2018) defines a leader as "anyone who takes responsibility for finding the potential in people and processes, and who has the courage to develop that potential" (p. 4). This process of becoming a brave leader begins with learning to be vulnerable and becoming more self-aware.

In 2015, I was hired to develop a nursing program at Siena College, a private Catholic college in upstate New York. This was a unique and amazing opportunity to take that leap of faith, be that woman in the arena, be vulnerable, to do my best to change the broken system of our oppressive patriarchal education that proliferates horizontal/lateral violence, and the old adage, "nurses eating their young." Where did that start? I remember times during my prelicensure nursing education being grilled on my patient's medications and shaking in fear. This was learning nursing within a behaviorist, fear-based, top-down transactional pedagogy which has been the norm in nursing for years. Students were afraid to speak in fear of error, and this continues to occur in many nursing programs to this day. This behaviorist approach to nursing education limits the student's perspective to that of the teacher/book/school and does not take into consideration the student's rational and constructive knowledge. With the benchmark of entry into nursing being the National Council Licensure Examination (NCLEX®), many schools of nursing continue to deliver education that is based primarily upon measurable outcomes. While this may be an important point of recognition, the educational philosophy surrounding this is often riddled with a pedagogy of control and conformity which by its very nature becomes oppressive. That being said, I question whether the oppression is coming from the teaching methodology, the teacher, or the nature of the profession of nursing. Not only does this occur in the school setting, it continues into the workplace where national quality measures are being set to assess how well nurses are doing in their job (Lally Flack & Thrall, 2019).

As noted in the 2011 Institute of Medicine (IOM) report, *The Future of Nursing: Leading Change, Advancing Health,* the Joint Commission believes that "the future state of nursing is inextricably linked to the strides in patient-care quality and safety that are critical to the success of America's healthcare system, today and tomorrow" (IOM, 2011). This, however, is only one measure of the worth of nursing. While it is extremely important to have standards of care for any practitioner, it should not be the say-all and be-all of a profession. The discipline of nursing must develop its sense of worthiness by virtue of knowledge, action, and voice. To this end, our discipline must include the theories, philosophies, and language of nursing (Smith, 2019; Watson, 2018). If a humanistic approach to education were consistently used in the classroom so that each individual student/nurse had a voice and ability to use it without oppression, I believe that would extend into the workplace and beyond.

Personally, I knew there had to be another way. In my doctoral studies I was assigned to develop a philosophy of nursing education which included my hopes of what it should be. Developing a personal philosophy of nursing education required an examination of the rich tapestry of philosophical ideologies while keeping in mind that nursing is a humanistic profession that should be nurtured in the academic world prior to its impact on the community. The way in which one is educated has the potential to alter the life experiences of the person so that they can have a voice and sense of worthiness and humanity to move forward in their profession. Looking into works of Piaget and Freire (2010), feminist pedagogy, and in particular, emancipatory pedagogy (Hills & Watson, 2011), along with Watson's theory of human caring, I knew there was alignment and a way to transcend this into the nursing education arena. While Watson's theory focuses primarily on the nurse/patient relationship, it can also be applied to the educational setting. Reducing oppression in the classroom and in the profession of nursing leads to the beginning of a process of liberation and emancipation. Nurse educators have a choice of how they choose to use power. By having power *with* instead of *over*, a caring community of learning can be developed and nurtured. This caring, humanistic curriculum/culture, whereby the students are active learners and partners with their teachers, allows for a liberating experience (Hills & Watson, 2011).

Up to this point in my professional life, I had unknowingly embraced a Caring Science philosophy as a clinical nurse and lived the pedagogical philosophy in my teaching. Once I had the theory and language to explain the methods of how I taught, I became passionate about learning more and applying it in a more direct way to my educational style. I strongly felt that there needed to be a change in the way we educate our nursing students and the way we treat each other as faculty. The original edition of this book *Creating a Caring Science Curriculum: An Emancipatory Pedagogy for Nursing* (Hills & Watson, 2011) became my guide to the realization that this way of educating is not only possible, but critical in the development of nurses. This opportunity to start a nursing program from the ground up found its way to me and I was able to instill these values that I held so dear. I took that leap of faith, and that brings me to where I am today. As discussed in depth in Chapter 14, the history and story of our program are shared, and we are very fortunate that the nursing department fully supports this pedagogy and way of being. From the development and implementation of our Caring Science curriculum (Hills & Watson, 2011), to creating a community of learning for both students and faculty, to the departmental structure, we are intentional in this integration.

With Chapter 14 as a foundation, the final nursing course, Transformational Nursing Leadership will now be reviewed and will describe in more depth the methods of educating and nurturing caring nurse leaders. The goal of our Caring Science curriculum and, in particular, the final leadership course, is to illuminate ways that nurses can lead with caring consciousness. The course description, student learning outcomes, highlighted class activities and assignments are now explored.

NURSING 415: TRANSFORMATIONAL NURSING LEADERSHIP

Nursing 415 is a capstone, clinical course, with the intention to provide an opportunity to assimilate the theoretical disciplinary knowledge of nursing with the core values of a Franciscan education within the context of the role of the professional baccalaureate-prepared nurse leader.

NURS 415 Course Description

This capstone course is designed to give the student the opportunity to assimilate the theoretical disciplinary knowledge of nursing with the core values of a Franciscan education within the context of the role of the professional baccalaureate-prepared nurse leader. This course prepares the nurse to be a Caritas-conscious leader through the application, synthesis, and evaluation of concepts and nursing issues. Experiences promote the development of knowledge and skills needed for leadership and management roles within a culturally diverse healthcare system. The caring nurse leader evaluates strategies to manage resources and apply transformational leadership principles to create compassionate, caring, work environments. The continuation of self-care strategies learned throughout the program is further explored to support lifelong integration both personally and professionally. Students are encouraged to reflect on how "being, doing, and becoming" a caring nurse transforms their role as a nurse leader.

NURS 415 Course Learning Outcomes

1. Synthesize the theoretical disciplinary knowledge of nursing with the core values of a Franciscan education to become a leader with caring consciousness.
2. Compare and contrast the role of leadership and management theories, including transformational leadership principles, in creating a caring, compassionate work environment.
3. Develop techniques to authentically communicate with nurse leaders, nurses, and staff to effectively lead a culturally diverse work setting.
4. Value the need for the nurse leader to provide a culture of mutual trust, teamwork, and open communication for effective delegation and creation of a caring workplace.
5. Examine how a nurse leader can use Caritas consciousness to contribute to the interprofessional team in order to better advocate for quality, safety, and improved patient outcomes.
6. Appraise current leadership trends and their impact on nurses, the practice of nursing, and healthcare.
7. Evaluate the role of the nurse leader as a driving force in the promotion of a dialectical relationship between theory and practice.
8. Demonstrate civic responsibility and leadership skills using a caring lens when engaging in professional and community service activities for a vulnerable or underserved population.
9. Compose a personal philosophy of transformative nursing leadership that reflects a synthesis of concepts learned in the baccalaureate program.

This is not a traditional nursing leadership/management course that educates nurses on the basics of management theory and group dynamics. It was with intention that a business management principles course is required as a nursing auxiliary course to cover this important content. This allows the Nursing Transformational Leadership course to delve into the critical theory and application of becoming a caring nurse leader at every stage of one's nursing career. Throughout the Caring Science curriculum, our nursing students are taught to be reflective thinkers and through our community of learning, to develop a strong voice. This course is intended to further develop a leader who embodies caring and empathy along with a voice which is essential in nursing. In addition, this course has a 45-hour clinical immersion where students identify a clinical setting and nurse leader to shadow. It is in this setting where the students assess the role of the advanced practice nurse as a leader and identify leadership traits.

Transformational Nursing Leadership Course Content

KNOW THYSELF, DEVELOPMENT OF CARING CONSCIOUSNESS

Self-reflection is a key component to discovery and leadership. As one of our course texts, *Mindful Leadership: A Guide for the Health Care Professions* (Johns, 2016), quickly points out, "leadership begins with leading self" (p. 1). Johns goes on to say that without a clear personal vision, self-awareness and reflection, it is impossible to become a leader. This deep work is important to identify one's strengths and limitations and learn how to develop them further. Without this awareness, it is difficult to be a strong leader (Johns, 2016).

Bennis (2009) in his book *On Becoming a Leader*, also speaks to the importance of "knowing yourself" in a chapter named as such. To gain a broader perspective on leadership, business leadership gurus such as Bennis and others are reviewed in this leadership course. In Bennis's chapter Knowing Yourself, he speaks to the importance of your personal experience in framing your leadership styles. Bennis believes that leaders must be reflective, self-directed, and have a clear vision of what is needed, and a passion and energy to get there (Bennis, 2009).

From the beginning of the curriculum in the Baldwin Nursing Program, we embrace and encourage deep reflection and self-assessment in the journey towards being a nurse leader with caring consciousness. As discussed in more detail in Chapter 14, reflection is done both during and after an action. This work goes back to the sentinel work of Schön (1987), where he defined this reflective work as having two dimensions: reflection "in-action" and "on-action." In our classes, we discuss this dance between reflective time as critical not only for enhanced clinical judgment (Tanner, 2006), but also to engage in creative tension (Senge, 1990) whereby one develops a reality and vision of a desirable practice. Senge's (1990) learning organization mirrors these reflective tenants through the importance of collaborative learning communities (similar to that of a Caring Science learning community), where leaders coach and mentor, engage in dialogue and listen, and build consensus (Johns, 2004).

Throughout the curriculum, students are asked to dig deep into self to learn more about themselves as people and nurses. In the leadership course, we begin with a repeat of the Keegan and Dossey, Holistic Nurse Consultants, Self-Care assessment (2004). They take this assessment during the first nursing course in the curriculum and repeat it once again during the last. This reassessment provides students an insight into any changes (positive or negative) in their self-care practices. Students then take time to reflect upon them and then journal about their discoveries. As noted in Chapter 14 of this text, self-care is an integral part of the curriculum and is discussed and promoted throughout. One student described this part of the education as such: "The program stressed taking care of yourself which is what is keeping me sane. Yoga and meditation have been instrumental in taking care of my personal health when I have been so focused in taking care of others. At times like these it is of utmost importance to take care of your physical and mental health to adequately take care of others" (Anonymous student narrative, April, 2020).

In addition to the self-care assessment, this course requires the students to look at other indexes to determine personality, strengths, emotional intelligence, and leadership styles. The Keirsey Personality Index is completed which identifies temperament traits. This free online assessment was created by educational psychologist Dr. David Keirsey and is a result of his work and research on human behavior. He identified four basic patterns of human behavior that have been noted throughout history (artisan, guardian, idealist, and rational). The assessment uncovers a greater understanding of "who you are, why you do what you do, and how to build effective relationships" (Keirsey, 2020).

Students also complete the HIGH5 Strengths Test (high5test.com). This tool is also a free online assessment that identifies a person's five highest strengths (HIGH5Test, 2020). Students use the results of both these indices to submit a personal reflection which is shared only between the faculty and student. These findings are used throughout the rest of the course to augment leadership discussion boards and the final reflection paper.

Students also take a self-assessment on their leadership style from The Foundation of Nursing Leadership (2015) titled What Is Your Leadership Style? (www.nursingleadership. org.uk/test1.php). This assessment identifies the prominent style(s) of leadership (transformational, transactional, laissez-faire) the student possesses. This assessment is very useful as we delve into the various styles of leadership found within themselves and those witnessed at work. Two other self-assessments that are completed throughout the semester are related to emotional intelligence and Brown's (2018) Daring Leadership assessment. All together, these self-assessments are pivotal in helping the students to look deeper into themselves to further their own understanding and growth into caring leadership.

LEADERSHIP THEORIES

Framed in nursing leadership, this course discusses the key importance of nurses being leaders at every stage of their careers from a student through all advanced practice arenas. As further highlighted and informed in the sentinel report *The Future of Nursing: Leading Change, Advancing Health* (IOM, 2011), nurses must be full partners on the healthcare team. As educators, we have a call to develop collaborative leaders at all levels of education and healthcare. In this course, we review this important "call to lead" in key message #3 of the IOM report. Mutual respect and collaboration have been found to lead to improved patient outcomes, decreased medication errors, and decreased staff turnover (IOM, 2011). To be respectful, collaborative leaders, students need to have an understanding of the different styles of leadership and how they not only identify with them, but how they impact their relational leadership. The self-assessments done early in the course begin to uncover these traits and styles and they can then learn more about themselves and how to improve their leadership styles. In Johns's (2016) text, he brings the reader to a better understanding of leadership styles through the narratives of nurses working in a healthcare system where all styles of leaders are present. This book gives a wonderful context to theory in a reflective way and resonates well with the students.

Transformational Leadership is the first theory that is discussed in depth. Students have multiple methods of learning this material including course texts, articles from both nursing leadership journals and business journals, and online videos/TED talks that they complete prior to class. Transformational leadership can be defined in many ways; however, the term was first used in 1978 by James MacGregor Burns who was a historian and political scientist. According to Burns (1978), transformational leadership occurs when "leaders and followers raise one another to higher levels of motivation and morality" (p. 20). This definition resonates with how one defines transformational, servant, and caring leadership styles in nursing today. It is inclusive of the very relational and moral experience that is fundamental in nursing (Johns, 2016). Watson's Caring Science theory clearly parallels the transformational leadership style with the integration of the ten Caritas Processes®. Nurses have a moral and ethical responsibility to care and that does not just include the relationship between the nurse and the patient. It transcends to all areas of one's life (Watson, 2008). Integrating both nursing and multidisciplinary leadership theories, students begin to incorporate their knowledge of transformational leadership into their results from their personal self-assessments. This leads to lively discussions as they share their individual findings to a discussion board assignment and begin to have dialogue with their peers. Through readings, discussions, and life experiences, students see the moral imperative this way of transformational leading possesses. It also leads to some unrest and internal angst as they witness leaders who do not exemplify this way of being.

The narrative stories within Johns's (2016) text are discussed to highlight differences between a transformational and transactional leader. The contrast between lived experiences in a transactional culture come to light immediately. Transactional leadership has been defined as "a means to an end," inflexible, reactive style of leadership (Johns, 2016). Bass (1990), a leadership scholar, further explains that the transactional leader uses rewards in exchange for accomplishments, passively manages by exception (looking for deviations from norms to be corrected and takes action only when standards are not being met), and finally, shifts responsibilities to others instead of making final decisions. Schuster (1994) discusses that while both styles of leadership are prevalent, the transformational leader can utilize some of the "tools" of transactional leadership; however, the transactional leader does not exemplify any components of a transformational leader. He goes on to say, "As a good volunteer leader, you earn your leadership and stewardship role by demonstrating an earnest desire to serve those people you lead. You can keep your ego enough in check to see issues from a higher level" (Schuster, 1994, p. 47).

Through online discussion boards and class dialogue, students share stories of leaders that exemplify both styles of leadership within their workplace. This is a very eye-opening experience as students talk about the cultures within healthcare, and at some level, the need to embrace many leadership styles to navigate the dynamic healthcare field. Students express dismay over trickle-down management, dictator leadership styles that they see in their units. Stating that when their voice is not heard, it leads to frustration and low self-esteem of the team. Students share their distress when the nurse manager implements change only when there are problems or shows up on the unit when there is an issue, and how this leads to the feeling of being alone and not having a leader. One eloquent student recently said, "those who are doing the caring, are not being cared for." In contrast, students who can identify leaders in their lives who possess a more transformational leadership style speak a different narrative where their voices are heard, power is shared, and they are empowered. One new nurse manager has found that the transformational style with which he is leading to be life altering to the team. He shared, "For example, when an error is made in relationship to patient care, I try to use this as an 'opportunity for learning' rather than making it seem punitive. When you are constantly pointing out fault but not providing the person an opportunity to learn from the mistake, it creates a negative environment for that person" (Anonymous student narrative, February 2020).

To further bring transformational leadership to life, we review Schuster's (1994) 13 qualities for the transformational leader to cultivate and how to apply them to nursing. Students immediately find a correlation between these qualities and the 10 Caritas Processes®. Schuster's qualities are based upon head (deep thinking), heart (empathy), and hand (congruent action). These qualities include key behaviors on which all leaders can reflect to further their leadership skills. Schuster makes clear that while these characteristics of a leader are significant, the deepest value is the relationship with others that leaders invest in. It cannot be overstated that a transformational leader begins and ends with the human relationship and collaboration between the parties (Johns, 2004). Students understand the alignment between these qualities to their personal journeys as a leader. See Table 15.1 for examples of our student's voices in their discussion boards and linkage to caring leadership. These qualities bring forth the needed attributes of a leader to embrace honesty, reflection, resilience, courage, and vulnerability in their roles.

Caring Leadership. The review of transformational leadership and its many attributes, along with Schuster's 13 qualities and the relationship to Caring Science carries the class directly into what it means to lead with caring consciousness. Much of what is discussed throughout the course and curriculum leads our nurses to see a way of *being* that is in distinct contrast to what they see in their workplaces. This can lead to increased dissatisfaction and frustration within their work environments. In our class dialogues and discussion boards, faculty and students are open and supportive of one another to discuss ways to improve their cultures with a caring transformational lens. During this capstone course, we spend two class sessions on the topic of caring nurse leadership and delve into the strategies one can take to integrate Watson's theory of Caring Science into leadership. During the first class, basic tenets of caring are reviewed as they relate to Watson's caring theory and application to leadership. The work of American philosopher Milton Mayeroff (1971) is shared to provide a link between the definition of caring and Caring Science leadership. He describes "to care for another person, in the most significant sense, is to help him grow and actualize himself" (p. 1). He acknowledges that it is in the "knowledge" of the other's needs, that one can help them by guiding their growth. In essence, this knowledge of another's needs reflects the power of a caring relationship. Watson (1999) in multiple works has beautifully discussed caring as love and energy and as a "moral ideal of nursing" (Watson, 1999, p. 29), which is inclusive of an obligation to protect another's human dignity. As beautifully summarized by Turkel, Watson, and Giovannoni (2017), "the core of the theory of human caring has love at the starting point for practicing caring" (p. 68). All of these components are necessary to become a leader with caring consciousness. The students take part in class activity where they review the 10 Caritas Processes® and discuss ways in which a caring nurse leader exemplifies these through a leadership role. They realize through this activity that there are tangible ways to lead with caring consciousness. Through their own self-discovery and group work, students begin to realize it is not as out of reach as it may seem. As previously mentioned, once students learn about transformational and caring leadership ideals, they often feel disillusioned with their current healthcare settings and feel this is not attainable. To help students see the reality of this in practice, a Watson Caring Science postdoctoral scholar is invited to share her lived experience as a nurse manager in a Neuro ICU unit. Dr. Marlienne Goldin brings to life all of the caring

TABLE 15.1 Transformational Leadership Qualities and Alignment to Caring Leadership

TRANSFORMATIONAL LEADERSHIP QUALITIES ADAPTED TO CARING LEADERSHIP	STUDENT NARRATIVE ALIGNMENT TO CARING LEADERSHIP
You embrace a personal and organizational view of the discipline of nursing that is authentic and sensitive to varying viewpoints.	It is impossible to be a leader of integrity and outside of work be a person who is without this character trait. Integrity is like a golden thread that should be visibly woven throughout our lives regardless of what hat we wear. Reflection, and learning from our everyday experiences, along with the knowledge garnered from this program will guide and direct us. I was not well mentored as a new nurse, but I feel that this was a generational flaw in the nursing curriculum and culture at that time. As Johns states in his article, "the value of investing in people and collaborative ways of relating" is significant for transformational leadership (Johns, 2004).
You are authentically present and develop compassionate, loving, and caring relationships with others.	The overarching theme that I took from the course is bringing the human aspect into leadership. Until I had the pleasure of working under a great transformational leader and learning the values taught in this course, I had always believed a strong leader had to have a cutthroat and sometimes merciless approach. This may be true in some fields which historically do not have a moral compass, but in most facets of life, being a leader must require the transformational and human aspect in order to truly be successful and empower those around you. Being a brand-new nurse is hard and scary. I had a lot of support from more veteran nurses when I first started, and it really made a difference in my growth and development as a new nurse not only professionally but also personally. It is hard for a new nurse to grow and learn if they spend all their time and energy worrying about how to not make a mistake because there will be little support when they need it.
You allow for various viewpoints and expressions of positive and negative feelings, beyond ego-self to transpersonal presence.	Helping your fellow nurses is what is important. When things go wrong, it's about who is standing there with you to help that makes a difference. All hands-on deck. I like to lead people, but I also just like to do my own thing. I like when others give advice or when I can ask for opinions on decisions. It's helpful in the nursing field, we don't know everything so being there to help each other is key. As a nurse leader, I have always considered myself to be largely on the transformational side of the continuum. For example, when an error is made in relation to patient care, I try to use this as an "opportunity for learning" rather than making it seem punitive. When you are constantly pointing out a fault but not providing the person an opportunity to learn from the mistake it creates a negative environment for that person.

(continued)

TABLE 15.1 Transformational Leadership Qualities and Alignment to Caring Leadership (*continued*)

TRANSFORMATIONAL LEADERSHIP QUALITIES ADAPTED TO CARING LEADERSHIP	STUDENT NARRATIVE ALIGNMENT TO CARING LEADERSHIP
You inspire and guide with compassion and equanimity, encouraging growth and development of your team.	Ultimately, at your job, you are listening, leading, encouraging, and teaching. Leaders listen, according to Johns, and "the leader comes to truly appreciate the situation and can respond rather than react" (Johns, 2016). This is a team-learning approach because you are starting with dialogue, gaining consensus via community, and offering positive feedback. Having positive and negative role models allows us to learn and grow as leaders ourselves. "All staff want to be valued for their contributions to the work of the team. When leaders fail to say 'thank you' or take the recognition for themselves, staff feel devalued. Successful people become great leaders when they shift the focus from themselves to others"(Sherman, 2012).
You are sensitive to the needs of yourself and your team as reflected in your creative problem-solving using all ways of knowing.	I have learned that you cannot truly be a transformational leader if you are not opening your heart and mind to your own needs along with the needs of the team. Allowing yourself to be vulnerable and to grow from that will only help make the team grow. Caring for the needs of others, including our nurses, takes all of Schuster's deep thinking, empathy, and congruent action—or as I love the analogous Head, Heart, and Hand (Johns, 2016).
You cocreate with others to equalize power to engage and empower your team.	Being a transformational leader means sharing power with your staff. As the Lessons from the Geese (McNeish, 1972) clearly articulate, when the leader gets tired, the others from the team come forward and take over to share the burden. A transformational leader guides from the side or behind, lifting others up. As written by J. Jackson et al. (2009), "Nursing Leadership Knowing" provides a forum for leaders to enhance their practice, as well as their relationship with their employees, which ultimately translates into optimal care for the patients we serve." That passage says to me that a leader in nursing has to inwardly reflect on their own practice and better themselves so they can do the same for others. A truly successful leader stands in the back and helps push forward the people around them to achieve goals and better practices.

You lead with courage and authentic presence with openness to the unknown.	The greatest barrier to courageous leadership is not fear—it's how we respond to our fear. Our armor—the thoughts, emotions, and behaviors that we use to protect ourselves when we aren't willing and able to rumble with vulnerability—move us out of alignment with our values, corrode trust with our colleagues and teams, and prevent us from being our most courageous selves (Brown, 2018). Reflecting on what I have learned about myself personally, and as a leader in this course thus far and in our readings, is that I have strengths and opportunities for growth. Brown (2018) speaks about choosing two core values in part II of her book. The two central values that mirror me are caring and courage. Going back to school was stepping into that arena. It was terribly uncomfortable, yet exciting at the same time. It was daring, and I faced the possibility of failing and I responded to the critics and cynics.
You nurture communication through your authentic presence while listening and speaking.	I am personally working on trying to be a better listener, and not multitasking as someone is speaking to me, and I am trying to take a deep breath and "think" about my words and my responses before the words roll off my tongue. When I'm having a face-to-face conversation with someone, I often will close my computer or set my phone aside, face down, so that I am able to give the person my full attention. Being a transformational leader takes a lot of hard work. You have to be always evaluating your role in order to be successful in this leadership style.
You appreciate accomplishments and celebrate the success of your team.	I really love how "Lessons from the Geese" stated how being part of a team helps the geese reach their goal quicker because they "travel on the trust of one another and lift each other up along the way" (McNeish, 1972). That is so beautifully yet powerfully stated. I never knew that the geese were honking at each other to offer words of support and encouragement. How we each need the power of the V formation and those cheerful words of encouragement along our own way! I try to always express gratitude to my peers/coworkers, because it is important to acknowledge their hard work and commitment. We need the power of positive reinforcement. I know for me, this is something I need to get through the day at times. Knowing I'm doing everything I can for my patients to the best of my ability and being recognized for it is nice. Even if it's a simple "thank you" for helping out when they didn't even have to ask for it. Words of encouragement go way further with someone than criticizing or argumentative behavior.
You maintain equanimity during difficult situations, having the courage to move through and rise above.	I feel that I have learned a lot about leadership and asking myself some really tough questions about my style. In the Brown's (2018) learning to rise section, the assessment states that I need to be brave enough to own my own story and rise after a mistake or failure. I recognize that I remain silent at times, out of fear, which is really what she calls "armoring up."

Source: Inspired by Brown, B. (2018). *Dare to lead.* Random House Inc; Hills, M., & Watson, J. (2011). *Creating a Caring Science curriculum: An emancipatory pedagogy for nursing* (1st ed.). Springer Publishing Company; Schuster, J. P. (1994). Transforming your leadership style. *Association Management, 46*(1), L39; Watson, J. (2008). *Nursing: The philosophy and science of caring.* University Press of Colorado; Watson, J. (2012). *Human caring science: A theory of nursing.* Jones & Bartlett Learning; Watson, J. (2018). *Unitary caring science: The philosophy and praxis of nursing.* University Press of Colorado.

leadership concepts studied in this course. Not only does she give the students hope for ways to embody caring leadership, she explains the importance of not shying away from the notion of nursing being love in action. In Goldin's (2019) research, she concluded that caring is a precursor of love and that connection cannot be separated in a truly authentic transpersonal relationship. To show a loving, caring presence in a leadership role to her staff, she has seen a highly reduced turnover rate and improved staff satisfaction (Goldin class presentation, 2020). Prior to the class, I ask our students to pose questions to Dr. Goldin for discussion. Following is a sample of the students' questions:

1. What do you think is the best approach as a leader to retain nurses and what is the biggest barrier to keeping them?
2. What is the best way a manager can directly discuss problems or situations that occur? What if the manager is not available to discuss this in person? Should the charge nurse handle the situation? In what way can this be done to minimize confrontation?
3. Being a nurse leader in a highly transactional culture, there must be days you have to recenter yourself back to the heart of the matter to be a transformational leader. How do you recenter yourself during difficult days? A transformational leader certainly cannot be without character and integrity in their inner person as the two personas intertwine: the work self and the out-of-work self.
4. Is there a process you take to refocus or recenter, and to build yourself up (fill your love bucket) either in your practice or in your personal life?
5. When you are new to management, it is easy to feel like you are on the job 24/7. What advice or tips would you give someone to help better balance work and life?
6. How do you apply Caring Science in the day-to-day workload with your staff?

The students leave this class experience with Dr. Goldin with an increased sense of hope for the future, and they further share that time with Dr. Goldin is incredibly helpful as she brings real-life stories of caring leadership in action. Students realize that there are leaders who exemplify caring consciousness and transformational leadership and it is not "just a theory" that cannot be put in action. It is amazing to witness that by their presence and eagerness to be caring leaders at every level, students bring this back to their workplaces and begin to change the culture from inside out.

The connection between the development of caring leadership is in alignment with the way we structure our curriculum and "presence" in the classroom. O'Connor's (2017) article, Creating Caring Connections Through Presence, speaks to the importance of having a leadership presence to create a caring connection between the leader and staff. This aligns to Watson's theory of human caring where there is a need for a person to be authentically present during the care for others and self (Watson, 2012). O'Connor discusses this connection and how a leader can use practices of check-in, mindfulness, meditation, walking the talk, and circle practice to enhance a leader's authentic presence in the workplace (2017). Students find this alignment to how they have been treated within our program and have life experience with the benefits of these caring practices. It is gratifying to see them take the concepts used in the curriculum and begin to apply them to the role of a caring nurse leader. These small but powerful tools that enhance a leader's presence can be used to improve teamwork, trust amongst members, feelings of being cared for, and in turn, change the work environment and satisfaction levels of all (O'Connor, 2017). Having experts in the field such as Dr. Goldin and others who integrate caring presence to their work environments, have given our nursing students tangible evidence and rationale with which to move forward into their practice.

COMMUNICATION, TEAMWORK, AND CIVILITY

Clear and open communication, teamwork, and civility are critical components in the creation of a healthy and caring work environment. Our curriculum embeds civility within the program from day one. As discussed in more detail in Chapter 14, it is imperative to create a culture that is civil and free from lateral or vertical violence in our community of learning. This is also the cornerstone of the development of an effective team, where there is respect, trust, and collaboration among members (O'Daniel & Rosenstein, 2008). A nurse leader is in an important position to establish a culture that fosters this open communication and collaboration. In alignment with Caring Science and leadership theories mentioned previously, the caring nurse leader must provide a safe harbor for their colleagues to express their ideas, concerns, and conflicts. The term "psychologically safe space" for open communication has been used to describe a work unit where staff can express both positive and negative emotions without the concern of retribution, punishment, or being made to feel less (Edmondson, 1999). Henderson (2015) elaborates that in this environment, leaders and the team at large can both give praise and offer constructive feedback to others safely. This is clearly linked to Caritas Process® #5 Allowing for expression of positive and negative feeling; authentically listening to another person's story (Watson, 2018). As caring nurse leaders, this must extend to our students and staff.

When we consider these important components of communication in the workplace, both Caring Science philosophy in education and practice come to light. As discussed in Chapter 14, ensuring a safe community of learning raises the voices of all, and I posit, does the same between a nurse leader and the staff. A trusting relationship between the student/staff and teacher/nurse leader must be based upon a shared ideology of power (Bevis & Watson, 1989; Hills & Watson, 2011). To foster growth in a nonjudgmental and nonthreatening climate, an educator or leader has the responsibility to give the student/staff the freedom to express their own experience and construct their knowledge freely. One way that Freire emphasizes this in his work is that of humanizing education (S. Jackson, 1997) and embodying the concept of power as energy rather than domination (Shrewsbury, 1993). The leader's role encompasses the ability to foster growth in others by drawing out knowledge and individual ideas (Gomez, 2008).

Teamwork and collaboration among the nurse leader and staff are foundational components of the transformational and caring nurse leader. To bring this to light in a powerful way, we use a leadership lesson called "Teamwork Lessons from the Geese." This lesson was first written by Dr. Robert McNeish in 1972 and has been adapted for use in many multidisciplinary arenas. He studied the patterns of geese and from these learned traits of geese, he created lessons for team building (improving sense of community, staying in formation to help the group move forward, sharing leadership with others, encouraging one another, and standing by each other in difficult times; McNeish, 1972). The alignment with Caring Science philosophy and transformational leadership is clearly depicted through the lesson. The students engage in the following discussion board to discuss how these lessons could be used in their clinical work environment.

Discussion Board: Communication, Teamwork, and Civility: Lessons From the Geese

Review "Lessons from the Geese" and discuss how this could be used to create and support an organizational culture that values and uses effective team communication and collaboration to improve both clinical and staff outcomes. Share an example of this lesson from your leadership clinical and/or your clinical experience.

In addition, reflect upon your work environment. Is it a welcoming civil workplace? How can what you have learned in this part of the course on leading change and managing conflict apply to the culture of your workplace? Give examples of what could change and how you as a leader can manifest that change.

The discussions among the students that evolve from this assignment further enhance the students understanding of leading with Caritas consciousness.

> *This video showcases how much we need each other. One's actions are for the greater good—in the case of geese, flying together in the same direction increases 71% greater flying range than flying on their own (McNeish, 1972). Who knew that our current COVID-19 crisis would emulate the need for this collective power of solidarity among individual citizens for the greater good of society? An apropos analogy to encourage us today! I really love how "Lessons from the Geese" stated how being part of a team helps the geese reach their goal quicker because they "travel on the trust of one another and lift each other up along the way" (McNeish, 1972). That is so beautifully yet powerfully stated. I never knew that the geese were honking at each other to offer words of support and encouragement. How we each need the power of the V formation and those cheerful words of encouragement along our own way!* (Anonymous student response, March 2020)

> *In the video, Lessons of the Geese, I believe there are many examples of transformational leadership and best practice lessons. One of the messages in the video spoke out to me. It said that when one goose starts to get tired, the ones in the back honk to motivate the goose in the front. Not only do the people I work with attempt to do this to motivate their peers, but I as a leader attempt to do the same. I believe in leading from the back, motivating the people ahead of me to keep going and do their best. Transformational leadership is about helping people realize their full potential while working together to achieve goals.* (Anonymous student response, March 2020)

FINAL REFLECTION PAPER

As noted in Chapter 14, students write a final reflection paper on nursing leadership and how their philosophy of nursing has evolved over their time at Siena College. It is a paper that is deeply reflective and includes how learning and living within a Caring Science curriculum and environment has changed their perspective on nursing and becoming a caring nurse leader. They start the curriculum with the development of their own personal philosophy of nursing using their personal experience and a limited knowledge of nursing theory. It is often eye-opening for the students to reflect on their first paper in the program and see how this has evolved over time with a Caring Science–infused curriculum. They discuss the role of becoming a transformative Caring Science nurse leader and how they see their roles moving forward with this knowledge. From the NURS 415 coursework, they have done much self-reflection and integration of personal traits into their individual roles as leaders. They can identify the positive impacts a transformational caring leader has upon their work and school environments. From this they further define caring through the lens of theory and their experience throughout the program. This culminating paper truly is the capstone of our curriculum and the student responses are extremely validating of the power of a Caring Science philosophy–infused education. Through their narratives and deep reflection, the outcomes of the integration of Caring Science philosophy into the curriculum are manifested. There is no better way to describe this than to allow the voices of our graduates be heard.

Reflection paper excerpts:

When I stop to think about how my nursing philosophy has evolved over time, I'm forced to smile inwardly. At the beginning of this nursing program, when asked about my philosophy, I simply did not have one. Soon after, I was introduced to the world of Jean Watson and my world exploded with possibilities. With the Jean Watson theory presented to me, I was finally able to articulate my thoughts and feelings in a way that represented my overall mindset in the field of nursing. "Caring Science is grounded in the ethics of belonging, which is greater than our being, expands beyond medical science, acknowledges the relational, life forces and the philosophical unitary field dimensions underlying all of humanity" (Turkel et al., 2017). With all of this now at my fingertips, I realized that I had found a nursing philosophy that I could embrace with my heart and mind. (Anonymous student paper, May 2020)

When I started my education at Siena, it took a while to ease into the groove of my new school. I was used to the "sink or swim" mentality and less of a nurturing environment. Self-care, what is that? It was such a relief to enter a program that prided itself on caring for the whole patient and ourselves. Siena's program aligned perfectly with my values, beliefs, and aspirations. I quickly realized I had made the right choice to become a nurse and found an institution that also fostered those values. (Anonymous student paper, May 2020)

Not only does Watson's theory provide the framework for my practice, but it also provides many tools to achieve a successful leadership role. Becoming a Caritas coach, attending events, and even enrolling in a doctoral program are all possibilities because of the Caring Science philosophy. Incorporating those Caritas Processes® into one's practice would hopefully help one develop into a better nurse leader. A leader can be described as "anyone who takes responsibility for finding the potential in people and processes, and who has the courage to develop that potential" (Brown, 2018). (Anonymous student paper, May 2020)

During my time in the Baldwin Nursing Program and my course work in the Caring Science curriculum, my vision of the art of caring in professional nursing and nursing leadership has been impacted positively. The foundation of the program and the curriculum is heavily based on Jean Watson's theory in nursing practice. One of the most important elements that has impacted my nursing profession is that of self-care. Self-care is an extremely important element in the caring sciences that is often overlooked by many professionals. In this current crisis, I have also learned that it is essential for the leader to take a break and let someone else step up to lead just like the geese do. If the leader is exhausted, then they are no longer able to take care of the flock. This rings true in my life at work and I'm grateful that I have a team that I can lean on so that I can be an effective nurse manager. The most important lesson I have learned is that keeping communication open and respectful is the key to success. (Anonymous student paper, May 2020)

In late 2017, I recognized that I was *not* getting *any better* as a nurse, and I *had stopped* improving, which was my impetus to seek change. Enrolling at Siena with the Baldwin Nursing Program gave me the opportunity to not only garner an excellent education, but I was taught, led, and encouraged. Most importantly, I was coached on self-reflection and mindfulness, which enabled me to access the deep recesses of myself. According to Christopher Johns, the first step to becoming a leader is knowledge of self (Johns, 2016). Taking what I have learned through this program and turning it into a demonstrable action has elicited a positive change in my practice and built a strong caring culture with my peers and team. This connectedness is also in accordance with Siena's mission, which strives to embody the vision and values of St. Francis of Assisi. (Anonymous student paper, May 2020)

My definition of caring in nursing has changed considerably in the past 2 years. My view of nursing care was a classic medical model centered around a nurse's most important role of providing direct care to the patients. There is no doubt that technical nursing has a crucial role but I have learned that a caring nurse knows not only how to provide hands-on care but also how to minister to spirit and soul and maintain a healing environment of safety. Additionally, a caring nurse leader is a role model in providing care to the patient by providing support and direction to the team, not dictating and establishing strict protocols to be followed. (Anonymous student paper, December 2018)

Caring is of utmost importance in leadership. I know how hard it is from experience to focus on caring when cost-saving requirements and efficiency demand results in value, instead of human values. It is shown that role-modeling and teaching the principles of caring mixed with the principles of leadership can change the culture of an organization (McDowell, Williams, & Kautz, 2013). (Anonymous student paper, May 2018)

REFLECTIONS ON LEADING WITH CARING CONSCIOUSNESS

The journey towards becoming a leader with caring consciousness has been both a personal and professional journey for me and now for our students in the Baldwin Nursing Program. Seeing the growth in our students personally and professionally speaks volumes to the importance of creating a community of learning that is immersed in Caring Science philosophy. When one looks at the alignment between Watson's theory of human caring and the theory of transformational leadership, there are direct and important correlations. Students recognize and appreciate the correlations and strive to become transformational caring leaders at every level of their professional work. This is so evident in the growth of the students over the years in our program as shown in their narratives in their written work and the implementation of changes in their workplaces.

Becoming a leader who exemplifies the values and ethics of caring consciousness is not only needed in our world at large, but also within the profession of nursing. We need to break down the patriarchal walls that have long been the foundation of our healthcare arena. I have no doubt that this begins with how we educate our young. I have seen first-hand the changes in these women and men who have been educated in a Caring Science pedagogy, where their voices are heard and equal to those of the faculty, where civility lives in the classroom and extends between students and faculty, where the heart of nursing and authentic presence exist in the students and the faculty, and where they learn new ways to become a leader who includes courage, vulnerability, heart-centered authenticity, and compassionate direction. The expression of "nurses eating their young" needs to be replaced with "nurses empowering their young." This new generation of nurses can be the change that we need to see in our profession, if given the opportunity and voice to feel empowered to do so.

I want to thank all my nursing students (many of whom have been showcased in this chapter) over the past 4 years who have demonstrated courage in finding their voices within the program and in their work settings. They have grown to embody caring consciousness and are living examples of the future of nursing.

REFERENCES

Bass, B. M. (1990). From transactional to transformational leadership: Learning to share the vision. *Organizational Dynamics, 18*(3), 19–31. https://doi.org/10.1016/0090-2616(90)90061-S

Bennis, W. G. (2009). *On becoming a leader.* Basic Books.

Bevis, E., & Watson, J. (1989). *Toward a caring curriculum: A new pedagogy for nursing.* National League of Nursing.

Brown, B. (2018). *Dare to lead.* Random House.

Burns, J. M. (1978). *Leadership.* Harper & Row.

Edmondson, A. (1999). Psychological safety and learning behavior in work teams. *Administrative Science Quarterly, 44,* 350–383. https://doi.org/10.2307/2666999

Foundation of Nursing Leadership. (2015). *Leadership development: Test one: What is your leadership style?* http://www.nursingleadership.org.uk/test1.php

Freire, P. (2000). *Pedagogy of the oppressed* (30th Anniversary ed.). The Continuum International Publishing Group.

Goldin, M. (2019). Nursing as love: A hermeneutical phenomenological study of the creative thought within nursing. In W. Rosa, S. Horton-Deutsch, & J. Watson (Eds.), *A handbook for caring science: Expanding the paradigm* (pp. 433–446). Springer Publishing Company.

Goldin, M. (2020). *Caring nursing leadership.* Class presentation in NURS 415: Transformational Nursing Leadership. Siena College.

Gomez, D. S. (2008). Women's proper place and student-centered pedagogy. *Studies in Philosophical Education, 27,* 313–333. https://doi.org/10.1007/s11217-007-9048-0

Henderson, A. (2015). Leadership and communication: What are the imperatives? *Journal of Nursing Management, 23,* 693–694. https://doi.org/10.1111/jonm.12336

HIGH5 Test. (2020). *Discover the best part of yourself.* https://high5test.com

Hills, M., & Watson, J. (2011). *Creating a Caring Science curriculum: An emancipatory pedagogy for nursing* (1st ed.). Springer Publishing Company.

Institute of Medicine. (2011). *The future of nursing: Leading change, advancing health.* The National Academies Press.

Jackson, J., Clements, P. Averill, J., & Zimbro, K. (2009). Patterns of knowing: Proposing a theory for nursing leadership. *Nursing Economics, 27*(3), 149–159. PMID: 19558075.

Jackson, S. (1997). Crossing borders and changing pedagogies: From Giroux and Freire to feminist theories of education. *Gender and Education, 9*(4), 457–467. https://doi.org/10.1080/09540259721196

Johns, C. (2004). Becoming a transformational leader through reflection. *Reflections on Nursing Leadership, 30*(2), 24–26, 38. https://www.researchgate.net/publication/8526598_Becoming_a_transformational_leader_through_reflection

Johns, C. (2016). *Mindful leadership: A guide for the health care professions.* Palgrave Macmillan.

Keegan, L., & Dossey, B. (2004). Self Care Assessment. In *Self care: A program to improve your life.* Holistic Nurse Consultants.

Keirsey, D. (2020). *Keirsey temperament sorter.* https://www.keirsey.com

Lally Flack, L., & Thrall, D. (2019). Values and philosophies of being. In W. Rosa, S. Horton-Deutsch, & J. Watson (Eds.), *A handbook for caring science: Expanding the paradigm* (pp. 243–256). Springer Publishing Company.

Mayeroff, M. (1971). *On caring.* Harper Collins Publisher.

McDowell, J. B., Williams, R. L. II, & Kautz, D. D. (2013). Teaching the core values of caring leadership. *International Journal for Human Caring, 17*(4), 43–51. https://libres.uncg.edu/ir/uncg/f/D_Kautz_Teaching_2013.pdf

McNeish, R. (1972). *Lessons from the Geese.* Unpublished.

O'Connor, M. (2017). Creating caring connections through presence. *Nurse Leader, 15*(5), 347–351. doi:10.1016/j.mnl.2017.06.004

O'Daniel, M., & Rosenstein A. H. (2008). Professional communication and team collaboration. In R. G. Hughes (Ed.), *Agency for healthcare research and quality* (Chapter 33). https://www.ncbi.nlm.nih.gov/books/NBK2637

Roosevelt, T., & Thomsen, B. (2003). *The man in the arena: The selected writings of Theodore Roosevelt; a reader.* Forge.

Schön, D. A. (1987). *Educating the reflective practitioner.* Jossey-Bass.

Schuster, J. P. (1994). Transforming your leadership style. *Association Management, 46*(1), L39.

Senge, P. M. (1990). *The fifth disciple. The art and practice of the learning organization.* Doubleday/Currency.

Sherman, R. (2012). What nurse leaders should stop doing. *Emerging RN Leader.* https://www.emergingrnleader.com/nurseleaderbehaviors

Shrewsbury, C. M. (1993). What is feminist pedagogy? *Women's Studies Quarterly, 3 & 4,* 8–16. https://www.jstor.org/stable/40022001

Sitzman, K., & Watson, J. (2018). *Caring science, mindful practice: Implementing Watson's human caring theory* (2nd ed.). Springer Publishing Company.

Smith, M. C. (2019). Regenerating nursing's disciplinary perspective. *Advances in Nursing Science, 42*(1), 3–16. https://doi.org/10.1097/ANS.0000000000000241

Tanner, C. (2006). Thinking like a nurse: A research-based model of clinical judgment in nursing. *Journal of Nursing Education, 45*(6), 204–211. https://doi.org/10.3928/01484834-20060601-04

Turkel, M. C., Watson, J., & Giovannoni, J. (2017). Caring science or science of caring. *Nursing Science Quarterly, 27*(2), 66–71. https://doi.org/10.1177/0894318417741116

Watson, J. (1999). *Nursing: Human science and human care: A theory of nursing.* Jones & Bartlett Learning.

Watson, J. (2008). *Nursing: The philosophy and science of caring.* University Press of Colorado.

Watson, J. (2012). *Human caring science: A theory of nursing.* Jones & Bartlett Learning.

Watson, J. (2018). *Unitary caring science: The philosophy and praxis of nursing.* University Press of Colorado.

Indigenist Nursing: Caring Keeps Us Close to the Source

Lisa Bourque Bearskin, Andrea Kennedy,
Leanne Poitras Kelly, and Christina Chakanyuka

INTRODUCTION

This chapter is an orature on caring in Indigenous contexts from a broad Indigenist (rather than Indigenous) stance as our action (Hart, 2007) to honour history and relationships with our global family. Our intention is to describe caring in keeping with Indigenous ways of knowing and collective responsibility. Caring practices are relational and rooted in authenticity, accountability, antiracism, and activism. Nursing has an important opportunity to cocreate wellness opportunities through relationships with Indigenous Peoples and respectfully engage with Indigenous knowledges.

WAYS OF BEING: RETURNING TO ORIGINAL TEACHINGS AS HOME FIRES

Opening Prayer

> We acknowledge our sacred Creator and give thanks for the breath of life and the wonder of this day and all the blessings contained within it. We are grateful for the opportunity to come together in our sacred space and for the opening to share our collective story. To the grandmothers and the grandfathers who are the keepers of our knowledge, keepers of our medicine, keepers of our healing: we want to express our deepest gratitude not only for being such amazing teachers but for keeping in trust, our wisdom and our knowledge. Thank you for imparting to us ancestral knowledge through the many aspects of nature and relationships when we need it and when we need to be reminded of who we are as human beings. Also, for others to seek and understand for themselves and their own caring practices. We ask for permission to impart our own knowing, from a place of truth, honour, and integrity. It is our hope that these words and thoughts will help to expand the consciousness and awareness of those who will one day read them, and think about how to act as a means to deepen our own understanding of Indigenous Peoples and the role Indigenous nurses play in helping and healing ways. We ask that our helpers and our guides be present to watch over us, to ensure that the information and knowledge that is conveyed is imparted with authenticity, integrity, and in accordance with our original instructions. Those laws of nature: land, waters, and sky, the laws of our language, the laws of our medicine, and the laws of our divine relationship with all things.

Beyond Land Acknowledgement

We humbly and respectfully acknowledge the ancestors, knowledge holders, and traditional territories where we live, work, and play.

We would like to acknowledge the traditional territories where this textbook is published. In Canada at Mississauga, Ontario, we recognize many nations including the Mississaugas of the Credit, the Anishnabeg, the Chippewa, the Haudenosaunee, and the Wendat People. In the United States at Sudbury, Massachusetts, we recognize the unceded lands of the Wampanoag, Nipmuc, and Narragansett People. In the United Kingdom at London, we recognize the unceded lands of tribal Indigenous Peoples whose names we cannot locate; we mourn this as a loss for our collective humanity.

Beyond this ritual of acknowledgement is a deep honouring. We honor this recognition as a signal of the urgent challenges we face in an era of Indigenous Sovereignty and COVID-19 where inequities are revealed and the acts of moral injustice are exposed. Such moral injustices require radical caring actions to foster reconciliation with Indigenous Peoples. According to the Truth and Reconciliation Commission of Canada (2015), it is time for Indigenous Peoples to assert self-determination, self-governance, and sovereignty principles guided by Elders and knowledge holders and led by the Peoples.

Intentionality

We come together as Cree-Métis nurses to describe caring in Indigenous contexts that is in keeping with our own ways of knowing. Sharing our own distinctive caring lessons that we each have inherited and experience in this space carries significant individual and collective responsibility. The term "Caring Science" conjures up the work of nurse scholars who have led the charge on carving out articulation for academic nursing work that reflects caring in the field. As nursing science continues to progress in society, it too becomes more socially conscious. Flaming (2003) describes how nursing moved from a primarily orally trained profession to one that relies heavily on literacy, and now public policy; we are cautioned to not be blindly pulled into the Western scientific vortex. Rather, we see Indigenous knowledges as decolonized Indigenous science (Indigenous Health Writing Group of the Royal College of Physicians and Surgeons of Canada, 2019). We believe this epistemological revolution is a global opportunity for nurses.

For years, we have read the works of legacy nursing leaders and reflected on the ways in which nursing is critical to the health journey that we see and experience in our nursing relationships. As Indigenous nurses, coming together to speak to this topic creates both excitement and caution. The opportunity to share inspires our collaboration and makes us revisit our core teachings. Equally important is the attention we must give to how these teachings are stewarded and represented. We honour these teachings in tension with the struggle to have Indigenous knowledges respected in the deeply entrenched colonial systems of nursing education and healthcare. It is sad that our typical state is to fight for equity while risking being overseen or co-opted in a health system with surface-level reform that treats inclusion as a "benevolent gift" (Stein & Andreotti, 2016, p. 373). We need to resist this approach, and reorient caring with ancient Indigenous philosophies based on our collective humanity.

Hawaiian author Manulani Aluli Meyer (2003) reminds us of the concept and philosophy of knowledge and its relevance to all nations. We return to the source of knowledge that we need for developing a deeper understanding of our experiences. To understand our own epistemologies, based on the beliefs, values, and practices of our peoples to be able to push the boundaries of what our experience means and what we can learn from them. In other words, to see, to know is to understand what caring is from our own unique lived experiences.

Indigenous caring knowledge is tied to those ancestral teachers and ultimately exists as "science" in its own right. This knowledge is held and passed on to use with respect and humility. We are not the original theorists, nor the final say on these matters. Caring is core to the work we do and is articulated from an Indigenous lens in parallel to larger conversations on Indigenous nursing ways of knowing. Dion Stout et al. (2001) discuss the central role of knowledge in health and how one "must maintain the integrity of traditional knowledge, and draw on it as a powerful lens which promotes health and well-being" (p. 2). Opening spaces in our academia that promote critical and reflexive thinking, writing, and acting on the topic of Indigenous Nursing Knowledge can help to push nurses to further explore the full meaning of caring within the context of relational practice.

Our collective perspective is not a subset of Caring Science, nor in any way subsumed into the body of theoretical work that is recognized as Caring Science. This chapter stands as distinct knowledge that predates nursing academia and will continue to guide those who take up this knowledge in pursuit of authentic Indigenous relationships. We are grateful for the space to share these teachings and know that the responsibility and obligations we hold are to our communities and our teachers who come from the land and have trusted us with hearing their words.

Process and Positionality

This chapter is an orature of our recorded conversations on how we bring life to caring within our own practices and within our own work environments. We developed this chapter first with our collective *direct quotes (in italics)* from these conversations; such quotes gave rise to paragraphs, and ideas were then connected back to existing literature to demonstrate respect, relevance, and validation of this as a scholarly process. We align our approach with that of Ngũgĩ Wa Thiong'o (1993), who describes orature as a means that goes beyond what Western academia may refer to as "storytelling" or "narrative." Ngũgĩ (1993) asserts that knowledge is actively recalled, assembled, consolidated, and transmitted through orature. It involves gathering input from the collective through oral interaction. It reflects a way of knowing and doing. This is active engagement and construction of a path forward that builds on sharing our collective teachings.

Orature is the method that is the link to the blood memory, a calling back. Métis scholar in Indigenous research and education, Cora Weber-Pillwax (2001a) refers to primary orality as "the reconnections with their own oral histories and in the expressions of these sacred reconnections that lie the healing and fulfilment of the individual and collective capacity to enter fully into the power of orality consciousness" (p. 163). Orature references foundational teachings that life is a ceremony which guides our relationships and abilities to act from our individual perspective in relation to the collective well-being of others; this is as important as Westernized peer review, and more relevant in Indigenous caring contexts. We are obligated to honour our teachers, particularly once knowledge is made public.

This chapter represents the crossroads at which we often find ourselves that acknowledge the gifts that we bring to this circle of nurses, as we respond to two main questions:

What do we mean when we talk about caring from our Indigenous worldviews?
How does care show itself in our practice and what can we do to help nurses to work more effectively with Indigenous populations?

In response, our orality consciousness is expressed in coming together within sacred spaces to consider how *ways of being and knowing* reflect what we mean when we talk about our Cree-Métis caring perspectives. We also connect *ways of doing* as reflexivity of how and why we understand the nature of caring in our nursing practice. Ways of being, knowing, and doing are interconnected and shared in successive sections, woven together as a whole. According to Cora Weber-Pillwax (2003), the centrality of orality is entrenched in Cree consciousness expressed as ways of being, knowing, and doing with interconnected actions and understood wholistically (mind, body, spirit) through language, ceremonies, songs, and relationships (place, self, kin, community, others).

The following viewpoints are shared mainly from our collective Cree-Métis worldview that is unique to our individual lived experiences. While our experiences are not generalized for all, we hope this shared narrative will highlight understanding Indigenous caring contexts through relationality, interconnectedness, and interdependence. With that said, it is also important to situate our self-understanding—who we are and where we come from—in relation to our collective consciousness. We come together, creating our own caring discourses and ethical space with good health and good minds to carry on the work that has been afforded to each one of us.

Christina. I was born and raised on Dene/Cree territory in the South Slave, Treaty 8 Region of the Northwest Territories. Growing up in the small community of Fort Smith, I was fortunate to connect strongly with my culture and the land in ways that have certainly shaped my sense of belonging as a Métis woman. I am fortunate to have strong family ties to both my father's Scottish relations as well as my mother's British and Dene/Cree-Métis relations. My father, Ian MacDonald, was born in Charlottetown, Prince Edward Island (PEI) to Helen and Don MacDonald and was a seventh generation settler-Canadian. He taught me to care through kindness, humility, and always choosing to see the best in people. My mother, Marie (Villebrun) MacDonald, was born in Hay River, Northwest Territories (NT) and is of British, Dene, and Cree-Métis ancestry. She taught me to care through showing up, through acts of service and compassion. My grandmother, Mary (Evans) Villebrun trained as a nurse/midwife in London at the Florence Nightingale School of Nursing and immigrated as a single woman to Canada where she met my grandfather, Earnest Villebrun. My grandmother loved nursing in the North. She inspired me with her love for people and rural/remote nursing stories of adventure, resourcefulness, and resilience. My mother's family was directly impacted by the colonial regulation of 'Indian' status by blood quantum and legislated gender-discrimination aimed at assimilating Métis people into the non-Indigenous population and taking away their claims to treaty rights. Prior to Bill C-31 being passed in 1985, my great-grandmother, Mary Gladue, lost her treaty status as a Denesuline woman when she married my great-grandfather, Frederick Villebrun, who was Cree-Métis. While my grandfather eventually regained his treaty status and rights, my mother has yet to regain her treaty status. My identity as an Indigenous Métis woman is not defined by blood quantum, but my unique position to see, experience, and value colliding worldviews of both the colonizer and the colonized (Little Bear, 2009). When I was young, an elder in my community once told me how he embraced his Métis situatedness as having "two eyes and one heart." I am thankful for this teaching as it resonates with my way of being in the world. While I live and breathe this situatedness, I have a heart for both my Indigenous and non-Indigenous relations. While my home fire will always be in the North, I consider myself blessed to be raising my family on the beautiful, unceded territory of the Coast Salish people whose relationships with this land remain unbroken to this day.

Leanne. Taanshi! Leanne dishnihkaashoon and I am the youngest of seven children born in Balcarres, Saskatchewan to Rose Amyotte and Alexander Poitras. Both of my parents are

Métis-Cree from Saskatchewan. My mother was born at home, in the area known as Katepwa, where I continue to return to feel whole, and my dad was born in the area known as Tullymet. Both were from Road Allowance families and like many Métis made a living travelling for the work and finding community among other Metis families. My maternal line of ancestor names include Racette, Cardinal, and Bellegarde. The women of my Poitras line had the family names of Jeaunotte, Ross, and Laverdure. I speak the names of my ancestral line as it reclaims and posi-tions Métis as present in this country for generations. It creates visibility in the face of invisibility. I acknowledge that I come from a complex life of love, laughter, family, racism, and shame. I am a cisgendered heterosexual woman with two sons, a husband, and have been a nurse for over 30 years. I have worked predominantly in First Nations health for my whole career, in particular with the Cowichan people on the Coast Salish territory of Vancouver Island for 25 of those. I gradu-ated from the University of Saskatchewan at a time when it was okay for an instructor to ask me: "But how would you describe your Indianness. . ..do you feel more White?" despite being visibly Indigenous and struggling with racism. I was rewarded when I behaved and disciplined when I spoke out. Nursing within colonized Canadian society taught me that being Métis was never Indian enough, nor was it quite good enough to compete with the Settler voice. Now I am older, wiser, and ready to disrupt. Many teachers have helped bring me into the light of self-love, some of whom are Indigenous knowledge holders, and others are settler coaccomplices. I have gratitude to the many wise Indigenous nurse colleagues who have shared themselves with me, Métis Elders, Cowichan Elders, and my friends and family who continue to guide my way. Maarsii.

*   **Andrea.** I am of European settler and Métis ancestry from Robinson-Huron Treaty territory in northern Ontario. My Métis grandmother Marie Girardit mainly hid her culture and fragile threads were passed to me. While I have held this thread since childhood, I did not engage in cultural reconnection until being welcomed as a guest in Treaty 7 territory about 10 years ago. I am so grateful to have my grandmother's thread, as now I am reconnected with my cousin Leanne from our Poitras family line. Being a welcomed guest in Alberta continues to be my own work with humility and respect, to look, listen, and learn with Elders and the community. I am blessed to learn with Elders Roy and Elaine Bear Chief (Siksika) and Grandmother Doreen Spence (Saddle Lake Cree Nation) who are deeply generous with their love, support, and guidance. I was traditionally adopted and named by bundle keeper Elder Fred Eagletail (Tsuut'ina) who has gone home, and I am honoured by my brother Elder Hal Eagletail who continues to acknowledge me as a sister. I am named and hanai (traditionally adopted) by Kupuna Francine Dudoit Tagupa (Hawai'i) who is a traditional healer and Indigenous community activist. Francine reminds me to be loving in my actions and connect with my ancestors—she says, "These things cannot be put on a shelf." She shows me how to bring my grandmothers' teachings forward as my kuleana (responsibility and privilege) to help the community. To be a strong helper, I must first love my whole self. She says, "You cannot give what you do not have." I am brought full circle to how I understand caring from my grandmothers, who showed up for the community as helpers and taught me to generously share kindness when we visited, cooked, served, cleaned, and comforted. Caring is about calling on my ancestors and opening my heart to ease suffering and nurture kindness.*

*   **Mona.** I am also known as Lisa, great grand-daughter of Miyoskipisim Alexia Bearskin and Margaret LaRocque of Beaver Lake Cree Nation in Treaty 6 Territory, Alberta. My family was born on the land with approximately 15,000 acres for about 1,200 Nation members who can no longer hunt as the animals are disappearing. They can no longer eat the fish from surrounding lakes due to worries of contamination. They can no longer find sacred medicines that were once plentiful. Despite these losses, our people have retained a close relationship with the land. This is where nohkum (my*

grandmother) Marianne Bearskin and nikawiy (my mother) were born. Due to the Indian Act, my grandmother and mother were removed from Nation membership because they "shacked-up" with nonstatus men. My nimosôm (grandfather) Oliver Bourque was Métis and raised seven children along the building of the Canadian railway at Mile 51 near Philomena, Alberta (AB). My father Raymond Langevin and grandmother Luicienne Langevin were settlers to the Lac La Biche Region, who immigrated from France and were cousins to Jacqueline Bouvier (Kennedy). The Langevin family is known for caring for the suffering. My grandmother Luicienne never forgot about me and tried to keep in contact with me as I grew up between homes. I was the only girl with five brothers, with an undeniable bond. My birth name evolved within the social context in which I was raised. Due to the deep-seated form of systemic racism and assimilation, I did not have a relationship with my father's family. He died when I was a baby. Growing up in the child-removal era, I remained connected to my brothers, returning to live with nikawiy and eventually back to our original home fires in Beaver Lake Cree Nation where I have embodied our historical connection to the land and original teachings to which I belong. I acknowledge my brothers as my protectors and my children (two sets of twins) as my teachers. Thanks to my nikawiy and nohkôm for gifting me breath, life, love, and belonging that lay deep in my blood memory. I have grown into a strong Cree/Metis woman who cannot be broken. I hold up my hands to Rose Martial and Cora Weber-Pillwax who picked me up when I was lost and who taught me that despite all the suffering there was something greater to come; and that was nikawiy's story where I learned to care for her whole being.

These introductions are a reminder that we are never alone and that this journey is not just about us individually, but rather it is about those whom we bring with us and those we have a responsibility for caring, protecting, nurturing, and supporting. Second, it serves as a reminder to the readers that we are accountable to our Peoples first and foremost. Through our collective experience within the nursing education and healthcare systems, we present our diverse yet unitary perspectives of caring in nursing.

Caring in Footsteps as a Lifelong Journey

Our Indigenous nursing caring journey starts with the self, with a deep introspection of our historic roots and lineage. This is a critical opportunity to acknowledge those who have gone before us and broken trail in a society that was not necessarily open to respecting Indigenous ways of being. This journey is a process of coming to know.

> Throughout this chapter, quotes in italics represent the collective authors' voices.
>
> *It starts with the self. If I do not know myself in my history and who I come from and who my family is in service to, it makes it really hard to be, to be holistic.*
>
> *We are walking in these footsteps with our knowledge holders and our grandmothers. We are following in the footsteps of the matriarchs and grandmothers of Indigenous nursing knowledge. It is more about what the work that we are doing will mean for the next seven generations coming behind us. For you know, our kids, our grandkids.*

We respect that we are living examples of this journey as a process, and not an achievable goal or outcome. We did not grow up in traditional ways and are now retracing our paths back to these old ways with the land, language, and ceremonies. We are expected to speak in this academic language because our traditional languages (and therefore cultures) have been disrupted. We have gone through genocide. Our families have been segregated and relegated to different social classes; we are facing these traumas and reclaiming our Indigeneity. Indigenous Peoples are not homogeneous; we are diverse Peoples based on kinship, teachings, and places of origin. It is crucial that caring in Indigenous contexts is not essentialized, tokenized, or romanticized. We understand and activate caregiving through our lived experiences to ease suffering as rooted in our collective humanity.

While retracing our footsteps along this path, we are never alone. We are guided by those who have gone before us. Our grandmothers give us strength and resolve for caring. We connect our practices to the many grandmothers who have been our teachers, who have taken in our families and welcomed us in ceremony as extended family. We have a responsibility to carry on their teachings for the well-being of future generations.

> *Indigenous philosophers and wise ones who give us some bread crumbs for the path or some you know, pieces of nourishment along the path that we can pick up, like berries to nourish us on the journey as we ourselves are involved in this process.*

Caring in Indigenous contexts is about nurturing connections and bringing people together in our shared paths. We have a responsibility to create and maintain good relations on the traditional territories where we live, work, and play. We are also grateful to have home fires where we can return, reconnect, and revitalize our culture.

> *And you know, speaking of the legislated identity of people you know, Métis who have dispersed and become invisible in many ways in the country, for me, having that land and a place to call a gathering space and a connecting space has been instrumental in being able to maintain connection to that family. And it forces us all to come together and, and say, "This is ours. What are we doing? Who are you?" and the next generation of children you know, gathering, again a gathering space.*

This is a wholistic journey of the body, mind, and spirit that honours footsteps over generations. We are part of a continuum of caring that will be passed on as our responsibility and privilege. Ways of being are woven with ways of knowing and doing as an interconnected whole; caring is central to this frame and understood through our hearts, minds, and spirits. As one of the most prominent Cree nursing leaders of our time would say: "*Indigenous knowledge must be well approximated by our own experiences to support the shift from 'ascribed' to 'achieved' wellness*" (Dion Stout, 2012).

WAYS OF KNOWING: CENTRALITY OF CARING

We believe that Indigenous ways of caring need to be reclaimed as part of our self-determination. We recognize the significant historic and social barriers that have tragically impacted our efforts to care as Indigenous nurses.

> *And that's not easy for me because I grew up in a family where you know, racism was so explicit that my parents rarely talked about our Métis identity overtly. Everything was translated or transmitted covertly or tacitly; implicitly there was so much shame around being Métis.*

> *I have witnessed and experienced inauthentic caring, anxiety, frustration, and fear of navigating a system that undermines the value of what I know as an Indigenous woman to be true. I have watched others suffer as my attempts to advocate have been dismissed.*

Globally, nursing and caring has been distorted by colonial historic, societal, and nursing disciplinary structures (Sweet & Hawkins, 2015). As Indigenous nurses, we are conscientiously disrupting this colonial process and reclaiming or recovering caring based on our Cree-Métis ways of being, knowing, and doing. We understand caring as a living philosophy that starts before we were born and extends through our childhood and is culturally shaped by our upbringing, lifelong learning, and socialization. Indigenous ways of being and knowing may be best understood by teachings from Cora Weber-Pillwax: "Indigenous knowledge is in our being as lived. It is at the intersection of ontology and epistemology where we need to begin to explore deeply our thoughts, because it is here where the people hold the knowledge" (2010, personal communication).

From this stance, Indigenous philosophies on caring are revealed in our experience and where the ethics about caring guide each of our actions. Values of authenticity, integrity, humility, respect, insight, and accountability are embodied. We see this as an enduring divine relationship and heart obligation that connects us to all beings. Indigenous ways of knowing are about caring that is embodied and experiential. This learning journey is rooted in place with ancestors and awakened memories. Along the way, we are nurtured by our grandmothers, mothers, aunties, sisters, and teachers.

> *Caring is modelled to us from a young age. I was walked to my first wake, 9 years old in a room of strangers and I was told to go and feed everybody, make sure everybody had a sandwich. I never understood how important that was to those people healing because here was this little child offering them food, As their grieving and celebrating the life of their loved ones. And even though it was a sad time for them, that act of caring, just to care, was unknown, right? Just to be present, caring is about being present, right? Caring and my ability to care has been cultivated from my own experience.*

Together, we honour our lived experiences and ask: What does caring mean? Caring is a way of being. It is about being human in those intimate, authentic moments when we sit with ourselves and each other in full presence, guided by our ancestors. Caring keeps us close to the source.

The Source

We need to stay close to the source of our spirit and knowledge by acknowledging our teachers and who we are. We draw on the wisdom of Winona Duke (2005) who speaks of the source as the sacred, which is "frequently based on the reaffirmation of the relationships of humans to Creation" (p. 12). Embodying the complexities is central to the spiritual foundations and sacredness of the land which is essential to our collective vitality (Duke, 2005). The further away from this original teaching, the greater the risk that this knowledge will be co-opted or appropriated because this is removed from the land and the Peoples. We need to connect ways of being and knowing with the community context that made those teachings come alive.

> *Where is the source of my knowledge and how do I position myself in relation to that knowledge and stay close to that? —you know, being really intentional about how I steward that. Whether it is who I am or teachings that others have given me—that's staying close to the source. That is the uniqueness of Indigenous Peoples—their source is spiritual within them. It starts within oneself; that is the initial source.*

Alice Reid, a well-known Métis nurse reminds us that "we are all creatures of Creation and from that sense we are all one with unique experiences. . . . It is always with us. It is a gift, and it is up to us to accept it or not. It is not something we claim; it is just being who we are and what we believe and how we behave" (Bourque Bearskin et al., 2016, p. 9). As Indigenous nurses, we are in tune with Western knowledge and Indigenous knowledges. Weaving these ways of knowing with the source is where nurses are going to fit with Indigenous Peoples. It is not about teaching everybody about the ceremonies and medicines; we need to learn how to hold the knowledge with which we have been gifted and pass it on with respect and permission from our teachers. Weaving is about honouring both systems that arise from biomedical and cultural sources. Indigenous nurses are uniquely invested and accountable for ancestral and spirit relations throughout our lifetime. We have a responsibility to care with our spirit and open heart, knowing that we stand on the shoulders of those who came before us. Indigenous nursing is shaped by those who were raised with traditional teachings, had a glimpse of it, or returned and engaged in years of learning that all lead to coming to their own self-knowing. We need to know who we are and where we come from so that we may care for others.

The source connects us to each other and back to the land. We need our Elders. We are at risk of losing a whole generation of old ones who were raised on the land, in traditional villages, and born in the igluvigak (snow house), tipis, or longhouse. We need to remember how close that act of caring is to who they are as people. Their everyday corporal acts of mercy remind us of the importance to be fully present in our everyday caring practices as nurses. Moreover, we need to stay connected to our old ones who have been there, who teach us how to stay close to the source, and respect this across the continuum of our life span.

> When you're born into the world, right? And if we could go back to some of those traditional ways, that birth was ceremonial. Birth as a caring being opens up a lifetime of these ways. It is self-discipline. It is knowing your body; it is being in relation to the moon. The connection of the physical human body to the world around us. It is the environmental connections to how we teach. The worldview, that connection to the environment, that connection to place and location.

> I feel I have become open to more of the messages that my ancestors have been giving me all along the way and now I'm seeing the value in these messages.

Caring keeps us close to the source. And we understand this way of being and knowing as an obligation of the heart.

Knowing From the Heart

According to Palmer (2011) the heart is the place in our bodies where those stories rest and calls us to respond to those events that have stimulated our senses. Our mentor Dr. Evelyn Voyageur from the Dzawada̱ʼenux̱w First Nation, is a retired RN and an Elder-in-residence at North Island College in Comox Valley, British Columbia. She teaches us that the "heart of community" is central to how one sees the world and that we can in fact change the heart of society one nurse at a time (Bourque Bearskin et al., 2016). Even the original Latin word for courage comes from the root word "cor" meaning heart (Skeat, 1963); in Cree, the word heart is "miteh" and the root word "mi" is a reference to the body. Heart knowledge as embodied is a sophisticated, intergenerational repository of knowledge that is core to our being (Gehl, 2012) and at the heart of what we hope to convey in this chapter. Heart knowledge is where ceremony lives and so, Indigenous caring is a heart obligation. We have a heart obligation to care for knowledge to perpetuate our collective well-being. Knowledge does not belong to us; we are responsible to care for knowledge with respect and wisdom.

> I have not thought up anything independently or out of the blue, everything comes to me from somewhere else, whether it be explicit, implicit or you know, through blood memory. And so, if I know that, then I have obligations from my heart to honour those teachers. They are ancestors, they are other professionals, they are friends, they are community. And that obligation extends beyond best practice as defined by my Professional Organization.

This commitment of the heart is quite different from Western worldviews, where often there is an individualistic seeking of accolades and knowledge generation. Indigenous caring ways disrupt this colonial approach and refocuses with our hearts to create good relations. Principles shared by Cora Weber-Pillwax (1999) on the importance of intention and caring are infused within our shared understanding and practice.

> What, what are my intentions? What language am I using to incorporate my acts of caring? What is our caring knowledge base, what are those acts? Again, it's rooted in each lived experience. And if we really do care in authentic ways in which we are true to our spirit and relational practice, it changes us because it's in the face of the "other" where we learn about ourselves.

We have much experience at a cellular level that we often call intuitive knowing. These visceral experiences resonate throughout our bodies and change our conscious awareness. As Elder Lionel Kinunwa (as cited in Steinhauer, 2002) explains:

> We have ancestral memories in our blood; they are in our muscles, they are in our bones, they're in our hair. . . . These memories come out of the molecular structure of our being. . . . your molecular structure picks up those vibrations, because each language has its own peculiar patterns. (p. 76)

Indigenous nurses, grounded in their Indigeneity, honour this as blood memory. This shared ancestral knowledge is the embodiment of caring in a morally authentic life and doing things in a good way for the people, as a responsibility and privilege. While caring is not rooted in our professional standards, in caring we have a unique contribution as nurses.

> This is about your intimate relationship caring. How did you learn to care? How do you care for others? I get to that bedside and I see a human being. I don't see an Indigenous client. I peel back and look at the very core aspects of humanity. Of one human being to the next. We get so over clouded with all these concepts and theoretical frameworks. Then we ask them "how are you? From a Western lens, how many times a day do we ask people how they are? From an Indigenous lens, from my Cree teachings, it's much more than, "how are you?". It's like pulling up a chair, you know, let's get into this. Being present is about being fully present.

Our heart obligation is to care for generations past, present, and future. This is our lifelong caring journey, walking in an ancient shared path with our own footsteps.

Knowing Through Authenticity

Full authentic presence requires nurses to deeply listen to our clients with cultural humility (First Nations Health Authority, 2020). We need to bear witness of our own experiences and engage in critical self-reflection of how we are connected/disconnected in Indigenous caring contexts (Ermine, 1995; Kovach, 2009; Tuhiwai Smith, 2012; Weber-Pillwax, 1999; Wilson, 2008). Seminal writing by Watson (2020) echoes these original unitary ideas that authentic caring is for the purpose of preserving the dignity and wholeness of humanity. The meaning of authenticity reasserts that relationality is essential to developing Indigenous knowledge that is constructed from a relationship with the people and the spiritual dimensions of Indigenous thought.

We are at risk for being lost in a veil of caring that abdicates our authentic caring presence. Authenticity requires nurses to be self-aware and relationally attuned to the Indigenous Peoples' reality within a complex context that is experienced at individual and broader societal levels.

So, if our nurses are very privileged, can they, what are the, what are the abilities to be authentic, authentic in your caring abilities if you don't have that understanding? If you, you haven't seen the racism and discrimination, right?

And so I do think that nurses are often comfortable, more comfortable to just deceive ourselves and look the other way because we are such a caring profession, full of nice people, you know, who have that burden of care on their hearts.

Authenticity is an ongoing journey of self-discovery from a place of humility and respect. We require genuine engagement with a fundamental respect for Indigenous ways. We have great capacity as nurses to care with courage and articulate the ongoing anti-Indigenous racism that persists in our healthcare system despite cultural safety training. Nursing needs to boldly and truthfully examine and address the truth of our collective colonization. While this work may lead to experiences of discomfort, shame, and vulnerability, this provides opportunity for growth, to reinvigorate teachings, and give voice to ancestors. While our collective history, social context, and reconciliation processes are unique to Canada, we hope this understanding may be extended to other colonized lands and Peoples.

Knowing Through Relational Ethics

The foundation of "knowing" is entrenched in relations and connections to one another. This foundation of knowing is what Ermine calls "ethical space": where distinct thoughts are brought together in a cooperative spirit, where new thoughts are generated, and where new actions emerge (1995; 2007). For us, we have come to know this as "relational ethics," the backbone to nursing care. This postmodern philosophy in nursing science reflects the old and ancient wisdom of Indigenous Peoples. Bergum and Dossetor (2005) extend these views further and explain how relational ethics shape a nurse's moral agency in relation to the client-nurse-healthcare environments. This relationship of mutual respect focuses on moral decision-making from a collective community perspective. Indigenous ways are deeply embedded in relationships, for creating and sustaining good relations. In Cree, we would call this *wîhchitawin* meaning "shared responsibility with everything." Caring is about being in relation to oneself, others, and all beings as a process: nursing shows up with community and the community flows back in return. Caring in Indigenous contexts is beyond cultural safety; rather we are advocates upholding Indigenous human rights and advancing Indigenous health equity (Bourque Bearskin, 2011). This is rooted in our own positionality and self-awareness as Indigenous nurses.

Behind every scholar, there's a community. There are old ones to have carried knowledge through ancestral lines.

We believe that authentic and relational care begins with self and extends as a cultural responsibility with clients. The context of Indigenous clients is defined from their worldview, and so, part of our duty as nurses is to not obscure their reality. This relational approach as the "ethics of care" focuses on the client's reality and the relationship with the nurse (Canadian Nurses Association, 2017). Indigenous caring contexts are understood from a wholistic perspective that recognizes how we are all relatives; relatedness requires genuine connection with our own struggles and strengths to support the struggles and strengths of clients.

Through this interconnection of relationships, we need to examine more deeply the fundamental need for authentic relationships in caring. We are accountable to all our relations.

We can't free ourselves, but we can understand Western domination. And constantly be able to check in and know what it is that we must capitulate for lack of a better term, and when we are being our authentic self. Because I think there's sort of systemic influences that are beyond our control and until the system changes, we cannot be free to operate the way that we want. But you know, the reality is there is going to be time pressures and hierarchies, egos, academic product management, all of those things. That is going to remain entrenched in the Western system and we must make those visible. Visible to ourselves, visible to the system, visible to our patients or clients and then you know, checking in—where and how can I exist authentically?

Nurses must engage in ongoing critical reflection of our relationships and how entrenched power and colonial systems of privilege influence caring practices. This requires us to be alert and attend to colonial threats that marginalize Indigenous ways of knowing and inextricably impair caring in Indigenous contexts.

Indigenous Nursing Knowledge

Indigenous ways of knowing/epistemology are complex knowledge systems based on multiple truths that shape our world and hold an integrity of their own. Ways of knowing are self-generating in the sacred; embedded and expressed through Indigenous cosmologies, epistemologies, and ontologies. This is observable through intergenerational oral communication systems that are inscripted into our blood memories and activated holistically in relationship between the human, nature, and spirit whereby Indigenous knowledge systems flourish (Aboriginal Nurses Association of Canada, 2005; Bourque Bearskin et al., 2016; Dion Stout, 2012; Ermine, 2005; Kovach, 2010; Lowe & Struthers, 2001; Little Bear, 2009; Tuhiwai Smith, 2012; Weaver, 2001; Weber-Pillwax, 1999; Wilson, 2008).

As Indigenous nurses, we embrace *kinanâskomânânak kâkînîkânohtêcik*, meaning that we are grateful to the first leaders. We honor the First Nations, Inuit, and Métis women who hold distinct and prominent roles within their societies, both as life givers and caregivers (Anderson, 2001; Aboriginal Nurses Association of Canada, 2016). Since time immemorial, Indigenous nursing knowledge has evolved from the traditional knowledge of healers to informing a unique body of nursing knowledge (Aboriginal Nurses Association of Canada, 2005; Burnett, 2010; Cashman, 1966; Drees, 2013). This historical representation of nursing was originally skewed by Nightingale who did not acknowledge the role of traditional healers. Nightingale's notes were absent on the "efficacy of Aboriginal health and healing practice such as caring for the sick, using traditional medicines, child bearing practices, healing the injured and caring for the frail ages and very young," and it is deeply concerning that her notes perpetuated the myth that Aboriginal people were uncivilized and savages (Best, 2018, p. 53).

In Canada, many First Nations, Inuit, and Métis nurses sought out the need to enhance meaningful inclusion of their own knowledge and caring practices. Early leaders such as Jean Goodwill and Jocyeline Bruyer advocated for a political platform to bring nurses together to discuss our personal responsibility and guiding ethical actions. Numerous leaders from the Aboriginal Nurses Association of Canada, now known as the Canadian Indigenous Nurses Association, contributed to this evolving and engendered description. Early definitions of Indigenous nursing knowledge were developed between Indigenous nurses in leadership roles. For example, the Aboriginal Nurses Association of Canada (1999) advocated that Indigenous health nursing include the domains of clinical practice, education, research, policy, and politics that are informed by the traditional Indigenous knowledges, values, and beliefs of Indigenous Peoples. Since then, much more research on Indigenous nursing knowledge has been completed and it is now through all Indigenous nurses that this unique body of knowledge is shared. It is the interrelated nature of identity as a Peoples, and as professional nurses, where cultural experiences centre the values we hold and provide the foundations for core beliefs of how nurses engage in caring practice and how Indigenous knowledges manifest in our individual practice (Bourque Bearskin et al., 2016).

> To be able to connect to those really fine aspects of nursing care that I learned in caring for my mother is why nursing was a really good fit for me. Or at least I thought it was a good fit because it espoused this holistic, whole person, it was all about the people but as I've grown in nursing it's not, it's become about the profession. It's become about our standards of practice; it's become about all of those legal biomedical guidelines that we're forced to follow. And I'm not saying that, we don't need that knowledge, but we've shifted to the other side of the continuum now where our attention is focused only on the biomedical and evidence-based practice knowledge.

Indigenous health education and care often focuses on the individual deficits and diseases that are prevalent in Indigenous populations while neglecting to consider the intersectional impact of colonization as a determinant of health (Crowshoe et al., 2019). Western theories of knowledge, science, and healing practices have been privileged within the discipline of nursing. We have seen and even experienced first-hand how Indigenous knowledges and healing practices have been snubbed and limited by both the legacy of colonial policies as well as present-day legislation (Richardson & Murphy, 2018). In order to create a counter-narrative to continued colonization in nursing, McGibbon et al. (2014) state that "although there are notable exceptions, examination of nursing's participation in colonizing processes and practices has not taken hold in nursing's consciousness or political agenda" (p. 179). Indeed, the historical role of nursing as an instrument of colonization in Canada is not often discussed in the academy of nursing.

> It's really important in nursing education that there are Indigenous nurses who are grounded in their Indigeneity. Who have come on their own healing journey or in the process of it can be there to speak to and teach nurses about how to care in a way that is not simply you know, the token PowerPoint slide at the end of a class on diabetes and Indigenous populations. But instead looking at the historical legacy and contemporary role of colonization on Indigenous health.

While nurses hold equity and justice as core values to the discipline, Indigenous Peoples in Canada still experience racism, stigmatization, and fear of judgement when accessing health services (Cameron et al., 2014; McGibbon, 2019; Richardson & Murphy, 2018; Thorne, 2019). Subsequently, many Indigenous people often do not feel safe when accessing healthcare and may therefore avoid the system altogether (Cameron et al., 2014; McGibbon, 2019; Richardson & Murphy, 2018; Thorne, 2019). Waite and Nardi, (2017) contend that, nurses often "deceive ourselves and think that because we are nurses we are, consequently, non-racist and non-oppressive, as our code of ethics and academic institutions declare they are staunch believers of this ideology" (p. 20). By accepting the uncomfortable truth about the role of nursing in advancing colonization, nurses may begin to explore what it means to support reconciliation in their practice. In recent years, an increasing number of both Indigenous and non-Indigenous nursing scholars have drawn attention to the urgent need to dismantle the dominance of Western knowledge and increase the "counter-narrative to continued colonization" in nursing education and practice (McGibbon et al., 2014, p. 179; McGibbon, 2019; Moffitt, 2016; Waite & Nardi, 2017).

To reconcile means to restore friendly relations and coexist in harmony (Oxford University Press, 2019). In considering how to reconcile Indigenous knowledges in education, Marie Battiste (2018) suggests the following:

> While many institutions are using a discourse of diversity to enlarge this agenda (to teach treaties, and Indigenous Knowledges (IK), and decolonize Eurocentric education) within human rights and social justice, there is still much that needs to be done to help them understand what IK is and how it can be used as a source of strength and motivation not just for Indigenous peoples but also for non-Indigenous peoples as a source of renewing connections to Aboriginal peoples and reconciling the colonial practices of the past and addressing larger issues of humanity and sustainability through holistic relationships. (pp. 138–139)

Nurses must learn how to embody relational ethics in their practice in order to provide culturally safe care that "honours Indigenous people's connection to self, others, the environment, and the universe" (Bourque Bearskin, 2011, p. 1). Nursing has already come a long way in creating cultural safety training programs for practicing nurses and even undergraduate courses that begin to explore the impacts of colonization on Indigenous health, but this is still not enough. We need to respect that it is up to Indigenous Peoples to determine what is safe and what is not, and how health and wellness are understood (Richardson & Murphy, 2018).

WAYS OF DOING: CARING IS ACTION

Caring is a verb, not a noun. Caring acknowledges ways of being and knowing through embodiment with congruent actions. These actions are guided by our mind, body, and spirit through every-day moments of visible activism for antiracist care that is grounded in humility, respect, and commitment to community. We need to resist actions that are limited to privileging physical caring; our mind-body-spirit as nurses needs to care for the mind-body-spirit of our clients and community. Caring is a wholistic action.

> *What the heart knows, is what the heart wants. And it keeps taking us there, as hard as it sometimes is to go there and you know, the physical aspect of caring, that's where I think our nursing profession has been focused, on that physical act of caring. There hasn't been any caring for the spirit.*

Cora Weber-Pillwax (2001b) speaks to the ways in which we generate and steward actionable knowledge within the academy. She states:

> If my work as an Indigenous scholar cannot or does not lead to action, it is useless to me or anyone else. I cannot be involved in research or scholarly discourse unless I know that such work will lead to some change out there in that community, in my community. (p. 169)

The premise of this statement demonstrates the responsibilities that Indigenous Peoples have in being accountable to their community through their work and their relationships. There is little room for discourse for the sake of discourse. Our ways of being and knowing as Indigenous nurses are ultimately in the pursuit of action that will result in change and betterment of our people and our communities. Our action reflects our ways of doing.

Many postcolonial nursing theories position the work of nurses and caring within a social justice lens that seeks to uncover and address oppressive societal systems. Action through activism, authentic communication, reciprocal relationships, patient-driven processes, equalizing power structures, and addressing racism all contribute to decolonizing work. Indigenous nurse ontology builds on the relationality that guides our practice. We engage in decolonizing work not because it is a nursing approach we have learned, but because we are accountable to our communities to work for change "out there."

For non-Indigenous nurses who work within Indigenous spaces, caring becomes about courage. It takes courage to place yourself within Canada's collective colonizing story and recognize your role. Confronting racism, inequity, and marginalization looks different when we situate ourselves within the history of the displacement of Indigenous Peoples from the land. Naming anti-Indigenous racism in Canada specifically, and owning the settler journey with this, takes courage. Cree education scholar and activist Shauneen Pete (2020) calls for "settler stamina" in which the fragility that often derails intentional engagement with anti-Indigenous racism is confronted. Maintaining the myth of settler innocence creates defensive positioning, complacency, and potential barriers to care.

> I think it needs to begin with, with an exploration of where we unintentionally or intentionally benefit from that history. As terrible as it might be, we are not to laying "White guilt" down because defensiveness and guilt are not helpful. What is helpful is being critically self-aware enough and accepting that this is what happened and that the narrative that we've been told since we were kids around our history is not the truth necessarily. Only then can the process of reconciliation begin.

To be an activist and be present in the doing means owning our own truths whether they be laudable or not.

Caring Is Humility and Respect

We need to engage in caring practices with humility and respect for our colleagues and clients. There are many important shifts that we can make towards positive change in our everyday actions. We need to begin with respect for the community and acknowledge the historic governance of Indigenous societies. We need to acknowledge that First Nations communities are communities; the term "reservation" was imposed by the government on Indigenous Peoples as a legislative label. Changing our language with a dignity-oriented approach is an important foundation for actionable change.

Caring practices are recognized in our communications; "What comes out of our mouths either hurts or heals people" (teaching gifted by Elder Roy Bear Chief from Elder Tom Crane Bear, Siksika Nation). Caring in Indigenous contexts is not realized through cultural competence which may continue to reinforce colonial power dynamics of the expert provider over the client. Rather, cultural humility (First Nations Health Authority, 2020) and respectful curiosity in communications may help nurses to better understand the client's world. This understanding is key to creating a trusting, caring space.

> *A simple question about traditional medicine can elicit a lot of, you know, different things. Even the act of asking somebody to self-identify is re-traumatizing for some people because it resurfaces that shame. So why on all our nursing forms do we have "which reserve are you from?"*

Patient and family-centred care is now a highly familiar approach within nursing and healthcare (Institute for Patient-and Family-Centered Care, 2020; McCalman et al., 2017). This approach is often spoken of, but not fully embraced in caring practices and environments. Again, we are concerned (similar to reconciliation efforts) that this is a token agreement. How do we engage in a meaningful way with Indigenous Peoples as partners in care? We need to respect how the client, family, and community are experts in their lived experiences and well-being. We need to bridge our nursing knowledge to the client's reality (Crowshoe et al., 2019).

Caring Is Anti-Racism

"Antiracism is the active process of identifying and eliminating racism by changing systems, organizational structures, policies and practices, and attitudes, so that power is redistributed and shared equitably." (NAC International Perspectives: Women and Global Solidarity, as cited in Alberta Civil Liberties Research Centre, n.d.). This is not about being politically correct—this is about authentically respecting human rights and dignity. Antiracism is a learning/practice journey that requires critical examination of communication, programs, and policies (National Collaborating Centre for Aboriginal Health, 2014). While antiracism may be realized in microinteractions, we need to advocate for positive change at department, disciplinary, and institutional levels. Nurses are part of the system and we all have a role to play in antiracism.

In contrast, anti-Indigenous racism is behaviours and processes that discriminate against Indigenous Peoples as "inferior to other groups in physical, intellectual, cultural, or moral properties" (Van den Berghe, 2007, as cited in Bond et al., 2019, p. 5). Anti-Indigenous racism is often played out through settler denialism that such racism exists and results from ongoing colonial domination in our society (Regan, 2010). Caring in Indigenous contexts requires nursing to address the deeply pervasive deficit-discourse that blames and problematizes Indigenous Peoples, when such harmful stereotypes are rooted in historic and social structures, and result in poor health outcomes and maintain system-wide inequity (Fogarty et al., 2018).

> *That discrimination experienced by my mom at one of the most vulnerable times in her life, losing a parent, it was that stereotype. So, there's my grandfather, the "drunk Indian," dying of self-inflicted alcohol-related disease of the liver. Meanwhile what they didn't know is that he'd been sober for about 15 years before he died. They didn't know that this broken family was finally coming together for the first time in years and beginning to reconcile. And for me, the caring context around all of that and what it means, is the reason why I'm so driven in this area of anti-Indigenous racism and responding to the TRC (Truth and Reconciliation Commission Calls to Action [Truth and Reconciliation Commission of Canada, 2015]) and*

UNDRIP (United Nations Declaration on the Rights of Indigenous Peoples [United Nations, 2008]). *Because, while these are useful tools, the action doesn't always follow in a real tangible way. There's health inequity—it still exists. There's racism in healthcare—it still exists. It's not something of the distant past.*

Sadly, within our profession, Indigenous nurses struggle with ongoing experiences of racism (Vukic et al., 2012). If Indigenous nurses experience racism, what is the deeper impact on the nursing care and health of Indigenous Peoples?

> *The caring piece for me is, is around the combination of that heart obligation, while becoming an anti-racist activist because at the end of the day that's the root of my understanding of this marginalization. In this racism that is so heavily embedded inside the history of our country and that we have all been impacted in some way, but been unable to articulate it because the act of articulating further pushes us out of being listened to. And so, as now, for the first time in our history I think the racism conversation is on the table and we, in my mind, that act of caring for us needs to include that in such an explicit way.*

Nursing's unexamined power and privilege may impair care that is shaped by unquestioned biases, attitudes, and beliefs. We cannot afford to ignore the conflicting power agenda of colonial domination with Indigenous self-determination in nursing.

While healthcare providers may be sympathetic towards Indigenous Peoples, there may be a "lack of tools to engage critically with questions of race and racialization and how these are manifested in the context of asymmetrical settler colonial power" (Sylvestre et al., 2019, p. 1). There are many ways to engage in meaningful antiracism education and actions to reorient caring practices with dignity and without discrimination towards Indigenous Peoples. Various strategies to address anti-Indigenous racism include:

- opening and facilitating candid nursing conversations on racism, including manifestations, extent, impact and compounding factors of White silence and privilege;
- designing human-centred antiracism as a common goal;
- developing antiracism priorities with indicators, goals, implementation strategies, and evaluation criteria;
- collaborating with Indigenous nurses and communities to develop antiracism resources, supports, and training programs;
- gathering and responding to feedback by Indigenous clients and stakeholders on cultural safety and quality of care;
- creating policies to support antiracism in nursing education and healthcare;
- creating nursing, interdisciplinary and community-based research programs focused on antiracism (Bond et al., 2019; The National Collaborating Centre for Aboriginal Health, 2014; Waite & Nardi, 2017).

Antiracism requires a critical approach where nurses need to lean in and engage in the messy and often uncomfortable process of decolonization. This requires understanding the colonial history of our discipline and self-locating with authenticity and without defensiveness. Again, as nurses we often self-identify as "caring" by the nature of our profession. However, we need to examine the authenticity of our caring practices and intentionally engage in antiracism approaches at individual-to-system levels. This requires a commitment to highly accountable caring practices that are free of discrimination.

Caring Is Activism

We agree that nursing is a political act (Canadian Nurses Association, 2009). As Indigenous nurses, this commitment to action is rooted in connection and accountability. We need the courage to keep walking in the path started by our ancestors with the steadfast intention to make things better than how we found them.

> *My experience awakens memories and whether or not I knew of things before, explicitly, I think when I'm living the journey it awakens in me the awareness, the memories that have been given to me by other people. And so, this heart obligation then, it allows me to relive those memories, it allows me to grow and act. It forces me to evaluate boundaries and trauma and find ways to navigate those and it positions me as activists.*

So how do nurses become activists? What will we do to show that we care? Indigenous author Thomas King (2003) memorably quotes in his book, *The Truth About Stories,* "But don't say in the years to come that you would have lived your life differently if only you had heard this story. You've heard it now" (p. 29). He is calling everyone who hears the history of Indigenous Canada to action. Once you know, you cannot pretend that you do not. Caring requires action. It may be something as simple as taking a few moments longer to listen to a family or make a call on their behalf. Activism may be disrupting racist interactions or challenging inequitable power structures. Activism can be recognizing for many Indigenous Peoples how the violence and trauma experienced due to racism is present as a potential backdrop to all interactions. Activism is learning about the local communities, the local language, and names of community lands where you live, work, and play. Activism can be unsettling. Settler colonialism scholar Lorenzo Veracini (2017) discusses how colonial studies support decolonization work. He states, "I am a settler, but indigenous resurgence is in my interest. It will make me a better human being and a worse settler" (p. 2). By this standard, becoming a "worse settler" through disrupting power systems in the pursuit of equity for Indigenous people constitutes activism and the direction for nurses working in Indigenous spaces.

To advance Indigenous rights-based, antiracist healthcare practices, we need to examine what we are doing to create and influence positive change. While we have all been impacted by collective colonization, we can resist and reshape this by considering the need for decolonial activism to advance our collective caring.

> *Advocacy and activism where sometimes we have to speak to the importance of caring with what the patient needs as central. Nurses and students need to be prepared to actually speak up to the policymakers and administrators. And it's a vulnerable place.*

We see this chapter as a form of activism. While there is obvious cultural tension in adhering to colonial scholarly writing, we hope that this orature brings us back to the source: ways of being, knowing, and doing that spring forth from original teachings, nurtured by our home fires. Activism may seem difficult, yet our footsteps on this path are eased with a loving approach that is congruent with caring.

CLOSING THOUGHTS

We ask nurses to bring these chapter teachings forward with respect and humility. Writing this chapter has been a difficult process: activism is not easy. Caring in Indigenous contexts may be introduced in written works such as this chapter. We are asking nurses to relate to this work as a heart obligation. This is not a gentle invitation—what are our actionable items? Nursing needs to step up in everyday moments with congruent beliefs and actions. Choosing silence is a form of unexamined privilege that is contrary to caring. We need to use this caring environment to advocate for Indigenous sovereign rights as heart work. This is about Indigenous human rights. Nurses have an opportunity to engage in authentic caring in Indigenous contexts; this collective approach is based on the principles of Peoples' active participation, gender equality, environmental and social justice, self-reliant and sustainable management systems while maintaining natural law and the assertion of sovereignty over the lands and resources.

> Speaking together is a collective expression of the concerns, thoughts, and aspirations that you hold for further generations of Indigenous people in Canada. Our contributions live in the manifestation of alternate approaches to life that come from the original inhabitants of this land. (Goodwill, 1975, as cited in Canada, Department of the Secretary of State, 1975, p. 1)

Understanding caring in Indigenous contexts requires authentic engagement in relationship with the Indigenous community. Wise caring practices are inextricably tied to our identities, history, traditions, language, land, and the "spirit" of place. Caring is a relational accountability to the self, to each other, to our profession, and to creation as a part of our humanness where we reside as nurses in caring for Indigenous Peoples. We hope this orature illuminates caring in Indigenous contexts so that all nurses may cocreate opportunities to build relationships with Indigenous Peoples and respectfully engage with Indigenous ways of being, knowing, and doing in our caring practices.

REFERENCES

Aboriginal Nurses Association of Canada. (1999). Aboriginal health nursing: A nursing specialty. *Aboriginal Nurse, 14*(2), 4.

Aboriginal Nurses Association of Canada. (2005). *30 years of community.* Author.

Aboriginal Nurses Association of Canada. (2016). *Ninanâskomânânak kâkinîkânohtêcik "We are grateful to the first leaders": Celebrating 40 years of unity in Indigenous Health.* Author.

Alberta Civil Liberties Research Centre. (n.d.). *Anti-racism defined.* https://www.aclrc.com/antiracism defined

Anderson, K. (2001). *A recognition of being: Reconstructing Native womanhood.* Sumach Press. (Original work published 2000)

Battiste, M. (2018). Reconciling Indigenous knowledge in education promises, possibilities, and imperatives. In M. Spooner & J. McNinch, (Eds.), *Dissident knowledge in higher education* (pp. 123–148). University of Regina Press.

Bergum, V., & Dossetor, J. (2005). *Relational ethics: The full meaning of respect.* University Publishing Group.

Best, O. (2018). The cultural safety journey: An Aboriginal Australian nursing and midwifery context. In O. Best & B. Frederick (Eds.), *Yatdjuligin Aboriginal and Torres Strait Islander nursing and midwifery care* (2nd ed., pp. 46–66). Cambridge University Press. (Original work published 2014)

Bond, C., Singh, D., & Kajlich, H. (2019). *Canada–Australia Indigenous health and wellness: Racism Working Group discussion paper and literature review.* The Lowitja Institute. https://www.lowitja.org.au/content/Image/Canada_Australia_Discussion_Paper-web_hi_res.pdf

Bourque Bearskin, R. L. (2011). A critical lens on culture in nursing practice. *Nursing Ethics, 18*(4), 548–559. https://doi.org/10.1177/0969733011408048

Bourque Bearskin, R. L., Cameron, B. L., King, M., Weber-Pillwax, C., Dion Stout, M., Voyageur, E., Reid, A., Bill, L., & Martial, R. (2016). Mamawoh kamatowin "coming together to help each other in wellness": Honouring Indigenous nursing knowledge. *International Journal of Indigenous Health, 11*(1), 5–19. https://doi.org/10.18357/ijih111201615024

Burnett, K. (2010). *Taking medicine: Women's healing work and colonial contact in Southern Alberta, 1830–1930.* UBC Press.

Cameron, B. L., Camargo Plazas, M. P., Santo Salas, A., Bourque Bearskin, R. L., & Hungler, K. (2014). Understanding inequalities in access to health care services for Aboriginal people: A call for nursing action. *Advances in Nursing Science, 37*(3), E1–E16. https://doi.org/10.1097/ANS.0000000000000039

Canada. Department of the Secretary of State. (1975). *Speaking together: Canada's Native women.* Author.

Canadian Nurses Association. (2009). *Position statement: Nursing leadership.* https://www.cna-aiic.ca/-/media/cna/page-content/pdf-en/nursing-leadership_position-statement.pdf

Canadian Nurses Association. (2017). *Code of ethics for registered nurses.* https://www.cna-aiic.ca/-/media/cna/page-content/pdf-en/code-of-ethics-2017-edition-secure-interactive.pdf

Cashman, T. (1966). *Heritage of service: The history of nursing in Alberta.* Alberta Association of Registered Nurses.

Crowshoe, L., Henderson, R., Jacklin, K., Calam, B., Walker, L., & Green, M. (2019). Educating for equity framework: Addressing social barriers of Indigenous patients with type 2 diabetes. *Canadian Family Physician, 65*, 25–33. https://www.ncbi.nlm.nih.gov/pmc/articles/PMC6347314

Dion Stout, M. (2012). Ascribed health and wellness, Atikowisi miýw-āyāwin, to achieved health and wellness, Kaskitamasowin miýw-āyāwin: Shifting the paradigm. *Canadian Journal of Nursing Research, 44*(2), 11–14. PMID: 22894003.

Dion Stout, M., Stout, R., & Rojas, A. (2001). *Thinking outside the box: Health policy options for NAHO to consider: Roundtable report.* National Aboriginal Health Organization.

Drees, L. M. (2013). *Healing histories: Stories from Canada's Indian hospitals.* University of Alberta.

Duke, W. (2005). *Recovering the sacred: The power of naming and claiming.* South End Press.

Ermine, W. (1995). Aboriginal epistemology. In M. Battiste & J. Barman (Eds.), *First Nations education in Canada: The circle unfolds* (pp. 101–112). UBC Press.

Ermine, W. (2005). *Ethical space: Transforming relations.* Paper presented at National Gatherings on Indigenous Knowledge, Rankin Inlet, NU.

Ermine, W. (2007). Ethical space of engagement. *Indigenous Law Journal, 6*(1), 193–203. https://jps.library.utoronto.ca/index.php/ilj/article/view/27669/20400

First Nations Health Authority. (2020). *Cultural humility.* https://www.fnha.ca/wellness/cultural-humility

Flaming, D. (2003). Orality to literacy: Effects on nursing knowledge. *Nursing Outlook, 51*(5), 233–238. https://doi.org/10.1016/j.outlook.2003.07.001

Fogarty, W., Lovell, M., Langenberg, J. & Heron, M. J. (2018). *Deficit discourse and strengths-based approaches. Changing the narrative of Aboriginal and Torres Strait Islander health and wellbeing.* National Centre for Indigenous Studies, The Australian National University. https://ncis.anu.edu.au/_lib/doc/ddih/Deficit_Discourse_and_Strengths-based_Approaches_FINAL_WEB.pdf

Gehl, L. (2012). Debwewin journey: A methodology and model of knowing. *AlterNative: An International Journal of Indigenous Peoples, 8*(1), 53–65. https://doi.org/10.1177/117718011200800105

Hart, M. (2007). *Cree ways of helping: An Indigenist research project.* Unpublished doctoral research. University of Manitoba. https://mspace.lib.umanitoba.ca/bitstream/handle/1993/8028/Hart_Cree_Ways_of_Helping.pdf?sequence=1

Indigenous Health Writing Group of the Royal College of Physicians and Surgeons of Canada. (2019). *Indigenous health primer.* Royal College of Physicians and Surgeons of Canada. http://www.royalcollege.ca/rcsite/health-policy/initiatives/indigenous-health-e

Institute for Patient-and Family-Centered Care. (2020). *PFCC best practices.* https://www.ipfcc.org/bestpractices/index.html

King, T. (2003). *The truth about stories: A native narrative.* Dead Dog Café Productions Inc and the Canadian Broadcasting Corporation.

Kovach, M. (2009). *Indigenous methodologies, characteristics, conversations, and context.* University of Toronto Press.

Kovach, M. (2010). Conversational Method in Indigenous Research. *First Peoples Child & Family Review, 5*(1), 40–48. https://fncaringsociety.com/sites/default/files/online-journal/vol5num1/Kovach_pp40.pdf

Little Bear, L. (2009). Jagged worldviews colliding. In M. Battiste (Ed.), *Reclaiming Indigenous voice and vision* (pp. 7–85). University of British Columbia Press.

Lowe, J., & Struthers, R. (2001). A conceptual framework of nursing in Native American culture. *Journal of Nursing Scholarship, 33*(3), 279–283. https://doi.org/10.1111/j.1547-5069.2001.00279.x

McCalman, J., Heyeres, M., Campbell, S., Bainbridge, R., Chamberlain, C., Strobel, N., & Ruben, A. (2017). Family-centred interventions by primary healthcare services for Indigenous early childhood wellbeing in Australia,

Canada, New Zealand and the United States: A systematic scoping review. *BMC Pregnancy and Childbirth,* *17*(1), 1–21. https://doi.org/10.1186/s12884-017-1247-2

McGibbon, E. (2019). Truth and reconciliation: Healthcare organizational leadership. *Healthcare Management Forum, 32*(1), 20–24. https://doi.org/10.1177/0840470418803379

McGibbon, E., Mulaudzi, F. M., Didham, P., Barton, S., & Sochan, A. (2014). Toward decolonizing nursing: The colonization of nursing and strategies for increasing the counter-narrative. *Nursing Inquiry, 21*(3), 179–191. https://doi.org/10.1111/nin.12042

Meyer, M. (2003). Hawaiian hermeneutics and the triangulation of meaning: Gross, subtle, causal. *Social Justice, 30*(4), 54–63. https://www.jstor.org/stable/29768223

Moffitt, P. (2016). Mobilizing decolonized nursing education at Aurora college: Historical and current considerations. *Northern Review,* (43), 67–81. https://thenorthernreview.ca/index.php/nr/article/view/593

National Collaborating Centre for Aboriginal Health. (2014). *Policies, programs and strategies to address anti-Indigenous racism: a Canadian perspective.* https://www.nccah-ccnsa.ca/Publications/Lists/Publications/Attachments/132/2014_07_09_FS_2426_RacismPart3_PoliciesStrategies_EN_Web.pdf

Ngũgĩ' Wa Thiong'o. (1993). *Moving the centre: The struggle for cultural freedoms.* James Currey.

Oxford University Press. (2019). *Definition of reconcile in English.* https://www.lexico.com/en/definition/reconcile

Palmer, J. P. (2011) *Healing the heart of democracy: The courage to create a politics worthy of the human spirit.* Jossey-Bass.

Pete, S. (May 6, 2020). *What does decolonization and Indigenization look like in the classroom?* Kikinoo'amaadawin Webinar Series. https://www.angelanardozi.com/webinars

Regan, P. (2010). *Unsettling the settler within: Indian residential schools, truth telling and reconciliation in Canada.* UBC Press.

Richardson, L., & Murphy, T. (2018). *Bringing reconciliation to healthcare in Canada: Wise practices for healthcare leaders.* HealthCareCAN Report. https://www.healthcarecan.ca/wp-content/themes/camyno/assets/document/Reports/2018/HCC/EN/TRCC_EN.pdf

Skeat, W. (1963). *A concise etymology dictionary of the English language.* Capricorn Books.

Stein, S., & Andreotti, V. D. O. (2016). Decolonization and higher education. In M. Peters (Ed.), *Encyclopedia of educational philosophy and theory* (pp. 370–375). Springer Science+Business Media.

Steinhauer, E. (2002). Thoughts on an Indigenous research methodology. *Canadian Journal of Native Education, 26*(2), 69–81.

Stout, M. D. (2012). Ascribed health and wellness, Atikowisi miýw-āyāwin, to achieved health and wellness, Kaskitamasowin miýw-āyāwin: Shifting the paradigm. CJNR: Canadian Journal of Nursing Research.

Sweet, H. M., & Hawkins, S. (2015). *Colonial caring: A history of colonial and post-colonial nursing.* Manchester University Press.

Sylvestre, P., Castleden, H., Denis, J., Martin, D., & Bombay, A. (2019). The tools at their fingertips: How settler colonial geographies shape medical educators' strategies for grappling with anti-Indigenous racism. *Social Science & Medicine, 237,* 112363. https://doi.org/10.1016/j.socscimed.2019.112363

Thorne, S. (2019). Genocide by a million paper cuts. *Nursing Inquiry, 26*(3), 1–3. https://doi.org/10.1111/nin.12314

Truth and Reconciliation Commission of Canada. (2015). *Truth and Reconciliation Commission of Canada: Calls to action.* http://trc.ca/assets/pdf/Calls_to_Action_English2.pdf

Tuhiwai Smith, L. (2012). *Decolonizing methodologies: Research and Indigenous peoples* (2nd ed.). University of Otago Press.

United Nations. (2008). *United Nations declaration on the rights of Indigenous Peoples.* http://www.un.org/esa/socdev/unpfii/documents/DRIPS_en.pdf

Veracini, L. (2017). Decolonizing settler colonialism: Kill the settler in him and save the man. *American Indian Culture and Research Journal, 41*(1), 1–18. https://uclajournals.org/doi/abs/10.17953/aicrj.41.1.veracini

Vukic, A., Jesty, C., Mathews, S. V., & Etowa, J. (2012). Understanding race and racism in nursing: Insights from Aboriginal nurses. *International Scholarly Research Notices, 2012,* 1–9. https://doi.org/10.5402/2012/196437

Waite, R., & Nardi, D. (2017). Nursing colonialism in America: Implications for nursing leadership, *Journal of Professional Nursing, 35*(1), 1–8. https://doi.org/10.1016/j.profnurs.2017.12.013

Watson, J. (2020). Nursing's global covenant with humanity – Unitary Caring Science as sacred activism. *Journal of Advanced Nursing, 76*(2), 699. https://doi.org/10.1111/jan.13934

Weaver, H. N. (2001). Indigenous nurses and professional education: Friends or foes? *Journal of Nursing Education, 40*(6), 252–258. https://doi.org/10.3928/0148-4834-20010901-05

Weber-Pillwax, C. (1999). Indigenous research methodology: Exploratory discussion of an elusive subject. *Journal of Educational Thought, 33*(1), 31–45. https://www.jstor.org/stable/23767587

Weber-Pillwax, C. (2001a). Coming to an understanding: A panel presentation: What is Indigenous research? *Canadian Journal of Native Education, 25*(2), 166–174.

Weber-Pillwax, C. (2001b). What is indigenous research? *Canadian Journal of Native Education, 25*(2), 166–174.

Weber-Pillwax, C. (2003). *Identity formation and consciousness with reference to Northern Alberta Cree and Métis Indigenous peoples.* (Unpublished doctoral dissertation). University of Alberta.

Wilson, S. (2008). *Research is ceremony: Indigenous research methods.* Fernwood.

Simulation, Narrative Pedagogy, and Caring Fidelity™ — The New Reality

Roberta Christopher

Because the cultural shift is rooted so deeply in our definition of reality (our metaphysics) and what is possible, a profound and comprehensive realignment of our mission and sense of self and other must be cultivated, sustained, and practiced.—Watson, 2002, p. 45

INTRODUCTION

Clinical placements and access to electronic medical records are challenges for nursing, allied health, and interprofessional education (Smith et al., 2010; Smith & Seely, 2010; Smith et al., 2013). Thus, academic programs integrate alternative experiences in curricula to augment knowledge, skill, competency, and literacy development. One frequent tool used to augment clinicals is simulation and narrative pedagogy. Three simulation categories commonly used include computer-based simulation, task and skill trainers (e.g., low to medium fidelity), and full-scale simulation (e.g., high fidelity), which may include aspects of the previous categories (Seropian et al., 2004). The aim of these alternative learning experiences is to recreate, or simulate, the clinical environment and caring experience. Simulation has strong theoretical and research evidence supporting its use in education and practice and has been endorsed by several professional organizations including the National League for Nursing (NLN) and the National Council of State Boards of Nursing (NCSBN; Hayden et al., 2014; NLN, 2015a, 2015b). Additionally, boards of nursing across the United States have approved for up to 50% of prelicensure clinical training hours to consist of clinical simulation (Florida Board of Nursing, 2020; Persico, 2018).

A key benefit to simulation is the learning and caring experience may be adapted and developmentally increased for the level of learner competence from novice to expert (Benner, 1984). Additionally, the experiential learning process offers the opportunity for cognitive development through active learning (the doing) and reflection (the caring experience; Kolb, 1984; Sewchuk, 2005; Waldner & Olson, 2007). Experientiality, as conceptualized by Fludernik (1996), is "the quasi-mimetic evocation of real-life experience" (p. 12). Narrative experientiality and storytelling facilitate the humanization of simulations, provide the foreground and evolving representational realities, and mimesis situated in human actionality (Fludernik, 1996; Kablitz & Neumann, 1998). Unfortunately, such experiential opportunities may narrowly focus on technical competency, the doing, without intentional emphasis on caring literacy (Sitzman & Watson, 2017), the transpersonal caring moment or experience (Blum & Locsin, 2010; Clark, 2016; Watson, 2018), or Caring Fidelity™.

Professions such as nursing have drifted toward the use of a medical model approach to competency development (Reed & Watson, 1994; Warelow et al., 2018). Competency and literacy development, however, must be grounded in pedagogy and praxis framed from the profession's ethical, ontological, epistemological, philosophical, and theoretical context (Hills & Watson, 2011; Watson, 2018). This dissonance and need for nursing curriculum transformation was first voiced by the National League for Nursing in the landmark publications on curriculum revolution, including the "Mandate for Change" (NLN, 1988) and the "Reconceptualizing Nursing Education" (NLN, 1989). The contracted emphasis on technical competency (the "doing") has continued in part due to (a) guidance of leading international competency models; (b) academic education and accreditation requirements; (c) professional regulatory requirements for licensure; and (d) the diversity and complexity of practice.

Reconciliation of such dissonance and knowledge development discourse was proposed by Watson and Smith (2002) through policy and practice recommendations. An example of this reconciliation in academia comes from the Christine E. Lynn College of Nursing at Florida Atlantic University (FAU) curriculum model, which seamlessly integrates Caring Science throughout the learning and practice continuum (FAU, 2019). An exemplar of reconciliation from practice is derived from the Kaiser Permanente—Northern California's Patient Care Services division's transformation of their professional practice framework and all aspects of clinical, operational, and administrative structures, processes, and outcomes through enculturation of Caring Science (Foss Durant et al., 2015).

As noted by Locsin (2005, 2009), human caring is foundational in simulated learning, curriculum, technological knowing, and interprofessional education. Thus, integration of caring literacy into curricula and simulated learning experiences is vital in keeping pace with innovation, advancing science, and technology disruptors (Tanioka et al., 2019; Waxman et al., 2019). Furthermore, the caring experience can no longer be limited to face-to-face acute, ambulatory, home, or long-term encounters (Schuelke et al., 2019). Pedagogy must include virtual care experiences *and* caring moments, whereby patient monitoring and caring interactions occur through telehealth or conferencing platforms, smartphone technology, simulated electronic medical records, and virtual nursing care. Innovative care models utilizing virtual nursing as "the new reality in quality care" are emerging (Schuelke et al., 2019, p. 322; Watson, 2002).

CARING FIDELITY™

Watson's (2008; 2018) Unitary Caring Science theoretical approach provides insights for humanism in the simulated caring moment throughout the caring study experience and provides a framework for the development of Caritas literacy and consciousness (Cara, 2003; Lee et al., 2017; Watson & Smith, 2002). From an axiological perspective, Unitary Caring Science provides a space to shift the healthcare simulation beyond the conventional approach of valuing technical competency to one of valuing (veritas) and centering (caritas) the learning experience on the "human-universe-health-healing process" and reality (Watson, 2018, p. 10). The aim of this approach is to move beyond task-consciousness to caring literacy consciousness (Lee et al., 2017).

According to Watson (2018), nursing praxis requires the "full depth of experience" (p. 20). Thus, learners must be able to appreciate and give attention to (caritas) and value (veritas) the caring moment that is being simulated to become caritas/veritas literate healthcare professionals. Caritas literacies, processes, and ethics, therefore, may be taught, acquired, applied, and critically reflected upon in the simulated caring experience. To keep pace with the evolving healthcare reality, a new form of fidelity, Caring Fidelity™, as conceptualized by Christopher (in progress), is an essential dimension of the simulated experience that must be integrated and cultivated with intention. To extend the simulated caring experience beyond conceptual (Dieckmann et al., 2007, 2009; Rudolph et al., 2007), equipment and environmental (Rehmann et al., 1995), physical (Alexander et al., 2005; Dahl et al., 2010; Dieckmann et al., 2007), perceptual (Alessi, 2000a, 2000b), phenomenal (Dieckmann et al., 2007, 2009), semantical (Dieckmann et al., 2007, 2009), and emotional or psychological types of fidelity (Beaubien & Baker, 2004; Dahl et al., 2010; Munshi et al., 2015), professional definitions, models, matrices, standards, and best practices in simulation (International Nursing Association for Clinical Simulation and Learning [INACSL], 2016a–h; 2017; Paige & Morin, 2013), must be revisited to include the Caring Fidelity™ dimension and Caring Science literacies. Otherwise, interprofessional teams will lack the needed caring literacies, processes, and language for their professional practice.

The Agency for Healthcare Research and Quality's (AHRQ) Healthcare Simulation Dictionary (Lopreiato, 2016) was developed by world-renowned simulation experts and provides globally accepted language for conceptualizing the Caring Fidelity™ dimension. Through etymological processes and understanding, fidelity requires "faithful adherence to truth or reality" (Lopreiato, 2016, p. 12). Thus, simulated learning experiences of care and caring moments require the same faithful adherence to the caring reality as to the technical reality. Some of the key aspects and dimensions of fidelity noted by the AHRQ experts included the

a. degree to which simulation replicates realism;
b. ability to reproduce relational attributes;
c. level of learner sense-making; and
d. dimensional factors (e.g., conceptual, physical, equipment, environmental, and psychological).

Despite the extensive etymological research and provided healthcare simulation language, no etymological or conceptual definitions for caring, caring moments or experiences, or caring fidelity in simulated healthcare experiences were provided by the experts. Additionally, the AHRQ cited nursing education competencies (Cronenwett et al., 2007; Cronenwett et al., 2009) used as instructional context do not include caring literacies.

According to Christopher (in progress), Caring Fidelity™ is conceptualized as the degree to which healthcare simulation-based educational methodologies and narrative pedagogies create mimetic-diegetic attunement through immersive caring/healing experiences by intentional cultivation of learner (a) caritas/veritas literacies and processes; (b) contemplation, action, reflection, and reflexivity; and (c) caring praxis. Moreover, Caring Fidelity™ further extends the 11 dimensions of simulation application proposed by Gaba (2004), and the NLN Jeffries simulation theory and framework (2016), and the potential for significant learning.

EXEMPLARS FOR THE NEW REALITY THROUGH SIMULATION, NARRATIVE PEDAGOGY, AND CARING FIDELITY™

Situating curriculum in Caring Science and the art of caring offers the opportunity to move beyond technical competencies. Simulation mimesis and corresponding thinking modes (physical, semantic, and phenomenal) provide theoretical insight into how this may be achieved (Dieckmann et al., 2007; Laucken, 1995). The INACSL Standards of Best Practice for Simulation (2017) and the NCSBN (2015) provide further structure, process, and outcomes through their professional standards and guidelines for simulation design and process. Discipline-specific frameworks that directly integrate Caring Science and interactive kinds of significant learning, such as Daley and Campbell's (2018) framework for simulation learning in nursing education, may aid educators in designing effective simulated learning and caring/healing experiences. Further, in high-tech teaching and learning environments, narrative pedagogy facilitates mimesis through the unfolding care studies. Such narratives foster caring literacy, complex decision-making, and clinical reasoning (Walsh, 2011).

Exemplar One: Interprofessional Programmable High-Fidelity Simulated Caring-Healing Experience

Jacksonville University's Keigwin School of Nursing (KSON) offers both ground-based and online programs. To ensure future professional nurses, nurse leaders, and advanced practice nurses are highly prepared, simulated computer-based electronic health record (EHR) systems are used. One such simulated electronic health record, EHR Go™, was chosen and integrated into the curriculum to augment clinical experience, electronic health record documentation exposure, and operationalize Caring Fideltiy™ in the nursing curricula. EHR Go™ provides simulated care studies as templates that may be adapted by faculty. Faculty and student guides, videos, narratives, and resources are provided. Additionally, the more than 600 care studies have corresponding virtual EHR charting specific to the care study that may also be adapted. Collections are provided by discipline, including interprofessional education (IPE), nursing, pharmacy, provider, therapy, assistants, health information technology and management, and informatics. Furthermore, caring studies are provided for a variety of settings encountered by patients across the care continuum, including adult and pediatric hospitals, clinic, emergency, long-term care, birthing center, rehabilitation/therapy center, and community pharmacy. Caring studies may also be sorted further by patient type, disease process, and social determinants of health to name a few. Finally, close to 50 programmable simulation caring studies are specifically provided to work with low- and high-fidelity manikins and with parallel, realistic EHR documentation.

The first EHR Go™ simulation caring study exemplar is designed to transform learning through reflective practice, centering on the caring experience, and application of a situation-specific theoretical approach. The caring study is designed for use across disciplines and IPE and for use with high-fidelity manikin simulations and electronic health record documentation. The Lee Geropalliative Caring Model is used as a structure for Caring Fidelity™ in this simulated caring/healing experience (Lee, 2018). Lee (2018) asserted that one of the key assumptions of the model is that patients who are at the end stages of disease and receiving palliative care can achieve well-being.

CENTERING-SELF

The centering-self stage of simulation in caring studies occurs during the prebriefing and briefing portions. This stage allows learners to develop Caritas literacy through centering both self and heart through caring consciousness and intentionality before entering the simulated, caring/healing experience via computer-based and high-fidelity manikin-caring studies. Watson (2018) noted that professionals and learners must be able to care for and treat themselves with loving-kindness before offering care to another in a professional caring/healing model. The centering process serves as the pause that allows for authentic presence of self by the student and educator. The process would be similar to centering-self outside of a patient's room before entering. Thus, the learners use Caritas Process #1 (Watson, 2018) of practicing and embracing loving-kindness and equanimity toward self and others. Educators further role-model centering of both self and heart in the simulation briefing. By centering self, learners and faculty enter into the simulated, caring/healing experience with a level of awareness described by Watson (2018) as "Caritas Consciousness." Additionally, learners get to know the one being cared for through the educator-provided briefing materials, rich caring narratives, and review of the EHR Go™ simulated electronic health record (e.g., spiritual, behavioral, physical, social, care needs). Such humanistic/altruistic processes, as proposed by Watson, support not only the Caritas process but provide the ethical foundation of caring. Learners also employ Caritas Process #2 by being authentically present before entering the simulated caring/healing experience. Through this process learners are enabled to nurture faith and hope. Learners also utilize Caritas Process #4 by entering into the experience of another and allowing the other (person being simulated) to enter the learner's experience. By doing so, human dignity and ethics nurture the authentic caring relationship.

Prior to the briefing narrative session with the educator, learners may complete a variety of instruments to measure caring behaviors, including self-rating of Caritas (Sitzman & Watson, 2019). One such instrument by Watson et al. (2012) is the Watson Caritas Self-Rating Score©. The instrument includes a five-item Likert-type scale with 1 meaning Never and 7 meaning Always. The instrument also includes a yes or no item asking if the nurse learner would recommend the hospital to someone they loved. This item would not be applicable. Finally, a qualitative item asks the nurse learner to share any notable caring or uncaring moments they have experienced. Reported reliability was Cronbach's α of .84 and exploratory factor analysis yielded a single factor which explained 61.6% of the variance. Use of such measures allow learners to be aware of and reflect upon their Caritas and to be sensitive to the development of self and others. Such cultivation and deepening awareness of self and then going beyond self is exemplified in Caritas Process #3 (Watson, 2018). Caring measures may be used pre- and postsimulation, at key intervals in the education program, and in professional practice for contemplation, action, reflection, and reflexivity to cultivate caring praxis.

One technique used by educators Cunningham et al. (2017) to center self and as a tool for learner centering is prebriefing mindfulness activities. One example is "Mindful Moments," a 2-minute guided mindfulness activity whereby learners are invited to the present moment by closing their eyes or lowering their gaze, entering into a period of relaxation, and focusing their intention to their thoughts, feelings, body sensations, environment, and breathing. Educators with experience in meditation use a standardized script to guide the mindfulness activity. Next the learners are provided a minute to transition into the simulated caring/healing experience (McKendrick-Calder et al., 2019). The 3-minute mindful moment process may then be incorporated as part of ongoing caring praxis.

Mindfulness to center self fosters situational awareness, reduction in performance anxiety, and healthy life skills beyond the simulation (Molloy et al., 2019). The Cognitive and Affective Mindfulness Scale—Revised (CAMS-R; Feldman et al., 2007) or other like instruments may be used by learners to self-rate mindfulness. The CAMS-R includes 12 items measuring the four domains of mindfulness (attention, present-focus, awareness, and acceptance/nonjudgement) and are calculated as one mindfulness score. Feldman et al. (2007) reported Cronbach's α between .81–.85, demonstrating acceptable internal consistency reliability, as well as evidence of convergent and discriminant validity.

CARING/HEALING EXPERIENCE

The caring/healing experience portion of the simulation, or implementation stage, shifts into the demonstration of Caritas processes, professional praxis, and technical competencies, skills, and attitudes. This stage allows learners to appreciate and give attention to (caritas) and value (veritas) the caring moment. Narrative storytelling, using evolving caring studies, guides the simulated caring/healing experience. The educator reads a portion of the caring study, and then pauses to ask learners guided questions aligned with the Caritas process, practices, and literacies. The evolving caring study continues with educator reading the narrative, pausing, and asking guided questions. As learners engage in the transpersonal caring/healing experience with the high-fidelity manikins or standardized patients, learners demonstrate Caritas/veritas processes and literacies as well as technical caring practices. Further the simulated electronic health record, EHR Go™, is to be used as a caring tool and facilitator versus a caring disruptor or barrier. Learning objectives, performance expectations, and outcomes value both technical caring practices and Caritas/veritas processes.

GUIDED REFLECTIVE PRACTICE

Reflection on one's practice is an essential step in the simulated experiential learning experience. Historically, debriefing has been approached from a judgmental perspective, focusing on errors, deficiencies, and failure. Learners can subsequently feel demoralized. Use of the Caring Science provides the opportunity to reframe the debriefing process from one of "judgmental debriefing to debriefing with good judgment" (Rudolph et al., 2007, p. 365). The good judgment model, developed by Rudolph et al. (2007) for debriefing, uses an advocacy/inquiry approach. Psychological safety is foundational to the debriefing process and includes meaning-making and sense-making systems. The debriefing process is further reframed with appreciative observations and insights by the educator. Rudolph et al. noted that the cornerstone of the good judgment approach is the inclusion of the learner's unique perspective as well as the expertise of the educator. The advocacy/inquiry approach includes transparent talking and guided reflection. Rudolph et al. conceptualized advocacy as an observation or statement and inquiry as a question. Additionally, educators guide the good judgment approach to ensure critical thinking, clinical reasoning, reflection and reflexivity of the caring/healing experience and the transpersonal caring process.

APPLICATION ACTIVITY: SIMULATED CARING/HEALING EXPERIENCE FOR MR. CHARLES BISHOP (ADVANCED)

The following simulated caring/healing experience application activity integrates Caring Science (Watson, 2018). The overarching goal of the activity is to move beyond the traditional focus on technical competence and medical models to Caritas processes and caring literacy (Watson, 2018). This is achieved through the incorporation of Caring Fidelity™. Readers are invited to experience the simulated caring/healing experience in EHR Go™ by visiting the following link: https://ehrgo.com/caringscience.

Application Activity Contextual Information

- Age of patient: 68-year-old African American male
- Clinical Focus: Transpersonal, interprofessional caring for a person experiencing congestive heart failure, severe decompensation: edema, dyspnea, tachycardia, and fatigue
- Works well with: Simulation manikins, standardized patients, and the NLN/Laerdal Case of Charles Jones

The application activity contains a summary of the EHR Go™ patient-caring study for simulation. This synopsis is shared only with you, the educator. If you would like your students to have a copy, you will need to provide it to them on paper or you can post it in your Learning Management System (LMS). The experience may be interprofessional or discipline specific. The application activity includes:

- A synopsis of the caring study
- Student expectations during simulation
- Learning objectives
- Summary of the problems, orders, and notes
- Electronic health record
- Simulated caring/healing experience
  - Centering-self (prebriefing and briefing)
    - Prebriefing information and suggested measures
    - Prebriefing centering-self mindfulness script
    - Briefing information
  - Caring/healing experience
    - Implementation
  - Guided reflective practice
    - Debriefing

After you have reviewed this document, go to Step 2, click on New Session and review the chart. When you are ready proceed to Step 3 to share the link to this chart with your learners as part of the briefing process.

SIMULATED CARING/HEALING EXPERIENCE: CENTERING-SELF STAGE (PRE-BRIEFING & BRIEFING)

Pre-Briefing Information

Prior to the Briefing Stage of the simulated caring/healing experience, provide learners with an overview of mindfulness principles and strategies that will be used to center self and heart through intention. Watson's (2018) Caritas/veritas literacies and processes are integrated throughout the experience. Reinforce that the centering process serves as a pause to allow for authentic presence of self in the caring/healing experience and is similar to pausing prior to entering a patient's room. Through the centering-self process, learners are invited to practice and embrace loving-kindness and equanimity toward self and others (*Caritas Process #1*). By centering on the present caring moment, learners employ *Caritas Process #2* by being authentically present before entering the Briefing Stage. Through Caritas Processes #3 and #4, learners enter into the experience of another and allow for the other (person being simulated) to enter into the learner's experience. This process promotes human dignity, ethical care, and self-awareness through authentic, caring/healing relationships.

Pre-Briefing Measures

Educators may elect to use valid and reliable instruments to measure self-rated Caritas and mindfulness. One such instrument, by Watson et al. (2012), is the Watson Caritas Self-Rating Score©. The instrument includes a five-item Likert-type scale with 1 meaning Never and 7 meaning Always. The instrument also includes a yes or no item asking if the nurse learner would recommend the hospital to someone they loved. This item would not be applicable. Finally, a qualitative item asks the nurse learner to share any notable caring or uncaring moments they have experienced. Reported reliability was Cronbach's α of .84 and exploratory factor analysis yielded a single factor which explained 61.6% of the variance. Use of such measures allows learners to be aware of and reflect upon their Caritas and to be sensitive to the development of self and others. Such cultivation and deepening awareness of self and then going beyond self is exemplified in Caritas Process #3 (Watson, 2018). Caring measures may be used pre- and postsimulation, at key intervals in the education program, and in professional practice for contemplation, action, reflection, and reflexivity to cultivate caring praxis. Refer to Sitzman and Watson (2019) for additional instruments for assessing and measuring caring in nursing and health sciences.

The Cognitive and Affective Mindfulness Scale—Revised (CAMS-R; Feldman et al., 2007) or other like instruments may be used by learners to self-rate mindfulness. The CAMS-R includes 12 items measuring the four domains of mindfulness (attention, present-focus, awareness, and acceptance/nonjudgement) and are calculated as one mindfulness score. Feldman et al. (2007) reported Cronbach's α between .81–.85, demonstrating acceptable internal consistency reliability, as well as evidence of convergent and discriminant validity. Mindfulness to center self fosters situational awareness, reduction in performance anxiety, and healthy life skills beyond the simulation (Molloy et al., 2019).

Centering-Self Mindfulness Script

[*Before you enter into the caring/healing experience with your learners, we invite you to center self through the same mindfulness process. Some educators attune the centering-self mindfulness experience through use of Tibetan singing bowls, relaxing music, nature sounds like ocean waves. We invite you to individualize the process for your learners and preferences.*]

Educator Reads:

1. I invite all of you to find a relaxed, comfortable position (e.g., seated in a chair or comfortable standing position). [pause]
   a. Keep your back upright but not rigid. [pause]
   b. Next, rest your hands wherever you find comfortable. [pause]
   c. Close your eyes or gaze downwards. [pause]
2. Now notice and relax your body. [pause]
   a. Notice any tight areas or tension. [pause]
   b. Relax them. [pause]
   c. Turn your attention to your breath. [pause]

    d. As you do this, you may notice your mind start to wander. This is natural. [pause]

    e. Be kind to your wandering mind, and gently redirect your attention back to your breathing. [pause]

    f. Instead of wrestling with your thoughts, practice observing them without reacting. [pause]

3. Come back to your breath over and over without judgement or expectation. [pause]

4. Take a few deep breaths. [pause]

    a. As you take a deep breath, feel the oxygen enlivening your body. [pause]

    b. As you exhale, feel your body relax. [pause]

    c. As you breathe, bring attention to the present moment without judgement. [pause]

    d. As you notice judgements arise, make mental note of them and let them pass. [pause]

5. Let your whole body be present as best you can. [pause]

6. Imagine yourself calm, peaceful, and focused. [pause]

    a. As you allow your mind calm, consider what you might be seeing [pause], hearing [pause], and feeling [pause] that shows you as calm, peaceful, and focused. [pause]

7. Now imagine receiving loving-kindness from another. [pause]

    a. As you allow yourself to receive loving-kindness from another, consider what you might be seeing [pause], hearing [pause], and feeling [pause] that shows you as calm, peaceful, and focused. [pause]

8. Now imagine giving loving-kindness to another. [pause] [*Caritas Process 1*]

    a. As you allow yourself to give loving-kindness to another, consider what you might be seeing [pause], hearing [pause], and feeling [pause] that shows you as calm, peaceful, and focused. [pause]

9. Take a deep breath. [pause]

10. Now turn your consciousness towards the caring/healing presence and transpersonal space you are entering with the person you will care for today. [pause] [*Caritas Processes #2 through #4*]

    a. Become aware of the authentic, sacred, healing space. [pause]

    b. Focus on your heart for a moment. [pause]

    c. Listen to your heart. [pause]

    d. Feel your heart open. [pause]

    e. Feel love for self and other. [pause]

    f. Feel the dynamic heart-centered vibration flowing throughout yourself and towards others. [pause]

    g. Appreciate, give attention to, and value the caring moment you are about to enter. [pause]

11. Take a deep cleansing breath. [pause]

12. When ready, allow your mind to be fully present for report and open your eyes.

    a. I invite you to return to intentionality, the heart space, as you immerse yourself in the caring/healing transpersonal experience. [*Caritas Processes #2 through #4*]

Briefing Stage

Now that learners have centered self, they are invited to enter into the simulated caring/healing experience. The briefing stage begins with the reading of the narrative patient-caring study synopsis.

EDUCATOR READS

The caring study begins with Mr. Bishop, a 68-year-old African American male, just having been admitted to the ICU. He has a medical history of congestive heart failure, hypertension, hyperlipidemia, atrial fibrillation and is a former smoker. He has been admitted to the hospital with complaints of a 12-pound weight gain, difficulty breathing, and edema in his lower extremities. Mr. Bishop is experiencing severe dyspnea, sinus tachycardia with an irregular rhythm, generalized edema, orthopnea, weakness, and fatigue.

CARING/HEALING EXPERIENCE (IMPLEMENTATION)

The caring/healing experience portion of the simulation, or implementation stage, shifts into the demonstration of Caritas processes, professional praxis, and technical competencies, skills, and attitudes.

Educator Reads
During the admission process and initial admission assessment, Mr. Bishop shared that his wife of 50 years had passed away last month, and he is having difficulty adjusting to this loss.

Educator Pauses & Asks
(Coach learners to respond as if they are the nurse in the narrative.)

1. What struck you about Mr. Bishop's clinical and emotional concerns? (Caritas Process #5)
2. How are you feeling as the healthcare professional in this caring/healing experience? (Caritas Processes #1 through #5)
3. How do you respond to Mr. Bishop? (Caritas Processes #5 through #7)
4. Which caring practices might you employ to be authentically present with Mr. Bishop in the caring/healing moment?
    a. Suggested learner responses (Adapted from Costello, 2018; Watson, 2018)
        i. Sit at eye level with Mr. Bishop (Caritas Process #2)
        ii. Be authentically present in the caring moment (Caritas Process #1)
        iii. Sit in silence and deeply listen as Mr. Bishop shares his life review, hopes, concerns, fears, preferences, values, needs, and beliefs
        iv. Get to know Mr. Bishop by cultivating a transpersonal caring relationship (Caritas Process #4)
        v. Resist the urge to interrupt and fix problems as Mr. Bishop shares
        vi. Be open to and supportive of the expression of positive and negative emotions (Caritas Processes #5)
        vii. When appropriate, ask questions to assess how spirituality plays a role in his life, such as "What gives you hope?" (Caritas Process #4)
            1. The caring moment provides an opportunity for spiritual assessment beyond the EHR, soul care for self and Mr. Bishop, and allowing and being open to miracles. (Caritas Processes #3, #7, #10)
        viii. Use caring/healing practices and creative use of self (e.g., therapeutic touch, music, guided imagery, etc.; Caritas Processes #6 and #7)

Educator Reads
Mr. Bishop begins to share that he is fearful about the potential for loss of autonomy and the ability to care for himself independently once he returns home. Both of his grown children live with their families in Florida and are not immediately available.

Educator Pauses and Asks
(Coach learners to respond as the nurse.)

1. Talk about your concerns. (Caritas Processes #4 and #5)
2. Respond to Mr. Bishop about what he is experiencing. (Caritas Processes #4 and #5)
3. What might you need to know about Mr. Bishop's fears and concerns? (Caritas Processes #4 and #5)
4. Talk about any fears or anxieties you feel at this point. (Caritas Processes #4 and #5)

Educator Reads
Mr. Bishop's initial admission assessment and the history and physical have now been completed. Orders have been entered into the patient's electronic health record. You re-enter the room. [pause] It has now been a couple of hours since the patient was admitted. Mr. Bishop will need a complete head-to-toe assessment, vital signs taken, intake and output, medications administered, and a review of his labs and diagnostics.

Educator Pauses and Asks
(Coach learners to respond as if they are the nurse in the narrative.)

- Prior to performing the technical caring practices, how would you:
  a. Engage in genuine teaching/learning experiences that attend to the whole person, their meaning, and within their frame of reference? (Caritas #7)
  b. Create a healing environment at all levels (physical, nonphysical, subtle environment of energy and caring consciousness) whereby wholeness, beauty, dignity, and peace are potentiated? (Caritas #8)
  c. Assist with comfort and basic needs with an intentional caring consciousness to allow for spiritual emergence? (Caritas #9)

Technical Caring Practices and Learning Outcomes
Use of high-fidelity manikins or standardized patients, and use of the EHR Go™ simulated electronic health record, create mimesis through immersive caring/healing experiences. Learners should achieve the following technical caring competencies and practices. Learning outcomes may be adapted for interprofessional education (IPE). Kaiser Permanente's NCAL Patient Care Services (2012) aligned the nursing process with Caring Science theory, Caritas processes, and caring literacy through development of the Caritas in Action nursing process framework. Caritas in Action serves as a best practice for operationalizing Caritas processes with supporting evidence and outcomes. Caring practices are further delineated by each phase of the nursing process. Kaiser Permanente's Caring Science: Caritas in Action website provides resources that educators may use during the stages of the simulated caring/healing experience. Some of the resources include videos, audio files, flyers, facilitator guides, and reflective exercise handouts. See provided link in the references for details.

Suggested Teaching Uses
Interprofessional Education (IPE)

- Pathophysiology of heart failure
- Cardiac measures and pulmonary assessments
- Decompensated heart failure
- Framingham risk-assessment tool
- Informatics competencies and skills

Nursing

- Abnormal respiratory assessment
- Medication review
- Abnormal peripheral vascular assessment

Pharmacy

- Polypharmacy and heart failure medications

Provider

- Management of heart failure
- Evaluation and management of chronic cardiopulmonary disease

Therapy

- Physical Therapy: Initial PT Evaluation for strengthening and fall prevention
- Occupational Therapy: Initial OT Evaluation for strengthening, balance, and fall prevention
- Mental Health Counselor: Grief counseling

Case Management

- Discharge planning

Suggested Technical Caring Practices and Learning Outcomes

1. Demonstrate caring literacy and Caritas processes. (IPE)
2. Create a plan of care that demonstrates Caritas in action. (IPE)
3. Effectively demonstrate the nursing process aligned with Caritas in action.
4. Recognize the pathophysiology contributing to the patient's current health status. (IPE)
5. Identify primary nursing diagnosis.
6. Identify relevant healthcare information in the patient's medical record. (IPE)
7. Complete a focused physical assessment to determine priority nursing interventions through critical thinking.
8. Demonstrate medication administration following the 5-Rights.
9. Identify indications, contraindications, and potential adverse reactions of administered medications.
10. Document assessment data and medication administration in patient chart.
11. Implement patient safety measures. (IPE)
12. Explain physical assessment findings and diagnostics related to patient condition. (IPE)
13. Interpret diagnostic findings to determine priority nursing interventions through critical thinking.
14. Implement provider orders. (IPE)
15. Prioritize interventions and document in the patient's care plan. (IPE)
16. Provide relevant patient and family teaching. (IPE)
17. Demonstrate therapeutic communication. (IPE)

18. Demonstrate accurate and professional communication with healthcare team members verbally and through EHR documentation. (IPE)
19. Demonstrate critical-thinking skills. (IPE)

Suggested Technical Caring Practices and Learner Performance Expectations

1. Document accurately and appropriately in the EHR using one or more of the following:
   a. Vital Signs tab
   b. Clinical Head to Toe Assessment
   c. Progress Note (IPE)
   d. Situation, Background, Assessment, Recommendation (SBAR) note (IPE)
   e. Care plan that demonstrates Caritas in action (IPE)
2. Perform focused assessment. (IPE)
   a. Cardio-respiratory
   b. Pain
   c. Risk
3. Administer medications as ordered.
4. Administer treatments as ordered. (IPE)
5. Provide care to maintain and/or improve respiratory status.
6. Provide care to maintain and/or improve cardiovascular status.
7. Complete patient teaching regarding diuretic therapy with Natrecor (Nesiritide). (IPE)
8. Demonstrate therapeutic communication with patient and/or family. (IPE)
9. Document accurately and appropriately in the EHR using specified documentation. (IPE)
10. Provide patient care in a safe manner using best practices. (IPE)
11. Communicate effectively with the interprofessional healthcare team. (IPE)
12. Demonstrate Caritas processes and literacies. (IPE)
13. Demonstrate complex decision-making and clinical reasoning. (IPE)

Electronic Health Record Chart Includes:

- Admission to intensive care unit
- Initial quick survey of patient
- Compression stocking
- Oxygen
- Fall precautions
- Full code
- Anticoagulation protocol
- Peripheral intravenous line
- Vital signs
- Daily weight
- Intake and output
- Urinary catheter
- Telemetry
- Low salt, low cholesterol diet
- Lab results
- Medication orders

- Physician history and physical
- Nurse admission assessment
- Chest x-ray report
- EKG report pending
- Echocardiogram report pending
- Consult for grief counseling
- Blank care plan

GUIDED REFLECTIVE PRACTICE (DEBRIEFING)

Reflection of one's practice is an essential step in the simulated experiential learning experience. Use of the Caring Science provides the opportunity to reframe the debriefing process from one of "judgmental debriefing to debriefing with good judgment" (Rudolph et al., 2007, p. 365). The good judgment model, developed by Rudolph et al. (2007) for debriefing, uses an advocacy/inquiry approach. Psychological safety is foundational to the debriefing process and includes meaning-making and sense-making systems. The debriefing process is further reframed with appreciative observations and insights by the educator. Rudolph et al. noted that the cornerstone of the good judgment approach is the inclusion of the learner's unique perspective as well as the expertise of the educator. The advocacy/inquiry approach includes transparent talking and guided reflection. Rudolph et al. conceptualized advocacy as an observation or statement and inquiry as a question. Additionally, educators guide the good judgment approach to ensure critical thinking, clinical reasoning, reflection, and reflexivity of the caring/healing experience and the transpersonal caring process.

Debrief—React
McDermott (2017) provided a practical approach to operationalizing the good judgment model and the advocacy/inquiry approach that will be adapted for the debriefing process. Guirguis and Cox (n.d.), with the University of Alberta, Faculty of Pharmacy and Pharmaceutical Sciences, developed a one-page debriefing tool using the advocacy/inquiry method adapted from the work of Rudolph et al. (2007; link is provided in the references). Begin by ensuring psychological safety and providing learners with an orientation to the debriefing process. The React phase encourages learner participation and allows the building of rapport and trust. Initial debriefing guided reflection might include:

- What went well?
- What might you do differently?
- Which caritas processes did you use?

Debrief—Understand
The purpose of the understand phase is to uncover thought processes and other factors that lead to a particular behavior or caring practice and to help learners find ways to improve Caring literacy and technical performance. The advocacy/inquiry method, proposed by Rudolph et al. (2007), is used by the educator to guide the process.

- Observe a caring/healing experience or technical caring practice.
- Comment on the observation.
- Explore the drivers behind the learner's thinking.

- Discover with the learner ways to attend to the Caritas process or the technical caring practices.

Guided Reflective Practice

The debriefing stage concludes with guided reflection. Learners are invited to reflect on the simulated caring/healing experience.

- How are you feeling?
- What did you learn from this caring/healing experience?
- How will you apply what you learned in your professional practice?

Reflection and reflexivity may be expanded further to deepen the development of Caring literacy and consciousness. Quinn (1992) proposed that when the nurse (or learner) enters into a sacred healing space, the nurse *is* the healing environment. Building upon this work, Watson (2004) provides additional reflective questions for further cultivation of Caritas. Example questions include:

- "If *I am the environment/community*, how can I *be* a more caring/healing environment/ self/community?
- How can I use my heart-centered awareness, my consciousness, my *Being*, my presence, my voice, my touch, *my face, my hands* for healing?" (Watson, 2004, p. 69)

Exemplar Two: Low Fidelity, Computer-Based Simulation and Narrative Caring Experiences[1]

EHR Go™ computer-based simulation application activities may also be used for small group or individual application activities outside of the simulation laboratory. Learners review the electronic health record prior to entering into the narrative caring experience. One interprofessional example is Ms. Tiffany Sutherland. Before entering into the electronic health record, learners are invited to center self through mindfulness practices as noted previously. This may be done through educator guidance or individual deep breathing and body-scanning techniques. Several smartphone and web-based applications are available for use by individual learners. Once the learner(s) have centered self, the caring study narrative is read.

Caring Study Narrative

Ms. Tiffany Sutherland is in the first trimester of an unintended pregnancy and comes to the women's health center today for her first prenatal appointment. She had a positive home test a few weeks ago, and a positive human chorionic gonadotropin (hCG) blood test in the clinic 1 week ago. She is taking Chantix to help her quit smoking and sertraline for mild depression. She had been on oral contraceptives until recently when she stopped taking them because she felt that the oral contraceptive pills (OCPs) and Chantix together were causing her to feel very depressed and "weird." This is an unintended pregnancy and Tiffany is not in a committed relationship. She is not sure if she wishes to terminate, have the baby and pursue adoption, or have the baby and raise it herself.

---

[1]Exemplars reproduced with permission from EHR Go. http://ehrgo.com/caringscience

The following probing questions may be used for individual reflection or small group Caritas/veritas discussions in the classroom.

1. After you have reviewed the provided context and electronic health record for Ms. Sutherland, how do you feel?
2. How is her lived experience similar or different to experiences from your life?
3. How will you practice loving-kindness in Ms. Sutherland's care?
4. How will you create a helping/trusting and empowering care experience as Ms. Sutherland self-determines her next steps?
5. How will you honor human dignity and respect for Ms. Sutherland?
6. Talk about some of the social, cultural, economic, and political issues that may have contributed to unintended pregnancy.
7. After appraising Ms. Sutherland's electronic health record, identify a Caritas process that you would use in the caring moment.
   a. Which Caritas process did you select and why?
8. Integrate your selected Caritas process into your nursing plan of care in the patient's electronic health record.
   a. Talk about the Caring literacies and practices you included in Ms. Sutherland's plan of care.

Exemplar Three: The Power of Narratives

Teaching with narratives empowers an educator to transform the learner's experience in meaningful and memorable ways. Dr. Patricia Benner (1984, 2009, 2011) has advocated for the use of narrative learning for decades because of their power to situate learners in real clinical contexts and to "experience" the unfolding story as if learners themselves were the nurse providing care. Kyriakidis (in progress) has followed Benner's urging and has adapted narratives for role-playing in a classroom to expose learners to experientially learn through narratives. The narratives can also be easily adapted for use in the clinical setting by practicing nurses.

According to Kyriakidis (in progress), in order to present prelicensure learners with the challenges that practicing, licensed nurses experience daily, parts of the narrative are shared with the learners, with pauses and probing questions at the pauses, to engage them to think and act like real nurses. Learners are coached to engage in and embrace first person responses as they respond to the "patient, family, or colleagues" in the narrative. Role-playing can be very effective as a learner can play the "patient, family, or colleague" to experience receiving differing interactions with "the clinician." Narrative learning can be adapted for small-group break-out discussions or for larger group responses and dialogue.

Following is an example of coaching learners based on narratives used by Kyriakidis (in progress). Dawn Simas shared her clinical story from practice about Keith and Paula (used with permission; names have been changed for anonymity). In this exemplar, the educator reads sections of the narrative and pauses to ask questions (several or few) for the learners to respond. Note that it is most effective to keep the probing questions in present, not future, tense in order to encourage deeper engagement. Examples of probing questions are interspersed between sections of the narrative as follows.

EDUCATOR READS

Narrative: She'll Be Okay by Dawn Simas

Keith was a patient in his 70s who was admitted to our floor with complications from acute myeloid leukemia (AML). Keith had been fighting AML for a couple of years, and now his disease was no longer responding to treatment. He came in with severe abdominal distension, and uncontrolled pain. Along with Keith was his wife of over 50 years, Paula.

The first night I had Keith, I had a feeling we had met before. Paula was asleep at the bedside, and Keith was in and out of wakefulness, sometimes drowsy after taking pain meds. Once Paula awoke and started talking, we realized that our families had attended the same church together, and their sons had played baseball with my older brothers. I made sure that Keith and Paula were comfortable with me being their nurse, and we laughed about what a small world it was.

As the days progressed, Keith was getting worse. His abdominal distension and pain worsened as his disease progressed. He wasn't stable enough to undergo testing, and he was also unsure if he wanted any further treatment.

EDUCATOR PAUSES AND ASKS

(Coach learners to respond as if they are the nurse in the narrative.)

1. What struck you about this situation?
2. How do you respond to Keith?
3. How are you feeling as the nurse in this situation?

EDUCATOR CONTINUES TO READ

Code status was broached multiple times with Keith, however he kept putting it off. One quiet night, while Paula slept for once, Keith expressed how afraid he was to die.

EDUCATOR PAUSES AND ASKS

(Coach learners to respond as the nurse.)

1. Talk about your concerns.
2. Respond to Keith about what he is experiencing.
3. What might you need to know about Keith's fear to respond well?
4. Talk about any fears or anxieties you feel at this point.

EDUCATOR CONTINUES TO READ

Keith explained that he was not afraid to die himself, but he was afraid to leave Paula alone.

EDUCATOR PAUSES & ASKS

(Coach learners to respond as the nurse.)

1. What nonverbal caring practices might you share with Keith? Talk about how you do that.

2. Talk about how you explore Keith's concerns.
3. Reflecting back, what might you have asked Keith differently after he expressed being afraid to die?
4. [Ask the person role-playing as Keith]: How are you experiencing the intimate questions and discussion?
5. [Ask the person role-playing as Keith]: Talk about what you are hoping for in the discussion, if you are Keith.

EDUCATOR CONTINUES TO READ

We talked for a long while that night, talking about all the things Paula was capable of doing for herself, and about how supportive their sons were towards their mother. After our conversation, he agreed to taking some pain meds, which he often stoically refused so he could be awake for his wife. The next day he made himself a Do Not Resuscitate, and his condition continued to deteriorate.

Two nights later, I was Keith's nurse again, and had gotten in report that he was in a lot of pain, and the meds didn't seem to be helping. Upon assessment, Keith appeared to be in distress. Keith was a Comfort Measures Only patient by this time, however I could see that Keith was struggling. His respirations were 30–32, he was diaphoretic, and he was pulling and moaning with every breath. I called the on-call doctor, and had his medications increased with little effect. Paula sat vigilantly at his bedside, tears in her eyes, and told me Keith would never want to be seen like this.

I promised her I would make Keith comfortable, and I called the on-call doctor a second time to get his medication increased. After a couple doses, Keith finally seemed comfortable. His respirations were back down to 14–16, he was no longer using all his accessory muscles to breathe, and he looked peaceful. Paula dozed off, with the promise I would wake her with any changes. On one of my frequent checks, I noticed immediately that Keith had taken a turn for the worse. He was having periods of apnea, was very pale, and was having mottling of his lower extremities. He also had tears slowly running from the corners of his eyes, down his face.

EDUCATOR PAUSES AND ASKS

(Coach learners to respond as the nurse.)

1. Talk about the significance of Keith's pallor and mottling.
2. What do you understand when you see tears running down Keith's face?
3. What do you do at this point in Keith's situation?
4. What caring practices do you provide?
5. What are you experiencing as Keith's nurse when you realize the change in his condition?

EDUCATOR CONTINUES TO READ

With my heart in my throat, I whispered in Keith's ear "She'll be OK," and then I woke up Paula to tell her about the change in Keith's condition. Paula and I sat at the bedside together for about 20 minutes, and then Keith took his last breath and passed away peacefully, holding his beloved wife's hand.

Paula was alone that night, her two sons having left earlier in the night. Paula called her old-est son, who said he would come right away, but it would take about 45 minutes to get there. I checked on my other patients, who were all comfortable, then asked my coworkers to keep an eye on them. I went back and sat with Paula, knowing Keith wouldn't have wanted her to be alone.

Educator Pauses and Asks

(Coach learners to respond as the nurse.)

1. What do you do or say as you are sitting with Paula before Keith passes?
2. How do you respond when Keith takes his last breath?
3. [Ask the person role-playing as Paula]: Talk about how helpful or supportive (or not) the responses from the learner(s) playing the nurse are to you.
4. How you are coping with Keith's dying and death?
5. What do you do or say when you return to stay with Paula, waiting for her son to arrive?

Educator Continues to Read

Paula shared with me stories of her and Keith's early marriage, of raising their children, and the joy of their grandchildren. She told me she was relieved that Keith went peacefully, and that she felt that he was trying to hold on for her. I shared with her the conversation that Keith had with me a few nights before, and told her what I had whispered in his ear before I had woken her. Paula cried with relief, knowing that some of the last words he heard were that she was going to be OK. Paula's son came, and gathered his mom to take home, sad at his dad's passing, but thankful that he was suffering no longer. Paula gave me a big hug before she left, and thanked me for not leaving her side.

Educator Pauses and Asks

(Coach learners to respond as the nurse.)

1. How do you respond to Paula and her son when they are ready to leave?
2. [Ask the person role-playing as Paula]: What other caring practices would you find help-ful or supportive?
3. What did you learn from this situation?
4. If you had this situation to do again, what might you do differently?

Educator Continues to Read

I left late that morning, catching up on all the charting I hadn't been able to do, but having made my patients passing easier on him and his family made it all worth it.
(Names have been changed for anonymity.)

Educator Pauses and Asks

1. Talk about the significance Dawn's story about Keith and Paula holds for you.
2. How might this situation and Dawn's thoughts and actions shape who you want to become as a nurse?

According to Kyriakidis (in progress), the diverse responses from learners, in the classroom, create rich learning from multiple emotional, caring, ethical, ethnic, interpersonal, and spiritual perspectives. This richness prepares learners with a deep understanding about possible ways of being a nurse in the caring situation. Imaginatively experiencing difficult and challenging situations, before actually entering clinical practice, helps learners gain embodied ways of being a good and caring nurse. This type of situated learning prepares, and helps in the formation of, inexperienced clinicians to know how they may engage in Caritas processes, and care for patients and their loved ones as they enter practice.

REFERENCES

Alessi, S. (2000a). Designing educational support in system-dynamics-based interactive learning environments. *Simulation & Gaming, 31*(2), 178–196. https://doi.org/10.1177/104687810003100205

Alessi, S. (2000b). Simulation design for training and assessment. In H. O'Neil, & D. Andrews (Eds.), *Aircrew training and assessment: Methods, technologies, and assessments.* Lawrence Erlbaum.

Alexander, A., Brunye, T., Sidman, J., & Weil, S. (2005). *From gaming to training: A review of studies on fidelity, immersion, presence, and buy-in and their effects on transfer in PC-Based simulations and games.* https://pdfs .semanticscholar.org/3475/e2b1a4093661fe4c82ef9b41fab549f3ea35.pdf

Beaubien, J. M., & Baker, D. P. (2004). The use of simulation for training teamwork skills in healthcare: How low can you go? *Quality & Safety in Health Care, 13*(Suppl 1), i51–i56. https://doi.org/10.1136/qshc.2004.009845

Benner, P. (1984). *From novice to expert: Excellence and power in clinical nursing practice.* Addison-Wesley Publishing, Nursing Division.

Benner, P., Kyriakidis, P., & Stannard, D. (2011). *Clinical wisdom and interventions in acute and critical care: A thinking-in-action approach* (2nd ed.). Springer Publishing Company.

Benner, P., Tanner, C. & Chesla, C. (2009). *Expertise in nursing practice: Caring, clinical judgment & ethics* (2nd ed.). Springer Publishing Company.

Blum, C. A., & Locsin, R. (2010). Teaching caring nursing to RN-BSN students using simulation technology. *International Journal of Human Caring, 14*(2), 40–49. https://doi.org/10.20467/1091-5710.14.2.40

Cara, C. (2003). *A pragmatic view of Jean Watson's caring theory.* https://www.watsoncaringscience.org/files/PDF/ Pragmatic_View.pdf

Christopher, R. (in progress). *Caring Fidelity™: The missing simulation fidelity and dimension.* Unpublished manuscript.

Clark, C. S. (2016). Watson's human caring theory: Pertinent transpersonal and humanities concepts for educators. *Humanities, 5*(21), 1–12. https://doi.org/10.3390/h5020021

Costello, M. (2018). Watson's caritas processes as a framework for spiritual end of life care for oncology patients. *International Journal of Caring Sciences, 11*(2), 639–644. http://www.internationaljournalofcaringsciences .org/docs/1_costello_special_10_2.pdf

Cronenwett, L., Sherwood, G., Barnsteiner J., Disch, J., Johnson, J., Mitchell, P., Sullivan, D., & Warren, J. (2007). Quality and safety education for nurses. *Nursing Outlook, 55*(3), 122–131. https://doi.org/10.1016/j .outlook.2007.02.006

Cronenwett, L., Sherwood, G., Pohl, J., Barnsteiner, J., Moore, S., Sullivan, D., Ward, D., & Warren, J. (2009). Quality and safety education for advanced nursing practice. *Nursing Outlook, 57*(6), 338–348. https://doi .org/10.1016/j.outlook.2009.07.009

Cunningham, R., Cleary, J., Dial, M., & Molloy, M. (2017). *Mindfulness tips for simulation: 2017 Simulation leader cohort.* https://sirc.nln.org/pluginfile.php/9/mod_forum/post/2641/Mindfulness%20in%20Prebriefing%20 .docx

Dahl, Y., Alsos, O. A., & Svanaes, D. (2010). Fidelity considerations for simulation-based usability assessments of mobile ICT for hospitals. *International Journal of Human-Computer Interactions, 26*(5), 445–476. https://doi .org/10.1080/10447311003719938

Daley, K., & Campbell, S. H. (2018). Framework for simulation learning in nursing education. In S. H. Campbell & K. Daley (Eds.), *Simulation scenarios for nursing educators: Making it real* (3rd ed., pp. 13–18). Springer Publishing Company.

Dieckmann, P., Friis, S. M., Lippert, A., & Ostergaard, D. (2009). The art and science of debriefing in simulation: Ideal and practice. *Medical Teacher*, 31, e287–e294. https://doi.org/10.1080/01421590902866218

Dieckmann, P., Gaba, D., & Rall, D., (2007). Deepening the theoretical foundations of patient simulation as social practice. *Simulation in Healthcare*, 2(3), 183–193. https://doi.org/10.1097/SIH.0b013e3180f637f5

Feldman, G., Hayes, A., Kumar, S., Greeson, J., & Laurenceau, J. P. (2007). Mindfulness and emotion regulation: The development and initial validation of the cognitive and affective mindfulness scale-revised (CAMS-R). *Journal of Psychopathology and Behavioral Assessment*, 29(3), 177–190. https://doi.org/10.1007/s10862-006 -9035-8

Florida Atlantic University, Christine E. Lynn College of Nursing. (2019). *Curriculum model*. https://nursing.fau .edu/academics/curriculum-model.php

Florida Board of Nursing. (2020). *Practical and registered nurse education program*. https://floridasnursing.gov/ licensing/practical-and-registered-nurse-education-program

Fludernik, M. (1996). *Towards a 'natural' narratology*. Routledge.

Foss Durant, A., McDermett, S., Kinney, G., & Triner, T. (2015). Caring science: Transforming the ethic of caring-healing practice, environment, and culture within an integrated care delivery system. *Permanente Journal*, 19(4), e136–e142. https://doi.org/10.7812/TPP/15-042

Gaba, D. M. (2004). The future vision of simulation in health care. *Quality & Safety in Health Care*, 13(Suppl 1), i2–i10. https://doi.org/10.1136/qshc.2004.009878

Guirguis, L., & Cox, C. (n.d.). *Debriefing using the advocacy-inquiry method*. University of Alberta, Faculty of Pharmacy and Pharmaceutical Sciences. https://sites.ualberta.ca/~hsercweb/viper/Advocacy_Inquiry_Method.pdf

Hayden, J. K., Smiley, R. A., Alexander, M., Kardong-Edgren, S., & Jeffries, P. R. (2014). *Journal of Nursing Regulation*, 5(2), Supplement S1–S464. https://www.ncsbn.org/JNR_Simulation_Supplement.pdf

Hills, M., & Watson, J. (2011). *Creating a Caring Science curriculum: An emancipatory pedagogy for nursing* (1st ed.). Springer Publishing Company.

International Nursing Association for Clinical Simulation and Learning Standards Committee. (2016a). INACSL standards of best practice: SimulationSM: Debriefing. *Clinical Simulation in Nursing*, 12, S21–S25. https://doi. org/10.1016/j.ecns.2016.09.008

International Nursing Association for Clinical Simulation and Learning Standards Committee. (2016b). INACSL Standards of best practice: SimulationSM: Facilitation. *Clinical Simulation in Nursing*, 12, S16–S20. https://doi. org/10.1016/j.ecns.2016.09.007

International Nursing Association for Clinical Simulation and Learning Standards Committee. (2016c). INACSL standards of best practice: SimulationSM: Outcomes and objectives. *Clinical Simulation in Nursing*, 12, S13–S15. https://doi.org/10.1016/j.ecns.2016.09.006

International Nursing Association for Clinical Simulation and Learning Standards Committee. (2016d). INACSL standards of best practice: SimulationSM: Participant evaluation. *Clinical Simulation in Nursing*, 12, S26–S29. https://doi.org/10.1016/j.ecns.2016.09.009.

International Nursing Association for Clinical Simulation and Learning Standards Committee. (2016e). INACSL standards of best practice: SimulationSM. *Clinical Simulation in Nursing*, 12, S48–S50. https://doi.org/10 .1016/j.ecns.2016.09.012

International Nursing Association for Clinical Simulation and Learning Standards Committee. (2016f). INACSL standards of best practice: SimulationSM: Simulation design. *Clinical Simulation in Nursing*, 12, S5–S12. https://doi.org/10.1016/j.ecns.2016.09.005

International Nursing Association for Clinical Simulation and Learning Standards Committee. (2016g). INACSL standards of best practice: SimulationSM: Simulation-enhanced interprofessional education (Sim-IPE). *Clinical Simulation in Nursing*, 12, S34–S38. https://doi.org/10.1016/j.ecns.2016.09.011

International Nursing Association for Clinical Simulation and Learning Standards Committee. (2016h). INACSL standards of best practice: Simulation[SM]: Simulation glossary. *Clinical Simulation in Nursing*, 12, S39–S47. doi. org/10.1016/j.ecns.2016.09.012

International Nursing Association for Clinical Simulation and Learning Standards Committee. (2017). INASCL Standards of Best Practice: SimulationSM: Operations. *Clinical Simulation in Nursing*, 13, 681–687. https:// doi.org/10.1016/j.ecns.2017.10.005

Jeffries, P. R. (2016). *The NLN Jeffries simulation theory*. Wolters Kluwer.

Kablitz, A., & Neumann, G. (1998). *Mimesis and simulation* [English translation]. Rombach.

Kaiser Permanente Nursing, NCAL Patient Care Services. (2012). *Caring science: Caritas in action*. https:// kpnursing.org/_NCAL/practice/caritas/action/index.html

Kyriakidis, P. (in progress). *Coaching learners in the development of engagement and caring practices: The power of narratives.* Unpublished manuscript.

Kolb, D. (1984). *Experiential learning: Experience as the source of learning and development.* Prentice-Hall.

Laucken, U. (1995). Modes of thinking: Reflecting on psychological concepts. *Theory & Psychology, 5*(3), 401–428. https://doi.org/10.1177/0959354395053008

Lee, S. M. (2018). Lee geropalliative caring model: A situation-specific theory for older adults. *Advances in Nursing Science, 41*(2), 161–173. https://doi.org/10.1097/ANS.0000000000000195

Lee, S. M., Palmieri, P. A., & Watson, J. (2017). *Global advances in human caring literacy.* Springer Publishing Company.

Locsin, R. C. (2005). *Technological competency as caring in nursing.* Sigma Theta Tau International.

Locsin, R. (2009). "Painting a clear picture:" Technological knowing as a contemporary nursing process. In R. Locsin & M. Purnell (Eds.), *A contemporary nursing process: The (un)bearable weight of knowing in nursing* (pp. 377–389). Springer Publishing Company.

Lopreiato, J. (2016). *Healthcare simulation dictionary.* Agency for Healthcare Research and Quality Publication No. 16(17)-0043. https://www.ahrq.gov/sites/default/files/publications/files/sim-dictionary.pdf

McDermott, M. (2017). *Debriefing with reflection: Best practice for learning in simulation in pre-licensure nursing education.* https://scholarship.shu.edu/final-projects/20

McKendrick-Calder, L., Pollard, C., Shumka, C., McDonald, M., Carlson, S., & Winton, S. (2019). Mindful moments – Enhancing deliberate practice in simulation learning. *Journal of Nursing Education, 58*(7), 431. https://doi.org/10.3928/01484834-20190614-09

Molloy, M. A., Cunningham, R., Cleary, J., & Dial, M. (2019). Enhancing situational awareness by using mindfulness during simulation. *Nurse Educator, 44*(6), 307. https://doi.org/10.1097/NNE.0000000000000669

Munshi, F., Lababidi, H., & Sawsan, A., (2015). Low-versus high-fidelity simulation in teaching and assessing clinical skills. *Journal of Tiabah University Medical Sciences, 10*(1), 12–15. https://doi.org/10.1016/j.jtumed.2015.01.008

National Council of State Boards of Nursing. (2015). NCSBN simulation guidelines for prelicensure nursing programs. *Journal of Nursing Regulation, 6*(3), 39–42. https://doi.org/10.1016/S2155-8256(15)30783-3

National League of Nursing Board of Governors. (1988). *Curriculum revolution: Mandate for change.* NLN Press.

National League of Nursing Board of Governors. (1989). *Reconceptualizing nursing education.* NLN Press.

National League of Nursing Board of Governors. (2015a). *Debriefing across the curriculum: A living document from the National League for Nursing, in collaboration with the International Nursing Association for Clinical Simulation and Learning (INACSL).* http://www.nln.org/docs/default-source/about/nln-vision-series -(position-statements)/nln-vision-debriefing-across-the-curriculum.pdf?sfvrsn=0

National League of Nursing Board of Governors. (2015b). *A vision for teaching with simulation: A living document from the National League for Nursing NLN Board of Governors.* http://www.nln.org/docs/default-source/ about/nln-vision-series-(position-statements)/vision-statement-a-vision-for-teaching-with-simulation. pdf?sfvrsn=2

Paige, J. B., & Morin, K. H. (2013). Simulation fidelity and cueing: A systematic review of the literature. *Clinical Simulation in Nursing, 9*(11), e481–e489. https://doi.org/10.1016/j.ecns.2013.01.001

Persico, L. (2018). A review: Using simulation-based education to substitute traditional clinical rotations. *JOJ Nursing & Health Care, 9*(8), 1–7. https://doi.org/10.19080/JOJNHC.2018.09.555762

Quinn, J. F. (1992). Holding sacred space: The nurse as healing environment. *Holistic Nursing Practice, 6*(4), 26–36. https://doi.org/10.1097/00004650-199207000-00007

Reed, J., & Watson, D. (1994). The impact of the medical model on nursing practice and assessment. *International Journal of Nursing Studies, 31*(1), 57–66. https://doi.org/10.1016/0020-7489(94)90007-8

Rehmann, A., Mitman, R., & Reynolds, M. (1995). *A handbook of flight simulation fidelity requirements for human factors.* Note No. DOT/FAA/CT-TN95/46. https://apps.dtic.mil/dtic/tr/fulltext/u2/a303799.pdf

Rudolph, J. W., Simon, R., Rivard, P., Dufresne, R. L., & Raemer, D. B. (2007). Debriefing with good judgment: Combining rigorous feedback with genuine inquiry. *Anesthesiology Clinics of North America, 25*, 361–376. https://doi.org/10.1016/j.anclin.2007.03.007

Schuelke, S., Aurit, S., Connot, N., & Denney, S. (2019). Virtual nursing: The new reality in quality care. *Nursing Administration Quarterly, 43*(4), 322–328. https://doi.org/10.1097/NAQ.0000000000000376

Sewchuk, D. (2005). Experiential learning: A theoretical framework for perioperative education. *AORN Journal, 81*(6), 1311–1318. https://doi.org/10.1016/S0001-2092(06)60396-7

Seropian, M. A., Brown, K., Gavilanes, J. S., & Driggers, B. (2004). Simulation – Not just a manikin. *Journal of Nursing Education, 43*(4), 164–169. PMID: 15098910.

Sitzman, K. S., & Watson, J. (2017). *Watson's caring in the digital world.* Springer Publishing Company.

Sitzman, K. S., & Watson, J. (2019). *Assessing and measuring caring in nursing and health sciences: Watson's caring science guide* (3rd ed.). Springer Publishing Company.

Smith, P. M., Corso, L. N., & Cobb, N. (2010). The perennial struggle to find clinical placement opportunities: A Canadian national survey. *Nurse Education Today, 30*(8), 798–803. https://doi.org/10.1016/j.nedt.2010.02.004

Smith, P. M., & Seeley, J. (2010). A review of the evidence for the maximization of clinical placement opportunities through interprofessional collaboration. *Journal of Interprofessional Care, 24*(6), 690–698. https://doi.org/10.3109/13561821003761457

Smith, P. M., Spadoni, M. M., & Proper, V. M. (2013). National survey of clinical placement settings across Canada for nursing and other healthcare professions—Who's using what? *Nurse Education Today, 33*(11), 1329–1336. https://doi.org/10.1016/j.nedt.2013.02.011

Tanioka, T., Yasuhara, Y., Dino, M. J. S., Kai, Y., Locsin, R. C., & Schoenhofer, S. O. (2019). Disruptive engagements with technologies, robotics, and caring advancing the transactive relationship theory of nursing. *Nursing Administration Quarterly, 43*(4), 313–321. https://doi.org/10.1097/NAQ.0000000000000365

Waldner, M. H., & Olson, J. K. (2007). Taking the patient to the classroom: Applying theoretical frameworks to simulation in nursing education. *International Journal of Nursing Educational Scholarship, 4*(1). https://doi.org/10.2202/1548-923X.1317

Walsh, M. (2011). Narrative pedagogy and simulation: Future directions for nursing education. *Nurse Education in Practice, 11*(3), 216–219. https://doi.org/10.1016/j.nepr.2010.10.006

Warelow, P., Edward, K. L., & Vinek, J. (2018). Care: What nurses say and what nurses do. *Holistic Nursing Practice, 22*(3), 146–153. https://doi.org/10.1097/01.HNP.0000318023.53151.33

Watson, J. (2002). Metaphysics of virtual caring communities. *International Journal for Human Caring, 6*(1), 41–45. https://doi.org/10.20467/1091-5710.6.1.41

Watson, J. (2004). Caritas and communitas: A caring science ethical view of self and community. *Journal of Japan Academy of Nursing Science, 24*(1), 66–71. https://doi.org/10.5630/jans1981.24.1_66

Watson, J. (2008). *Nursing: The philosophy and science of caring* (rev. ed.), University Press of Colorado.

Watson, J. (2018). *Unitary caring science: The philosophy and praxis of nursing.* University Press of Colorado.

Watson, J., Brewer, B. B., & D'Alfonso, J. (2012). *Watson caritas self-rating survey* (WCSR) ©. Watson Caring Science Institute. http://www.watsoncaringscience.org/wp-content/uploads/2012/09/WCPS-_Self-Rating_Final1.pdf

Watson, J., & Smith, M. C. (2002). Caring science and the science of unitary human beings: A trans-theoretical discourse for nursing knowledge development. *Journal of Advanced Nursing, 37*(5), 452–461. https://doi.org/10.1046/j.1365-2648.2002.02112.x

Waxman, K. T., Bowler, F., Forneris, S. G., Kardong-Edgren, S., & Rizzolo, M. A. (2019). Simulation as a nursing education disrupter. *Nursing Administration Quarterly, 43*(4), 300–305. https://doi.org/10.1097/NAQ.0000000000000369

UNIT IV

Beyond Evaluation to Authentication

In this unit, we explore different aspects of evaluating students' performance and progress. From a Caring Science perspective this becomes an onerous task because the evaluation strategies used must be congruent with the Caring Science paradigm. Although it is recognized that teachers have the responsibility to assess students' abilities, competencies, and knowledge, among other attributes, there have been very few significant developments in this area.

This unit contains one chapter that offers a connoisseurship model of evaluation. We describe this model, explore the issue of grading, and provide some examples of alternative strategies for assessing both classroom and clinical evaluation.

Connoisseurship: An Alternative Approach to Evaluation

One can create an exquisite Caring Science curriculum and use innovative emancipatory pedagogical practices and then undermine all the advances by making inappropriate choices about methods of evaluating students' practice and progress. If the evaluation methods used do not embrace or are not congruent with Caring Science, the previous work will be eroded.
—Hills & Cara, 2019, p. 206

INTRODUCTION

Evaluating student performance is an intrinsic aspect of being a teacher. Within a Caring Science curriculum, this task becomes extremely important because, if the evaluation strategies that are implemented are not congruent with the Caring Science paradigm, the evaluation process has the potential to undo all the work that preceded it. Because of the value base of a Caring Science curriculum, nurse educators must pay diligent attention to how students are evaluated. The evaluation strategies to be used cannot undermine the efforts of the faculty members to establish equitable, respectful, caring relations throughout a program of studies. The purpose of this chapter is to explore the issues of evaluation, grading, and assessing practice (clinical) performance and to describe some evaluation strategies that we believe are congruent with the Caring Science perspective.

EVALUATION

Generally, evaluation is used to provide landmarks or points of reference for teachers and students. Evaluation provides indicators that let teachers and students know where they are in relation to where they want to be or where they are trying to go.

Also, evaluation is a method that is used to determine worth or value, and it provides clues about progress, performance, achievement, or the lack of it. Unfortunately, all too often, evaluation becomes the most important aspect; it becomes the *ends* instead of the means, and as the ends "it surfaces as the energy system that drives the whole education" (Bevis, 2000, p. 264)—in other words, the *driver* of the educational pursuit rather than *markers* for learning progress. When this occurs, as it often does, everything else becomes less important and the entire learning process becomes consumed with the evaluation of learning rather than the learning itself. Because of our tendency to think of learning as behavioral change, our evaluation strategies tend to reflect this focus by attempting to measure changes in behavior. When we do this, we automatically and sometimes unknowingly endorse a very narrow view of learning that basically says that all learning is behavioral and therefore measurable. But much of learning in nursing is *not* behavioral and therefore cannot be measured this way.

In a Caring Science curriculum based in a relational emancipatory pedagogy, we are interested in cultivating a disciplined scholarship that is necessary for developing expertise. For example, we are interested in students

> *acquiring insights, seeing patterns, finding meanings and significance, seeing balance and wholeness, making compassionate and wise judgments while acquiring foresight, generating creative flexible strategies, developing informed, skilled intentionality, identifying with the ethical and cultural traditions of the field, grasping the deeper structures of the knowledge base, enlarging the ability to think critically and creatively, and finding pathways to new knowledge.* (Bevis, 2000, p. 265)

As Hills and Cara (2019) explain,

> So many aspects of nursing practice—compassion, empathy, thoughtfulness, consideration, perceptual awareness, discretionary decision-making, touch, listening for understanding warmth, respect, authenticity, and others—are not easily measured. Nevertheless, they are critical aspects of caring for people and they are essential to Caring Science curriculum and pedagogy. (p. 206)

Therefore, we need to develop new evaluation strategies that can access students' thinking and that can capture more of the essence of the essential attributes of a Caring Science curriculum.

CONNOISSEURSHIP

Bevis (2000) created an interpretative-criticism model of evaluation. In Bevis's model, students are engaged with teachers in the process of criticism as a way to assist them to use knowledge and experience to make comparisons and be critics.

We have developed this model of evaluation further and emphasize a connoisseurship model of evaluation but rather than criticism, we think of it as critique. Inspired by the work of Eisner (1972, 1985), Bevis (2000) expands the notion of evaluation. Eisner (1985) speaks of the art of appreciation that he labels "connoisseurship." As he explains, "a connoisseur goes further than generalizations or classifications by perceiving the unique attributes of phenomena that distinguish one thing from another even within a category" (quoted in Bevis, 2000, p. 286). For nurse educators to use this approach to evaluation, they must have an expert grasp on: the meaning of the experience in the field; the deeper structures of the subject; the history and historically significant issues of the field; both classical and the current literature of the field; the characteristics of the educated expert nurse; the educative processes that shape the expert professional nurse; and the modes of inquiry appropriate to the field (Bevis, 2000). This evaluation model of connoisseurship focuses on developing skills of observation, critique, and authentication. These skills of connoisseurship encourage students to grow professionally and improve their expertise in nursing.

Our connoisseurship model of evaluation requires a certain level of expertise and scholarship in order to provide the rich descriptions, interpretations, comparisons, and judgments that are inherent in the model. Indeed, it is precisely this experience and scholarship that distinguishes the one who is learning from the one who is evaluating the learning. So, a critical aspect of the connoisseurship approach to evaluation is the ability to teach the process of connoisseurship and criticism to the colearners by providing them with experiences and working with them to hone their abilities to recognize good practice. It is not possible for students to become connoisseurs while they are students; however, as Bevis (2000) suggests, what they can do is begin an apprenticeship in the art of perception, appreciation, and comparison. "It is the very lack of experience on the part of students that handicaps them in developing 'taste' and sophistication in perceiving and interpreting events of care" (Bevis, 2000, p. 284).

Influenced by Bevis (2000), we adapt a five-part evaluation model of interpretive-critique. This model consists of five parts by combining looking and seeing as observing. The five components of our connoisseurship model of evaluation are:

- *Observing*—Observing requires that we both look and see. Looking at something is quite different from seeing something. Seeing is looking with attention and focus. Seeing is attending to the details, the context, the situation, the environment, the parts, and the whole. It also involves recognizing what is being looked at.
- *Perceiving and Intuiting*—Perceiving and intuiting involve our personal sensing and interpreting. It means paying particular attention to the unique and particular, both of the person and the situation. This type of perceiving requires intuition and imagination. It is similar to what Benner (2001) observed in expert nurses' practices. These nurses were able to perceive whole situations and know what to do in a given situation without breaking the situation down into component parts. Perceiving and intuiting in this way involves an ability to perceive what is significant and what is trivial in a given situation, a judgment that can be made only in the light of experience. Given the limited experiences that students may have, nurse educators have a significant part to play in helping students "unpack" these situations. Working with learners to examine the significance of what they see educates them in developing their perceiving and intuiting abilities and enhances their expert judgment.
- *Rendering*—Rendering is a way of describing the indescribable . . . it has virtual rather than actual meaning and depends upon symbolic language such as metaphor or simile. These are thick, rich descriptions that are situation based, contextual, and subjective. They rely on the observer's ability to use metaphor, prose, imagery, and simile to give accounts of human experiences. Rendering is subjective with the meaning of the experience being honored.
- *Interpreting Meaning*—Meanings are our personal interpretations of events. As discussed in an earlier chapter, they are deeply personal, and based on our assumptions, beliefs, values, and ethics. It challenges the old adage "seeing is believing" and turns it on its head to *believing* is *seeing*. We see certain things because of our belief systems. In evaluation situations, accessing students' meanings assists nurse educators in understanding what students are doing with information, knowledge, and experiences. A wise teacher can be heard asking their students to "think out loud." This nurse educator is trying to access the meanings that students are making internally.
- *Authenticating*—Authenticating requires that you have the context and knowledge for comparisons. It is in this aspect of the model that the critique is made about the value or

significance of the nursing situation being assessed. Authentication requires knowledge of how students learn, as well as education and nursing theories so that it is grounded in the reality of nursing and learning.

LEARNING ACTIVITY: USING THE CONNOISSEURSHIP MODEL TO ACCESS LEARNING

ENDS IN VIEW

In this learning activity, you will use the critique and connoisseurship model to access learning.

READ

After reading Chapter 18, complete this learning activity.

WRITE

Consider your recent clinical experience. Using the critique and connoisseurship framework just proposed, assess your clinical experience. Consider each component and evaluate your learning in your clinical experience.

DIALOGUE

Share your assessments of your learning experiences with your classmates. Consider the following questions:

- How does this model of evaluation fit with your views of evaluation?
- To what degree is this model congruent with Caring Science and a relational emancipatory pedagogy?

REFLECT

In your journal, write about how you might do your practicum differently if you were to start over. Use the critique and connoisseurship model to describe the aspects that you might focus on differently.

LEARNING ACTIVITY: DEVELOPING CRITERIA FOR EVALUATING LEARNING

ENDS IN VIEW

In this learning activity, you will have opportunities to develop criteria to assess learning.

WRITE

Read the following situations and choose one to work on, or you may choose a situation from your own experience if you wish. Develop criteria to assess learning, and describe how you would evaluate the situation that you have chosen. Consider how you will know that learning has taken place. What will you take as evidence that learning has occurred?

SITUATIONS

1. You are a nurse teaching prenatal classes. This is your final session.
2. You are in charge of continuing education and have organized a teaching/learning session on continuous patient records.
3. You are a nurse on a maternity ward and are teaching a first-time mom to bathe her baby.
4. You work on a cardiac unit, and you are doing discharge planning with a 65-year-old male who has experienced a myocardial infarction.
5. You are a community health nurse making a home visit to an elderly gentleman living with diabetes.
6. You work with the Ministry of Health and have just completed a health promotion session on community participation in healthcare with the regional health officers.

DIALOGUE

Share the situation you chose, the criteria you developed, and the evaluation process you described with your classmates. What important points need to be remembered when developing criteria for assessing learning? What patterns emerged from the discussion of your evaluation processes? Discuss any discrepancies and explore these in relation to the Caring Science framework outlined in Chapter 4.

REFLECT

In your journal, reconsider the criteria you developed and the evaluation process that you described in light of your discussions with your learning partners or study group. Are there any changes you would make?

ASSESSING STUDENTS' PERFORMANCE: THE DILEMMA OF GRADING

Grading is perhaps the most difficult aspect of teaching/learning within a Caring Science curriculum. The notion of a person assigning grades to another person's work without that person being involved in the decision-making violates the basic assumptions upon which the Caring Science curriculum rests.

Yet, you may find yourself in situations in which you are required to *grade* someone else's work. Usually, institutions require teachers to assign grades to students' work and to submit them.

Learning and grading are often confused. It is often assumed that a grade that a student received in a course is a reflection of the learning that the student experienced in that course. Yet, we have all had experiences where we have learned a great deal but were unable to demonstrate that learning in the specific tasks (assignments) that we were asked to complete! We believe that it is important to separate learning from grading. In our opinion, learning is a deeply personal experience that has to do with the discovery of personal meaning.

As difficult as it is for many nurse educators, they have no control over what students learn. Students are self-determining human beings and have complete control over what they learn. Grading, in contrast, is an assessment that teachers are required to make about students' performance on a set of specific tasks at a given moment in time. We are committed to having assignments relate to students' learning as much as possible, that is, to making them practical and relevant. However, in the end, it still comes down to the judgment that the teacher must make about each student's ability to meet certain criteria. In a book on curriculum development within Caring Science, it seems even more critical that the evaluation methods be congruent with and reflect the philosophy of this perspective. Conditions must be such that the evaluation methods used do not sabotage the integrity of the learning within a course. This means the evaluation process must be transparent and certain conditions must exist, including the following:

- Power differences between teachers and learners are discussed and negotiated.
- Criteria for evaluation are consistent with Caring Science and a relational emancipatory pedagogy.
- As much as possible, students and teachers negotiate the evaluation process.
- Evaluation criteria integrate lived experiences, theoretical understandings, and critical reflection.
- Peer and self-evaluation are valued.

TIME OUT FOR REFLECTION

Think about different ways that you have been evaluated in an education system. Answer the following questions:

- What methods of evaluation stand out for you as being participatory?
- Have you had an experience in which you felt that the power differential between you and the nurse educator was negotiated? Describe this experience.
- What was your most rewarding evaluation experience?
- What would you recommend as the most appropriate strategies for evaluating nursing students in a Caring Science curriculum?

It has become popular for nurse educators to develop rubrics. Most rubrics are reductionistic and quantitative but as we have already suggested, this method of measurement is antithetical to the philosophy and desires of a Caring Science curriculum that is trying to develop insights, pattern recognition, intuition, and creativity. So what are the alternatives? Let us discuss some.

Using Descriptive Rather Than Numerical Grading Scales

Table 18.1 is an example of a descriptive grading scale. Yes, eventually you may need to give a numerical grade but you can begin by deciding if a paper for example is an "A," "B," or "C." It is worth mentioning that it matters if you are grading undergraduate or graduate students. The level of the student brings particular contextual issues such as safety for prelicensed undergraduate students. This issue may not be of concern for graduate registered nurses.

Contract Grading: An Alternative to Traditional Evaluation Strategies

Contract grading is an interesting strategy for evaluating students' performances that recognizes the power differences between students and teachers and then attempts to negotiate that

TABLE 18.1 Descriptive Grading Scale

GRADE	GRADE POINT VALUE	PERCENTAGE	DESCRIPTION
A+ A A-	9 8 7	90–100 85–89 80–84	An A+, A, or A- is earned by work which is technically superior, shows mastery of the subject matter, and in the case of an A+ offers original insight and/or goes beyond course expectations. Normally achieved by a minority of students.
B+ B B-	6 5 4	77–79 73–76 70–72	A B+, B, or B- is earned by work that indicates a good comprehension of the course material, a good command of the skills needed to work with the course material, and the student's full engagement with the course requirements and activities. A B+ represents a more complex understanding and/or application of the course material.
C+ C	3 2	65–69 60–64	A C+ or C is earned by work that indicates an adequate comprehension of the course material and the skills needed to work with the course material and that indicates the student has met the basic requirements for completing assigned work and/or participating in class activities.
D	1	50–59	A D is earned by work that indicates minimal command of the course materials and/or minimal participation in class activities that is worthy of course credit toward the degree.
COM	Excluded Grade	N/A	**Complete** (pass). Used only for 0-unit courses and those credit courses designated by the Senate. Such courses are identified in the course listings.

power by allowing students to be involved in the grading process. Contract grading allows students to make important choices about what, how, and when to learn, thereby facilitating the development of a partnership learning/teaching environment. As an evaluation strategy, it is consistent with a Caring Science curriculum and a relational emancipatory pedagogy.

Contract grading can take many forms. Typically, teachers outline expectations for students for each grade level and students enter a contract for the grade that they want to achieve in the course (Table 18.2). For each grade, the number and the quality of the assignments vary. For example, if a student negotiates for a "B," they do the work required for a "B" grade, and it must be in keeping with the quality description of a "B" assignment. Usually, teachers retain the discretion of assigning the plus or minus of the grade to the work produced.

To be successful, contract grading requires an up-front investment by the nurse educator and is initially time consuming to implement. Students are not usually familiar with this evaluation strategy and can be leery of it. Nurse educators need to provide as much information as possible and spend the time required to allow the students to make an informed decision about whether or not they want to participate in the contract-grading evaluation. Ultimately, it is the students' collective choice that determines whether or not contract grading will be used

TABLE 18.2 Example Description of Teacher's Expectations for Each Grade Level

TASK	C	B	A
1. Regular attendance	required	required	required
2. Journal notes	required	required	required
3. Completion of two typescripts including analysis and feedback from your partner	required	required	required
4. Audio or videotaped demonstration of helping interview	required	required	required
5. Class presentation		required	required
6. Personal guidelines for helping		required	required
7. Research paper			required
8. Option: (except for number 4). You may propose a substitution for any of the tasks listed. This must be negotiated with the instructor. Such negotiation must be completed by July 22.			

to assess their performance. It often surprises us how students are reluctant to engage in this evaluation method. However, when you have an open discussion about the underlying power issues involved, while making it clear that if you evaluate them in the traditional way you have all the power, they typically engage quickly. Grade contracts do shift the power difference and help students to have more responsibility for their grades. In most cases, the teacher will have them sign an actual contract that does not have any weight per se but instead is a symbolic act.

One criticism of contract grading is the belief that all students should be striving for an "A." Obviously, for an undergraduate program, we do not want to encourage students to strive for a "D" or an "F" as both of these are below average and failing. However, when the consequences of this choice are described to the students, they usually do not choose to be unsuccessful or fail. Allowing students to retain control and responsibility for their actions is a powerful experience that enacts a Caring Science and relational emancipatory pedagogy. Putting control in the students' hands often results in their delivering better quality work. As a nurse educator, you need to consider the composition of your class recognizing that this might in fact give some students permission to do less. However, at the same time, other students who feel disempowered by grading might become motivated by the control they receive through grade contracts and make a better grade.

When using contract grading, a clear description of each task must be provided, and the precise criteria for grading must be described fully.

A similar but slightly different strategy described by Zander and Zander (2000) is to give everyone an "A" and have them describe what they will do to earn the "A." Zander and Zander suggest that using this strategy moves students and teachers from a "measurement" world to a "world of possibility." "The A is not an expectation to live up to but rather a possibility to live into" (p. 25). Of course, there are many educational institutional barriers to using these creative approaches. We are confident that in the future, "mastery" will become more important in nursing education than "grades" as a measurement of knowledge.

Also, it is worth noting that because of the extensive exploration and discussion that is needed to endure this type of grading is well understood, it is difficult to do with online courses. When you are face-to-face, you can "read" the students' comfort levels better.

LEARNING ACTIVITY: DESIGNING EVALUATION CONSISTENT WITH A CARING SCIENCE CURRICULUM

ENDS IN VIEW

In this learning activity, you will have an opportunity to develop your own evaluation methods that are consistent with a Caring Science curriculum and a relational emancipatory pedagogy.

WRITE

In your journal, based on your learning to date, make a list of the characteristics that you consider to be essential to quality evaluation practices in a Caring Science curriculum.

DIALOGUE

Share your list of characteristics of quality evaluation practices with your classmates. Compare and critique your lists and search for common characteristics. Discuss any characteristics that do not seem to fit with your understanding of a Caring Science curriculum.

REFLECT

In your journal, illustrate how evaluation relates to other aspects of your relational emancipatory pedagogy.

PRACTICE (CLINICAL) EVALUATION: ACCESSING STUDENTS' LEARNING

Historically nurses' practice competence has been assessed using behavioral objectives and professional competencies. Basically, we relied on the students' ability to recite signs and symptoms of diseases, develop nursing care plans, and recall on demand the nursing care required for a particular disease. However, behavioral objectives as guides to evaluation support a philosophy of evaluation that is "reductionistic, mechanistic, control and predictive-oriented, empirical, and manipulative" (Bevis, 2000, p. 275).

As we embrace a Caring Science framework as the foundation for a Caring Science nursing curriculum and a relational emancipatory pedagogy, we need to develop new ways of evaluating students that are congruent with this theoretical/philosophical position. Practice evaluation presents particular challenges because we need to feel comfortable that our students and graduates are safe. In the past, we tended to assume that behavioral objectives that were measurable ensured safe nursing practice. However, with only a moment's reflection, it is apparent that the tool that has always been used to assess students' practice (clinical) performance is the nurse educator. We rely on our judgment to assess students' abilities to practice safely.

> Safety is more than performing the technical task without error and harm to the patient. Safety also resides in being able to depart rule-driven behavior quickly, to cut through distractors to the heart of a problem and to solve it creatively. In this way, knowledge, understanding, insights, and intuition wisely used also determine safety. (Bevis, 2000, p. 276)

In other words, it is to these attributes that we must turn to appraise students' performances. We turned our attention to these attributes in a study (Hills, 2001) that was designed to develop a way of evaluating practice performance that was consistent with a Caring Science curriculum with a relational emancipatory pedagogy. We began by considering Benner's (1984, 2001) domains of practice and competencies and massaged those to be more congruent with our curriculum. We ensured that all domains and competencies were: nursing concepts, not biomedical ones; included community settings as well as acute-care settings; reflected health promotion; and, finally, concentrated on developing competencies that reflected what *could* be rather than what *is*. Thus, began the development of a Clinical Appraisal Form. Table 18.3, from Hills (2016, p. 304), describes Benner's domains of practice, how they were changed, and the rationale for the change.

TABLE 18.3 Benner's and CNPBC Domains of Practice With Rationale for Changes

BENNER'S DOMAINS OF PRACTICE	CNPBC DOMAINS OF PRACTICE	RATIONALE
Helping Domain	Health/Healing Domain	to include health
Teaching-Coaching Function	Teaching/Learning Domain	to include learning from client
Diagnostic and Patient-Monitoring Function	Clinical Judgment Domain	combined as each involved aspects of clinical judgement
Effective Management of Rapidly Changing Situations		
Administering and Monitoring Therapeutic Interventions		
Monitoring and Ensuring the Quality of Health Care Practices	Professional Responsibility Domain	to capture essence of the domain in language more congruent with curriculum
Organizational and Work-Role Competencies	Collaborative Leadership Domain	to incorporate language that more accurately reflected a Caring Science philosophy

CNPBC, Collaborative Nursing Program of British Columbia.

Source: With permission from Hills, M. (2016). Collaborative and emancipatory: Leading from beside. In W. Rosa (Ed.), *Nurses as leaders: Evolutionary visions of leadership* (p. 304). Springer Publishing Company.

With consultations from several nurse scholars (Dr. Jean Watson, Dr. Em Bevis, and Dr. Chris Tanner), five domains of practice were identified: health and healing, teaching/learning, clinical judgment, professional development, and collaborative leadership. Within each domain, several quality indicators were identified with specific indicators developed for each domain that reflected changes in course themes. For example, in semester two the focus is on people's experience with chronic health challenges; thus, all of the quality indicators reflect this theme. The five domains of practice remained constant in every semester throughout the program. The quality indicators changed in each semester reflecting the semester focus and the increased complexity of learning nursing practice.

Initially, nurse educators experienced difficulty using this appraisal form. "They reported a tendency to use the quality indicators . . . in the practice appraisal form as if they were behavioral objectives" (Hills, 2001, p. 340). Given that this form was developed specifically to replace behavioral objectives, more faculty development was needed.

This experience led us to develop what we called the "Iterative review and dialogue process" (Hills, 1993, 2001; Hills et al., 1993). Through our discussions, we realized that we needed to have learning and evaluation connected. Rather than *testing* students in clinical situations, we needed to access their thinking about their practice. We needed to access students' thinking and the way that they processed information. We know that telling stories, or narrative accounts from patients' lived experiences, is an effective way of accessing students' thinking about practice situations. Having them reflect on these narratives develops insight and reflective practice.

The group reached this watershed moment when one member of the group reminded us that "students have to have insight into their practice. Students must be able to critically reflect on their experience and derive insight from that reflection. Students are not *safe* [author's emphasis] if they cannot do this" (Hills, 2001, p. 342). This revelation transformed our thinking about clinical evaluation by reframing what it means to be a *safe* nurse: it was the culmination of our past experiences, our critical dialogue, and our raised consciousness that permitted us to see this link between insight and safety as the key to transform our evaluation practices.

As a result of these discussions, we conceptualized the following evaluation process, named the Iterative Review and Dialogue Process (IR&DP; Hills, 2001).

ITERATIVE REVIEW AND DIALOGUE PROCESS

- Students write a narrative account of practice in their journal.
- Students analyze this "story" using a framework designed for this purpose: Practice Appraisal Form (PAF).
- The story and analysis are submitted to faculty members for review.
- Faculty members respond to students' critiques by posing questions that encourage the students to further reflect on the experiences they described.
- These notes, questions, and comments are returned to the students.
- The students respond to the faculty's comments.

This iterative process is repeated.

An example of this iterative process is reflected in the journal of a first-year student who, in her second semester (people's experience with chronic health challenges), is working with a woman who is living with Parkinson's disease. She states:

Another quality indicator of the health and healing domain is beginning to develop an open caring approach. I think this was illustrated when I took a seat near my client's bed so that we could communicate openly and comfortably with each other. She welcomed this. She very much guided the communication, willingly telling me her stories of her family and her disease. I contributed by listening. A question posed to me [by my faculty member] was "what is it like to listen to another?" Well in this case it was very easy because I was deeply interested in her story. I tried to remain aware of my posture, keeping it as welcoming to communication as possible, which I found a little difficult to do upon the first time meeting someone. However, my client made it easier for me because of her openness, sincerity, and her willingness to teach. I very much appreciated this. This made it extra interesting and intrigued me to listen very actively—with all my senses. I truly empathized with this woman and I could feel her frustration, her sadness, her happiness, her acceptance. I was drawn in by her knowledge, and her experience—her life. I learned so much. I tried to understand as much as I could. I did not judge or jump to conclusions. She led the way, and I followed willingly down her life's path. I was very involved.

This excerpt demonstrates how the domains of practice and the quality indicators prompt students to reflect on their clinical experiences and identify specific ways they engaged in those clinical situations. It also demonstrates how the nurse educator prompts the student to reflect further by asking critical questions. The iterative process is also well demonstrated in this excerpt.

Another quality indicator in the health and healing domain is that it "focuses on the person not the disease." In this case, the student states:

I see my client just like anyone else. She is conscious of her weight, her appearance—how her hair looks. She has good days and bad days. She has interests of her own—reading. She is a person, a whole person, her own unique person, and I feel lucky to have gotten to know her the way I have. It is a wonderful, connecting experience. [My faculty member] asked "What made you mention that you see your client just like everyone else?" [the student responds:] The reason that I touched on the fact, in my story, that I see my client like anyone else is because I have heard all too often, in the past, clients being seen or known as their disease and nothing else. I have heard caregivers referring to patients as "the leg" or "the arm," depending on the client's condition. These caregivers are neglecting to see the whole person. Some may wonder why with all those problems, such as a progressive disease, one would worry about their appearance. Again, they are neglecting to tend to the whole person, and neglecting to support their client's coping mechanisms, values, interests, and worth. I just wanted to make it clear that I don't think that way, or conduct my practice that way. Even though my client has a disease, she is more than that. She cares, hopes, copes, and dreams. She has her own special interests, and each person living with a disease has their own story. You cannot treat every Parkinson patient the same, because they are more than a Parkinson patient, they are their own unique person.

Again, the domains and competencies provide a structure for students to describe their experiences and reflections. Nurse educators gain access to the students' thinking and can prompt further insight and reflection by asking questions and sharing their perceptions.

New ways of appraising practice performance must be developed if we are to successfully shift to a Caring Science paradigm. Benner's (1984, 2001) revolutionary work on excellence in clinical expertise could make a remarkable contribution to the evaluation of nursing students' clinical performance. If the concepts revealed in much of her research, but particularly in her book, *From Novice to Expert* (1984, 2001), were experimented with as guides for clinical evaluation, this contribution would be realized. As she explains:

> Perceptual awareness is central to good nursing judgment and . . . this begins with vague hunches and global assessments that initially bypass critical analysis; conceptual clarity follows more often than it precedes. (Benner, 2001, pp. xxi–xxii)

You can often hear experienced nurses describing their sense of something not being quite right. They often have a gut feeling about something. They can be heard saying things like, "the patient was just going sour." They usually cannot explain the signs and symptoms, they just have an intuition that is usually later confirmed.

As Benner explains:

> Expert nurses know that in all cases definitive evaluation of a patient's condition requires more than vague hunches, but through experience they have learned to allow their perceptions to lead to confirming evidence. (Benner, 2001, pp. xxi–xxii)

Imagine if we began to create evaluation strategies that concentrated on assessing students' abilities to recognize salient contextual aspects of a given practice situation and assisted them to link this perceptual awareness to nursing actions. We would be on a new path of practice evaluation: one that would mean that nurses were learning how to be experts and connoisseurs of their own practice, and evaluation would encourage this development, rather than act as an impediment to it.

REFERENCES

Benner, P. (1984). *From novice to expert: Excellence and power in clinical nursing practice.* Addison Wesley.

Benner, P. (2001). *From novice to expert: Excellence and power in clinical nursing practice.* Prentice Hall.

Bevis, E. (2000). Accessing learning: Determining worth or developing excellence: From a behaviorist toward an interpretive-criticism model. In E. Bevis & J. Watson (Eds.), *Toward a caring curriculum: A new pedagogy for nursing* (pp. 261–303). Jones & Bartlett.

Eisner, E. (1972). Emerging models for education evaluation. *School Review, 80*(4), 573–589. https://doi.org/10.1086/443050

Eisner, E. (1985). *The educational imagination* (2nd ed.). Macmillan.

Hills, M. (1993). Clinical evaluation: Creating a practice appraisal form. In M. Hills (Ed.), *Collaborative Nursing Project: Development of a generic integrated nursing curriculum in collaboration with four partner colleges.* Report to the Ministry of Advanced Education, Centre for Curriculum and Professional Development.

Hills, M. (2001). Using Co-operative Inquiry to transform evaluation of nursing students' clinical practice. In P. Reason & H. Bradbury (Eds.), *Handbook of action research, participatory inquiry and practice* (pp. 340–347). Sage.

Hills, M. (2016). Collaborative and emancipatory: Leading from beside. In W. Rosa (Ed.), *Nurses as leaders: Evolutionary visions of leadership* (pp. 293–309). Springer Publishing Company.

Hills, M., Belliveau, D., Calnan, R., Clarke, C., Greene, E., & Tanner, C. (1993). *An iterative dialogue process for clinical evaluation.* In M. Hills (Ed.), *Collaborative Nursing Project: Development of a generic integrated nursing curriculum in collaboration with four partner colleges.* Report to the Ministry of Advanced Education, Centre for Curriculum and Professional Development.

Hills, M., & Cara, C. (2019). Curriculum development processes and pedagogical practices for advancing caring science literacy. In W. Rosa, S. Horton-Deutsch, & J. Watson (Eds.), *A handbook for caring science: Expanding the paradigm* (pp. 197–210). Springer Publishing Company.

Zander, R., & Zander, B. (2000). *The art of possibility.* Penguin Books.

Ensuring the Future of Nursing: Embracing Caring Science

In this last unit, we enter into new space where we reflect and revision education generally. We offer another level of philosophical and ethical critique grounded in another turn of whole person, unitary consciousness—bringing the parts and whole together; bringing the heart and mind together—*educare*—the soul of education with caring. We introduce the notion of *Caritas* education—of learning and teaching, as an evolved ethic, epistemology, and pedagogy, which unites caring and love (Palmer, 2004).

Here we ask new questions, rhetorical and otherwise, such as what kind of curriculum can sustain *Caritas*: Love and epistemology and pedagogy as ethic? How do we break the dominant mindset of separation and put the parts back into the whole?

We seek to reconcile and unify educational, epistemological, and ethical models of caring as pedagogical and curricular reforms now and in the future—for nursing education, science, and society alike.

In this closing unit we consider transformational learning concepts and introduce broader energetic symbolic notions of "words"—words we use in teaching, learning, theories, and interpretations, in communicating our Knowing, Being, Doing. We reveal how "words" and language carry energetic power to influence others, for better or for worse.

Language, combined with the power of personal experiences, possesses the energy of love and caring. Thus we seek to address the "ethics of face" of the individual, as unique "other," whether in the classroom or clinical setting, near or afar, real time or virtual, reaffirming that Caring Science is not a unitary singular rule-bound approach. Rather, Caring Science invites all the diversity and synergistic emergence of science, arts, philosophy, and humanities, with personal meaning, growth, and evolving consciousness—awakening to an expanding and changing worldview that is upon us.

Finally we conclude by proposing "authentication criteria with examples of 'Disciplinary Evidence' relevant for a Caring Science curriculum"; for example, what would be/could be some operational and philosophical guidelines for anyone considering taking this disciplinary Caring Science curriculum perspective seriously?

These new authentication criteria can be the rhetorical overriding evidentiary directions for all futuristic programs. They incorporate distinct Caring Science disciplinary criteria as an evolved standard and evidence-guide to help assure and sustain nursing as a distinct *Caring-Healing-Health* discipline and profession for another century.

Palmer, P. (2004). *A hidden wholeness: The journey toward an undivided life.* John Wiley and Sons.

Reflecting and Revisioning: Bringing the Heart and Mind Together

If nurse educators continue to describe nursing using medical language of diseases, diagnosis and treatment, nursing risks remaining trapped in the medical paradigm. On the contrary, when nurse educators use the language of health, healing, people's experiences, suffering, caring, "being with," being present, or authentically listening, they are allowing the invisible work of nursing to emerge ontologically for nursing students.
—Hills and Cara, 2019, pp. 202–203

BRINGING THE HEART AND MIND TOGETHER FOR CARING SCIENCE EDUCATION

Introduction

It is acknowledged that it takes about 100 years for a profession to mature as a distinct separate entity and come of age in its own right. As we complete the revision of this book, we honor and acknowledge this year, 2020, as the 200-year anniversary of Florence Nightingale's birth, the founder of modern nursing in the world, who died in 1910. Thus, we are here together 200 years later, to make the right choices for this historic timeline and to reignite the enduring light and love of the heart and soul of nursing's human caring knowing/being/doing/becoming in the world.

PARTS AND WHOLES: THE RHETORICAL AND HAUNTING QUESTIONS FOR NURSING EDUCATION

As we face an unknown new world yet to be defined, there remains in nursing and science and society alike the rhetorical question about parts and wholes, Love and shared humanity, a shared world. Although we are challenged to work with whole, unitary human beings and whole knowledge systems, our dominant mythologies have tended to focus on parts. As such, there is a provocative "wondering"—are we to remain helpless and even destructive to ourselves and to our knowledge of human caring, healing, health, and humanity? Or, are we now mature enough to question, critique, and address the other side of the epistemological mythology—that is, to put the parts back into the whole and vice versa?

We are ethically challenged to address new questions, especially for professional nursing education and curricula that invite wholes and Love and all of human experiences into our relational emancipatory pedagogies and disciplinary knowledge matrix.

We each are invited to ponder the following rhetorical questions as a reflective self-guide toward evolutionary transformative teaching and learning:

- How do we/you put the parts back into the whole?
- How do we/you integrate facts with meanings?
- How do we/you acknowledge that the personal is also the professional?
- How do we/you allow our/your ethics to become our/your epistemology rather than perpetuating epistemological myths that deform our ethics?
- How do we/you honor ontology-of-spirit-filled relationship and caring relationship as ethic, as epistemology, as pedagogy and praxis for advancing professional nursing and healing?
- How do we/you cocreate, develop, and practice Caring Science, rather than the dominant biomedical-technological science model?
- How do we/you create communities of caring in our classrooms and clinical settings?
- How do we/you create opportunities for authentic dialogue whereby all questions are considered sacred?
- How do we/you integrate, honor, and sustain humanity and relational Human Caring-Love in the midst of technological advances?
- How do we/you create a Caring Science curriculum for nursing in the next century and for healing healthcare systems?

Caring Science serves as a guide toward answering these rhetorical, haunting questions for a shared future. Because nursing and nursing education are at a critical turning point for survival, due to all the conflicting demands, nursing and nurse educators are invited to make the hard turn toward its disciplinary foundation, in what we have posed as Caring Science. This work both honors the past and opens a new horizon for an inspired future of nursing for sustaining human caring around the globe throughout time.

Without making the hard turn to be directly accountable to the public for its Caring Science disciplinary foundation, as a continuous, constantly evolving guide to mature caring-healing-health knowledge and practices, nurses may succumb to being very good technicians of a totally transformed healthcare system. If that were to occur, nursing will have lost its way, disconnected from its ancient and noble history. In continuing the evolutionary turn toward Caring Science as the disciplinary foundation to guide future practices, nursing continues to evolve in harmony with the evolution of human consciousness and its global covenant with the planet, society, and humanity itself.

As we bring closure to this work, we also open our hearts to timeless and rhetorical questions which haunt us through the ages. As nursing educators and as a caring profession, where are we to learn the ultimate, the last test and proof of the work of humanity with which we deal: Human Caring/*Caritas*/Love and our shared human conditions? Native Americans and Indigenous cultures around the globe offer insights and wisdom beyond our extant mythic Western epistemology. Their unitary, whole-worldview approach to knowing is by honoring human life within the context of a comprehensive cosmology that informs views of life and death, living and dying, and humans' place in the universe. In their cosmology, life and death, knowledge, and all of life's events are one great sacred circle of the web of life. Real life, health, and illness stories of healing, survival, changing, dying are beyond humans' full control; they have to be considered within the web of life itself, from a wiser knowledge system, a larger cosmology, a larger ethic than our rational, ego, cognitive lens. This shift to a larger cosmology that integrates Caring and Love and Healing is essential if we are to sustain humanity for both human and planetary survival at this point in history (Levinas, 1969/2000).

This is a time in our human history to put the parts back into the whole, toward a living ethic, epistemology, and ontology of wholeness, relationship, and human caring–healing. It is a time for education, for curriculum, for teaching and learning to serve the evolution of our shared humanity and our common tasks for surviving and thriving in an unfolding and dramatically changing world and planet.

We can say that Caring Science is a model of thought and practice in which biomedical science and technical evidence alone are not simply blended with *Caritas,* but Caring Science is an evolved view of science itself, which both holds and transcends biomedical science and evidence per se.

Caring Science holds an expanded unitary worldview of oneness and an ethic of *belonging* as the prime consideration; a dimension that recognizes "the face of other," beyond "any case."

As Chinn and Falk-Rafael (2018) explain,

> The dominant biomedical discourse fails to account for the intersecting personal, social, cultural, and political structures that come into play in the experiences of health and illness, and fails to address the urgent need for care that supports dignity, humanization, and human flourishing. (p. 688)

In this respect, we assert that Caring Science can be defined as "an evolving ethical-epistemic field of study that is grounded in the discipline of nursing and informed by related fields; as such, it incorporates Love as a core element of human-human-divine connections" (Watson and Smith, 2002, p. 456).

The fact that nursing deals with phenomena of human caring, relationships, health-illness, health promotion, healing, living, dying, pain, suffering, and all the vicissitudes of human existence and lived experiences, forces nursing education and practice to acknowledge and further develop an expanded view of science. We offer a science model that can accommodate Love and all of humanity. You may ask: How can we dare to put an elusive concept such as Love in a model of science? On the other hand, we reply: how can we dare not to include Love in its fullest sense in our science, since Love is core to sustaining humanity, human caring, teaching, and learning.

This view has obvious implications for the future of nursing education and practice and indeed invites challenges for nursing as a caring profession and discipline. It also offers a fresh futuristic vision for an educational ethos that would seek to promote this ethic of "face," of Love, of relation and interconnectedness oneness with all. To reference Levinas (1969/2000), "the face" of other answers to "the unquenchable desire for infinity" (p. 150). At the same time, this separate other yet "presence of 'the face' [of other] includes all the possibilities of the transcendent relationship" (p. 155). This understanding helps us make new connections between Levinas's notion of "the face" and the transcendence of transpersonal caring—a welcoming of "the face" in a caring moment, connecting with the infinite field of universal Love in the moment (Watson, 2018), whether in the classroom or clinical setting. With this understanding, Levinas's views take us, in education and practice, beyond the purely biomedical model back to the face and the inexhaustible dimensions of our shared humanity in teaching and learning in a new way.

In practical and pedagogical terms, it invites constant reflecting, questioning, and revising of educational programs, curricula, healthcare policies, institutional regulations (where one size fits all), assessment procedures, and use of only one form of "evidence." It leads us beyond nursing as a subset of medical sciences, while still being part of them and indeed merging and transcending them, but also informing them.

This leads to the question of what kind of curriculum can sustain such a *Caritas-Love Ethic* as an aspiration and inspiration. As this book describes,

> [T]he curriculum would be framed around knowledge of nursing theories, exploring all ways of knowing about a given clinical-human phenomenon—for example, the phenomenon of suffering, healing, transpersonal human caring relations, patterns, community, consciousness, unitary wholeness, and the relational ethics of belonging—as a guide to knowledgeable, informed moral practices. (Watson, 2018, p. 67)

A Caring Science/Caritas orientation to nursing education for now and our future intersects with arts and humanities and related fields of study, beyond the conventional, clinicalized, and medicalized views of the person as well as health/healing. For Nightingale, "[N]ursing involved a sense of presence higher than the human, a 'divine intelligence that creates, sustains, and organizes the universe—and our awareness of an inner connection with this higher reality'" (Macrae, 2001, quoted in Watson, 2005, p. 63). Her views, along with Levinas and his philosophy, invite us to "face our humanity" and our connectedness with the greater, infinite dimensions of our life and work.

In embarking upon Caring Science/*Caritas* education, we invite others to cocreate open space to allow an evolved/transformed caring consciousness to enter our phenomenal field—opening to notions of *Caritas/Love and Infinity* of the human spirit and creativity beyond our imagination of today's standards (Levinas, 1969/2000; Watson, 2005, 2018; Watson & Smith, 2002).

As Smith (2019) recommends,

> Students should be guided to practice from the knowledge and values of the discipline: seeing patients through the lens of wholeness and interconnected with family and community; appreciating how the social, political, and economic environment influences health; attending to what is most important to well-being; developing a caring-healing relationship; and honoring personal dignity, choice, and meaning. This is the disciplinary perspective that transcends individual nursing theories. (p. 13)

As we invite Love back into our hearts, our minds, our classrooms, and our practices, we invite the original *Primordial Love* back into all of life and all living things. For Levinas (1969/2000), and for us, this inviting Love back into our lives, our work as nurse educators, our world, "is not meant to be anti-intellectual" (p. 109) but rather to lead to the very development of intellect. Thus, this perspective makes a case for an underlying theoretical-philosophical-ethical foundation for nursing rather than reverting to classical assumptions of science and knowledge and the technologies of teaching and learning. This view also reflects an evolutionary perspective for the nursing profession, especially nursing education, and the nature of knowledge itself.

As Chinn (2019) claims,

> If we grapple with the ontological meaning these theories have for us, and search for the meanings and realities that lie beyond their theoretical reach, then we can begin to close the gap between nursing science and art. We can recognize the significance of epistemologic

knowledge, and how ontological perceptions of reality can change how nurses practice nursing [and learn in nursing education]. (p. 8)

As we reconsider nursing education within a broader ethos proposed here, we realize that our approaches to our learning and teaching and practices have been too small and limiting to allow for respect of the deeper aspects of our life and work as nurse educators. In other words, our jobs as educators have been too small with respect to the deep nature of the work of nurses and teachers, who are here to lift up the human spirit, to return to Love as foundation for being/becoming whole (Watson, 2005). As Chinn and Falk-Rafael (2018) explain, "practices of teaching and learning grounded in nursing perspectives will prepare nurses to practice with a firm nursing theoretical foundation and advance the discipline of nursing as one that supports dignity, humanization, and human flourishing" (p. 693). Thus, we extend a moral invitation to create new or at least different educational and pedagogical options for science and society alike.

AFFIRMATIONS OF CARING SCIENCE CONSCIOUSNESS FOR NURSING EDUCATION

- Every way of knowing becomes a way of being; thus, epistemology becomes ontology.
- Epistemology as ethic is a set of values to live by, a way to conduct our lives.
- Behind this reframed ethic is a way of knowing that is personal, promoting personal meaning.
- Truth is personal, radically personal, not abstract, at arm's length, propositional, "out there"—that is, to call upon Einstein: "every fact is theory-laden."
- Knowledge and knowing are cocreated; movement toward truth is a mutual movement, with conflicts, dialogue, debates, and dialectical movement toward consensus.
- Knowing emerges between and among us.
- Knowledge and knowing are about mutuality and reciprocity; meaning seeks us from our heart-center, rather than us seeking truth (Einstein talked about "listening to the universe speak"; there is a reciprocal dance between the knower and the knowing).
- Knowing, teaching, learning, and caring transform one's own knowing, teaching, and learning if they are guided by a higher dimension of caring consciousness.

The transformation-learning literature (Bache, 2001) has noted that words we use in teaching-learning, theories, and interpretations carry much power to influence others. Words not supported by the energy of personal experiences have much less power than words grounded in personal experiences that possess the energy of love and caring.

[B]eing conscious of the words used to describe nursing's domain of practice becomes a critical aspect of nursing education. So, when using language that *emphasizes* the biomedical, physiological, technical, and skills aspects of nursing, there is the risk of making the compassionate, caring, relational, and spiritual aspects of the discipline of nursing less important and, often, invisible. (Hills & Cara, 2019, p. 202)

In this book, we consider that higher energy thoughts and words, such as love and caring, bring higher frequency energy into the learning space. Although the power of the teacher is significant to create the consciousness of a community of scholars and colearners, the more important power is the power of the group, the community, and the learning circle. For example, the word "Caritas" conveys high-vibration energy of caring and love.

Accordingly, Chinn and Falk-Rafael (2018) recommend,

> [W]hen we as educators ground our practice in nursing, we teach nursing in powerful ways that show nursing values and ideals through action, revealing deeper meanings of the words that form texts, lectures, and objectives set forth in a curriculum outline. (p. 688)

The current intellectual evolutions in caring-healing-health knowledge and practices and Caring Science frameworks are right in front of us in society and science alike. We have to face the fact that whether we like it or not, whether we agree with it or not, there is evidence of an evolved global awareness of our shared humanity and our shared environment: the fact that we metaphorically and literally "hold another person's life in our hands." As nurse educators, we are personally involved in transforming live encounters with the world through our scholarship, our knowledge, and our forms of teaching and learning—hence, a call for this new Caring Science curriculum framework, grounded, and informed/transformed as prevailing ethos and ethic is worthwhile.

Caring Science is not a unitary thing, a singular and rule-bound belief system. It engages with the diversity of the sciences and arts, philosophy, humanities, and with notions of personal growth, and of transformative caring consciousness. This takes time, or, put more forcefully, it takes courage by nurse educators to enliven the importance of human relationships and Caring Science, as the epicenter of what nursing actually means, as its first and necessary condition.

Such an approach applies also to our students so we can see their "faces" and our "faces" can be seen by them, and we are seen to practice what we teach. This is not easy. As noted, it takes a certain aspiration, courage, and inspiration, what is ultimately a metaphysical worldview that recognizes and accommodates the tensions that will be met along the way. This applies to all relationships, educator–student and student–educator, student–student, educator–educator relations. If we treat our relations with others merely as roles, there is a danger of collapsing back into a universally objectivist mode of thinking in which the educative relation has no face—this student, this lecturer, this patient, this nurse, this doctor, but no face, no "other," no unique individual. In the field of bioethics, these matters are often framed as issues of race, ethnicity, and power, and so on.

> Thus, what is central in my role as a teacher to the student as other is responsibility. I have an obligation more primary than any freedom. In fact it might not be too strong to argue that my singularity as a teacher comes into existence through my exposure to the student as other. Here the otherness of the student can be characterized as uniqueness, something that transcends my categorization. The uniqueness of the student is actually a call to me for assuming responsibility to that person. I am responsible to her [sic] precisely because s/he is irreplaceable in the pedagogical relationship, regardless of how many others there are. At this moment, to that person, I am responsible. That student, whose face I see, is irreplaceable, calling me to respond. This obligation is mine, personally. (Joldersma, 2001, pp. 186–187)

From a Caring Science lens, Riane Eisler (2007) makes a case for "caring economics" and the need for a "caring revolution" with respect to the values, politics, and policies of socioeconomic justice. She highlighted the fact that our economic values are guided toward reward, conquest, exploitation, and domination; this global political worldview toward social justice threatens the very survival of our species and our environment and spills over into our classrooms and our student–student, student–educator, and educator–educator relationships. Indeed, the survival of humans and our planet is now up close and personal as never before with respect to these foundational issues that are embedded in the politics and economics of our globe.

Caring Science calls into question and offers a challenge to seek our way through the political, economic, and techno-rational infrastructures that increasingly weigh us down in the name of quality that searches for universal standards; whether in learning and teaching, research, administration, or curriculum planning and implementation. These same infrastructures also weigh on students in terms of assessments, progress reports, and research or project proposals.

> [A] caring lens must underline the respect and uniqueness of all individuals, as well as the mutuality, trust, and equity throughout the relationships (among administrators, colleagues, staff, and students) taking place within the nursing education workplace . . . Nurse educators must embrace their Human Caring literacy and their political skills along with their power of influence in order to move from a biomedical paradigm into a humanistic perspective, hence transforming the working environment to endorse Human Caring relationships across the nursing school. (Brousseau & Cara, 2021, p. 171)

There is no easy way out; we are all invited to enter into this new space together and cocreate what might be, rather than succumb to what is and no longer works for us, for students, for patients, for humanity. As we make this turn together, we can engage in some of the lingering questions that may serve as value and intellectual guides for curriculum reform/transformation.

TIME OUT FOR REFLECTION

- How would you define a Caring Science curriculum?
- What does Caring Science offer for nursing education and practice?
- What is the difference between the discipline of nursing and the profession of nursing? Why is this difference important to understand?
- What are the characteristics that distinguish a Caring Science curriculum from another type of nursing curriculum?
- How can epistemology be/become an ethic?
- How will you incorporate Caring Science into your curriculum-development process?
- How can one justify having Love and Caring within its framework for education?
- How would you describe issues of social-moral justice operating in your personal life world? Your experience as a nurse educator? As a nursing student?

In Closing, We Offer Quality Indicators to Authenticate Your Caring Science Curriculum"—Philosophical and Operational Guidelines

In reviewing your current curriculum, ask yourself, your faculty, your students, your system, the following questions about your curriculum:

- **Ethic:** Is there evidence of an Ethic of Belonging in the curricular structure/organization/content and teaching/learning experiences: Is there evidence of experiences to learn and live out Human Caring, starting with Self-Caring, radiating in concentric circles to Other—Community—Environment—Planet—Universe? Is there evidence of a cosmology of connectedness with All? Is it obvious that the worldview is such that it is understood that each person resides in a larger pattern of infinite oneness with the environment/universe?

- **Ontology:** Does the curriculum have evidence indicating that the development and implementation is based on the nature and substance of the discipline of nursing as well as a relational ontology? That is: Are nursing philosophies, theories, research, and practice models of nursing phenomena and caring-as-a-way-of-being, embedded within the curriculum throughout?

- **Epistemology:** Will the curriculum guide emancipatory pedagogies and teaching/learning strategies that engage students in all ways of knowing within the discipline, congruent with and located within the domain of nursing and human phenomena? Does the curriculum invite and validate all ways of knowing, acknowledging Caring as a serious epistemic endeavor, and not simply a soft nice way of being?

- **Practice/Praxis:** Does the curriculum guide students to learn the practice of nursing from the perspective of nursing values, theories, and philosophies that incorporate caring and healing? Is there attention to the dialectic of knowing-being-doing, helping the student to critique conventional practice? Is practice approached as Praxis, that is, practice that originates from moral reflection, contemplation, and critique that is informed by the ethics, philosophies, values, and theories of caring and healing and human health/illness phenomena?

- **Relational Emancipatory Pedagogy:** Is there evidence of caring pedagogies as emancipatory teaching/learning experiences, including arts, humanities, and human vicissitudes, based upon nurse educator's consciousness of the need for meaningful personal and professional educational and practice experiences? Do nurse educators and curricular content, structure, relations, and diverse learning experiences bring forth the students' voice, restoring the heart of nursing education?

- **Teaching/Learning Focus:** Does the curriculum guide the teaching/learning experience from the foundation of nursing's disciplinary knowledge? Is there evidence of honoring all the vicissitudes of the human lived experiences for both students and patients? Is there evidence of passion for scholarship and the love of nursing? A love of humanity? Of self and other? A commitment for scholarship and knowledge of caring, health, and healing embedded within the students' personal/professional relations and classroom/practice experiences?

- **Distinguishing Disciplinary Knowledge:** Does the curriculum orient students to distinguish nursing's sphere of knowledge development from other disciplines and professions, especially medical science, through diverse forms of scholarly pursuit and critique?

- **Interdisciplinary Scholarship and Practices:** Is there evidence of respecting and incorporating other forms of knowledge and other professions within the sphere of learning and practice? Is it evident that Caring Science is transdisciplinary? Are there learning and teaching experiences and practices that demonstrate complementary, harmonious relations and learning with diverse theories, and fields of knowledge, science, and technology?

- **Social Justice and Equity:** Is there curricular evidence of classrooms and embodied experiences that demonstrate intersectionality as well as communities of caring and equity, embracing and celebrating diversity, be it ideas, social, economic, gender, race, lifestyle, ethnicity, customs, and beliefs?
- **Caring Scholarship:** Is there evidence in the curriculum of scholarship that embraces multiple forms of inquiry toward research and creative knowledge development; forms of Inquiry which contribute to generation of new disciplinary knowledge of nursing phenomena and human caring-health-healing?

We offer these reflective *authentication quality indicators* of a Caring Science curriculum—an authentic intellectual blueprint and value-based guide for assessing present and future caring curricula that are grounded in the discipline of nursing. These guides represent *authentication quality indicators* and point toward new goals and standards for nursing education.

As nursing education enters into this evolved disciplinary foundation to prepare the coming generations of nursing professionals, then it fully comes of age. Likewise, with this disciplinary foundation for nursing education, nursing will be sustaining its authentic commitment to, and Love of, humanity and the unknown, unfolding future. As it does so, it is positioned to fulfill its mission and covenant with society worldwide for the next 100 years.

We close with the words of Nigerian writer and poet Ben Okri and his perennial wisdom for our shared future:

In a world like ours . . .

Individual authenticity lies in what we can find that is worth living for. And the only thing worth living for is Love . . . The Love that can make us breathe again, Love a great and beautiful cause, a wonderful vision. A great Love for one another, or for the future. (Ben Okri, 1997, p. 57)

REFERENCES

Bache, C. (2001). *Transformative learning*. Noetic Sciences Institute.

Brousseau, S., & Cara, C. (2021). Nurse educators' political caring literacy and power to promote caring relationships in nursing education. In C. Cara, M. Hills, & J. Watson (Eds.), *An educator's guide to humanizing nursing education: Grounded in caring science* (pp. 161–182). Springer Publishing Company.

Chinn, P. L. (2019, March). *Keynote Address: The Discipline of Nursing: Moving Forward Boldly*. Presented at "Nursing Theory: A 50 Year Perspective, Past and Future," Case Western Reserve University Frances Payne Bolton School of Nursing. https://nursology.net/2019-03-21-case-keynote

Chinn, P. L., & Falk-Rafael, A. (2018). Embracing the focus of the discipline of nursing: Critical Caring Pedagogy. *Journal of Nursing Scholarship, 50*(6), 687–694. https://doi.org/10.1111/jnu.12426

Eisler, R. (2007). *The real wealth of nations: Creating a caring economics*. Berrett-Koehler.

Hills, M., & Cara, C. (2019). Curriculum development processes and pedagogical practices for advancing caring science literacy. In W. Rosa, S. Horton-Deutsch, & J. Watson (Eds.), *A handbook for caring science: Expanding the paradigm* (pp. 197–210). Springer Publishing Company.

Joldersma, C. W. (2001). Pedagogy of the other: A Levinasian approach to the student-teacher relationship. In *Philosophy of Education Yearbook*. University of Illinois at Urbana-Champaign.

Levinas, E. (2000). *Totality and infinity*. Duquesne University. (Original work published 1969)

Macrae, J. A. (2001). *Nursing as a spiritual practice*. Springer Publishing Company.

Okri, B. (1997). *A way of being free*. Phoenix.

Palmer, P. (2004). *A Hidden Wholeness: The Journey Toward an Undivided Life*. John Wiley and Sons, Inc.

Smith, M. (2019). Regenerating nursing's disciplinary perspective. *Advances in Nursing Science, 42*(1), 3–16. https://doi.org/10.1097/ANS.0000000000000241

Watson, J. (2005). *Caring science as sacred science.* F. A. Davis.

Watson, J. (2018). *Unitary caring science: The philosophy and praxis of nursing.* University Press of Colorado.

Watson, J., & Smith, M. (2002). Caring science and the science of unitary human beings: A transtheoretical discourse. *Journal of Advanced Nursing, 37*(5), 452–461. https://doi.org/10.1046/j.1365-2648.2002.02112.x

Index

Printed in the United States
by Baker & Taylor Publisher Services